MOLECULAR BIOLOGY AND IMMUNOLOGY IN HEPATOLOGY

Advances in the Treatment of Intractable Liver Diseases

Molecular Biology and Immunology in Hepatology

Advances in the Treatment of Intractable Liver Diseases

Edited by

Takao Tsuji, MD, PhD
Professor and Chairman, Department of Medicine and Medical Science (Gastroenterology, Hepatology and Infectious Disease), Okayama University Graduate School of Medicine and Dentistry, Okayama, Japan

Toshihiro Higashi, MD, PhD
Vice President, Chief of Gastroenterology and Hepatology Division, Okayama Citizen's Hospital, Okayama, Japan

Mikio Zeniya, MD, PhD
Associate Professor, Division of Gastroenterology and Hepatology, Department of Internal Medicine, Jikei University School of Medicine, Tokyo, Japan

Karl-Hermann Meyer zum Büschenfelde, MD, PhD, MDh.c., FRCP
Emeritus Professor of the Johannes Gutenberg University, Mainz, Germany

2002

ELSEVIER

Amsterdam – Boston – London – New York – Oxford – Paris
San Diego – San Francisco – Singapore – Sydney – Tokyo

ELSEVIER SCIENCE B.V.
Sara Burgerhartstraat 25
P.O. Box 211, 1000 AE Amsterdam, The Netherlands

First edition 2002

Library of Congress Cataloging in Publication Data
A catalog record from the Library of Congress has been applied for.

ISBN: 0-444-50653-5

⊗ The paper used in this publication meets the requirements of ANSI/NISO Z39.48-1992 (Permanence of Paper).
Printed in The Netherlands.

Contents

Preface

The 20th century was a period of remarkable technological revolutions in medicine. According to the development of molecular biology and immunology, there was a great progress in my research field, gastroenterology, hepatology and immunology. I graduated from Okayama University School of Medicine in 1961 and began to study hepatology. Soon after that, Dr. Blumberg discovered hepatitis B surface antigen and was awarded a Nobel prize. A new era began after his discovery.

Professor Karl-Hermann Meyer zum Büschenfelde and I were studying non-B hepatitis and proved the etiological importance of liver specific protein and liver membrane antigen in active chronic hepatitis or autoimmune hepatitis. Virological advancement was also remarkable. The emergence of mutant virus in hepatitis B and C results in the immune escape from the neutralizing antibody as is observed in HIV infection and this escape turned out to be a cause of chronic viral infection. Although we have been piling up new knowledge and new drugs have become available, we still have intractable liver diseases. Both Professor Meyer zum Büschenfelde and I felt that integration of the recent knowledge of virology, molecular biology and immunology is necessary to reveal what we can do now and what we should do to treat liver diseases.

This book consists of chapters that focus on many intractable liver diseases. I selected important topics in hepatology from meetings that I organized. These include both clinical research, e.g. the treatment of interferon resistant hepatitis C virus or hepatocellular carcinoma and basic research, e.g. transgenic mice models. Some readers may not be familiar with some fields of the contents; however, all of them are unavoidable topics to overcome the intractable liver diseases. The authors are all front runners in current hepatology research and give us proper information on each topic. I hope this book will prove useful to all readers and become a guide to hepatology research in the 21st century.

I would like to sincerely thank Dr. Kazuhiro Nouso, assistant professor of our department, for his efforts in planning and editing this book.

Takao Tsuji

Contributors

Yoshio Aizawa
Division of Gastoroenterology and Hepatology, Department of Internal Medicine, Jikei University School of Medicine, Tokyo 3-25-8, Nishishinbashi Minato-ku, Tokyo 105-8461, Japan

Hubert E. Blum
Department of Medicine, University of Freiburg, Hugstetter Strasse 55, D-79106 Freiburg, Germany

J. Ch. Bode
Em. Professor of Medicine, Honoldwag 18, D-70193 Stuttgart, Germany

Janos Feher
Second Department of Internal Medicine, Medical Faculty, Semmelweis University, Szentkiralyi str 46, H-1088 Budapest, Hungary

Kenji Fujiwara
Third Department of Internal Medicine, Saitama Medical School, 38 Morohongo, Moroyama-cho, Iruma-gun Saitama 350-0495, Japan

Hiroshi Fukui
Third Department of Internal Medicine, Nara Medical University, 840 Shijo-cho, Kashihara-city, Nara 634-8522, Japan

M. Eric Gershwin
Division of Rheumatology, Allergy and Clinical Immunology, University of California at Davis, One Shields avenue, TB 192, Davis, CA 95616-8660, USA

Norio Hayashi
Department of Molecular Therapeutics, Osaka University Graduate School of Medicine, 2-2 Yamadaoka, Suita-city, Osaka 565-0871, Japan

Toshihiro Higashi
Okayama Citizen's Hospital, 6-10 Amase, Okayama-city, Okayama 700-8557, Japan

Takafumi Ichida
Third Department of Internal Medicine, Niigata University, 757 Ichiban-cho, Asahimati-dori, Niigata-city, Niigata 951-8122, Japan

Hiromi Ishibashi
Institute for Clinical Research, National Nagasaki Medical Center, Kubara 2-1001-1, Omura-city, Nagasaki 856-8562, Japan

Tetsuya Ishikawa
First Department of Internal Medicine, Reserch Center for Infectious Disease, Aichi Medical University School of Medicine, 21 Yazako, Nagakute, Aichi-gun, Aichi 480-1195, Japan

Satoshi Kaihara
Department of Transplantation and Immunology, Graduate School of Medicine, Kyoto University, 54 Jawahara-cho, Shogoin, Sakyo-ku, Kyoto-city, Kyoto 606-8501, Japan

Shinichi Kakumu
First Department of Internal Medicine, Reserch Center for Infectious Disease, Aichi Medical University School of Medicine, 21 Yazako, Nagakute, Aichi-gun, Aichi 480-1195, Japan

Shuichi Kaneko
First Department of Internal Medicine, Kanazawa University School of Medicine, 13-1 Takara-machi, Kanazawa-city, Ishikawa 920-8641, Japan

Akinori Kasahara
Department of General Medicine, Osaka University Graduate School of Medicine, 2-2 Yamadaoka, Suita-city, Osaka 565-0871, Japan

Kozo Kayano
Department of Gastroenterology and Hepatology, Yamaguchi University School of Medicine, 1-1-1, South-Kogushi, Ube-city, Yamaguchi, 755-8505, Japan

Kenichi Kobayashi
First Department of Internal Medicine, Kanazawa University School of Medicine, 13-1 Takara-machi, Kanazawa-city, Ishikawa 920-8641, Japan

Yoshiyuki Kobayashi
Department of Medicine and Medical Science, Okayama University Graduate School of Medicine and Dentistry, 2-5-1, Shikata-cho, Okayama-city, Okayama 700-8558, Japan

Kazuhiko Koike
Department of Infectious Diseases, Internal Medicine, Graduate school of Medicine, University of Tokyo, 7-3-1 Hongo, Bunkyo-ku, Tokyo 113-8655, Japan

Margaret J. Koziel
Department of Infectious Diseases, Beth Israel Deaconess Medical Center, and Harvard Medical School, Room 223A, 4 Blackfan Circle, 330 Brookline Ave, Boston, MA 02215, USA

Shigeki Kuriyama
Third Department of Internal Medicine, Kagawa Medical University, 1750-1 Ikenobe, Miki-cho, Kita-gun, Kagawa 761-0793, Japan

Gabriella Lengyel
Second Department of Internal Medicine, Semmelweis University, Szentkiralyi str 46, H-1088 Budapest, Hungary

Michael Manns
Division of Gastroenterology and Hepatology, Medical School of Hannover, Carl-Neuberg Str. 1, 30625 Hannover, Germany

Karl-Hermann Meyer zum Büschenfelde
Em. Professor of the Johannes Gutenberg University, Mainz, Trabenerstrasse 8, D-14193 Berlin, Germany

Hiroshi Miyakawa
Fourth Department of Internal Medicine, Teikyo University School of Medicine, 3-8-3 Mizonokuchi, Takatsu-ku, Kawasaki-city, Kanagawa 213-8507, Japan

Satoshi Mochida
Third Department of Internal Medicine, Saitama Medical School, 38 Morohongo, Moroyama-cho, Iruma-gun Saitama 350-0495, Japan

Minoru Nakamura
Medicine and Biosystemic Science, Kyushu University Graduate School of Medical Sciences, 3-1-1, Maidahsi, Higashi-ku, Fukuoka-city, Fukuoka 812-8582, Japan

Shin-ichiro Nakamura
Department of Medicine and Medical Science, Okayama University Graduate School of Medicine and Dentistry, 2-5-1, Shikata-cho, Okayama-city, Okayama 700-8558, Japan

Toshiya Nakatani
Third Department of Internal Medicine, Nara Medical University, 840 Shijo-cho, Kashihara-city, Nara 634-8522, Japan

Kazuhiro Nouso
Department of Medicine and Medical Science, Okayama University Graduate School of Medicine and Dentistry, 2-5-1, Shikata-cho, Okayama-city, Okayama 700-8558, Japan

Kiwamu Okita
Department of Gastroenterology and Hepatology, Yamaguchi University School of Medicine, 1-1-1, South-Kogushi, Ube-city, Yamaguchi, 755-8505, Japan

Masao Omata
Department of Gastroenterology, University of Tokyo 7-3-1 Hongo, Bunkyo-ku, Tokyo 113-8655, Japan

Morikazu Onji
Third Department of Internal Medicine, Ehime University School of Medicine, Shitsukawa, Shigenobu-cho, Onsen-gun, Ehime 791-0295, Japan

Isao Sakaida
Department of Gastroenterology and Hepatology, Yamaguchi University School of Medicine, 1-1-1, South-Kogushi, Ube-city, Yamaguchi, 755-8505, Japan

Hirohisa Shigematsu
Medicine and Biosystemic Sciences, Kyushu University Graduate School of Medical Science, 3-1-1, Maidashi, Higashi-ku, Fukuoka-city, Fukuoka 812-8582, Japan

Shinji Shimoda
Medicine and Biosystemic Sciences, Kyushu University Graduate School of Medical Science, 3-1-1, Maidashi, Higashi-ku, Fukuoka-city, Fukuoka 812-8582, Japan

Hiroki Takahashi
Division of Gastoroenterology and Hepatology, Department of Internal Medicine, Jikei University School of Medicine, Tokyo 3-25-8, Nishishinbashi Minato-ku, Tokyo 105-8461, Japan

Koichi Tanaka
Department of Transplantation and Immunology, Graduate School of Medicine, Kyoto University, 54 Jawahara-cho, Shogoin, Sakyo-ku, Kyoto-city, Kyoto 606-8501, Japan

Gotaro Toda
Division of Gastoroenterology and Hepatology, Department of Internal Medicine, Jikei University School of Medicine, Tokyo 3-25-8, Nishishinbashi Minato-ku, Tokyo 105-8461, Japan

Hirohisa Tsujinoue
Third Department of Internal Medicine, Nara Medical University, 840 Shijo-cho, Kashihara-city, Nara 634-8522, Japan

Masayuki Uemura
Department of Medicine and Medical Science, Okayama University Graduate School of Medicine and Dentistry, 2-5-1, Shikata-cho, Okayama-city, Okayma 700-8558, Japan

Arndt Vogel
Department of Gastroenterology and Hepatology, Medical School of Hannover, Carl-Neuberg Str.1 30625 Hannover, Germany

Akiharu Watanabe
Third Department of Internal Medicine, Faculty of Medicine, Toyama Medical and Pharmaceutical University, 2630 Sugitani, Toyama-city, Toyama 930-0194, Japan

Kazuhide Yamamoto
Department of Medicine and Medical Science, Okayama University Graduate School of Medicine and Dentistry, 2-5-1, Shikata-cho, Okayama-city, Okayama 700-8558, Japan

Michitami Yano
Institute for Clinical Research, National Nagasaki Medical Center, Kubara 2-1001-1, Omura-city, Nagasaki 856-8562, Japan

Hiroshi Yatsuhashi
Institute for Clinical Research, National Nagasaki Medical Center, Kubara 2-1001-1, Omura-city, Nagasaki 856-8562, Japan

Makoto Yoshiba
Division of Gastroenterology, Department of Medicine, Showa University Fujigaoka Hospital 1-30, Fujigaoka, Aoba-ku, Yokohama-City, Kanagawa 227-8501, Japan

Hitoshi Yoshiji
Third Department of Internal Medicine, Nara Medical University, 840 Shijo-cho, Kashihara-city, Nara 634-8522, Japan

Mikio Zeniya
Division of Gastoroenterology and Hepatology, Department of Internal Medicine, Jikei University School of Medicine, Tokyo 3-25-8, Nishishinbashi Minato-ku, Tokyo 105-8461, Japan

Hepatology in 21st Century

Molecular Biology and Immunology in Hepatology
Edited by T. Tsuji, T. Higashi, M. Zeniya and K.-H. Meyer zum Büschenfelde

CHAPTER 1

General Aspects of Molecular Biology and Immunology for the Treatment of Intractable Liver Diseases

Karl-Hermann Meyer zum Büschenfelde

Johannes Gutenberg University, Mainz, Germany

INTRODUCTION

During recent years, cell biology, biochemistry, molecular biology, immunology, immunogenetics, and gene technology have led to a better understanding of the physiologic functions of the different cellular components of the liver. The importance of the structural–functional relationships and interactions between liver cells and matrix components also have been realized. In particular, cytokines, chemokines, adhesion molecules, hormone-like factors, metabolites etc. released by parenchymal and non-parenchymal liver cells have been identified that play a crucial role in maintaining liver-related functions and liver homeostasis. Disturbances of the balance of the various regulatory factors may change the phenotype and numbers of different liver cells, and lead to abnormalities in liver structure and function as well as liver injury.

One of the most important physiologic functions of the liver is the maintenance of immunologic homeostasis. The liver as an immune-privileged organ favors the induction of peripheral tolerance rather than induction of immunity. How the immune response is regulated locally in the liver and which cell types and molecular mechanisms are involved in shaping the hepatic immune response is content of this contribution.

1. THE LIVER AS IMMUNE PRIVILEGED SITE

1.1. Microenvironment and the role of liver cells

Parenchymal and non-parenchymal cell populations form a unique microenvironment. Liver sinusoidal endothelial cells (SEC) constitute a wall between hepatocytes and the cells as well as components within the sinusoid [1]. Kupffer cells (KC) and liver-associated lymphocytes (LAL) are found in the sinusoidal lumen adhering to the SEC. KC are located mainly in the periportal area, a strategic position for phagocytosis and elimination of antigens or pathogens entering the liver via portal-venous blood.

1.1.1. Hepatocytes

Hepatocytes not only serve as target cells of immune reactions, but may also play an active role in initiation and perpetuation of immune processes, as shown by the upregulated expression of major histocompatibility complex (MHC) class I antigens and the de novo expression of MHC class II antigens in acute and chronic hepatitis [2,3]. Furthermore, hepatocytes express important accessory molecules at inflammatory sites, such as intercellular adhesion molecule-1 (ICAM-1), lymphocytes function-associate antigen-3 (LFA-3) and CD36 OKM5 antigen, which may replace or bypass professional antigen-presenting cells [4]. The binding of ligands to accessory molecules augments the biochemical signals provided by the antigen-specific T-cell receptor (TCR) and therefore appears to be necessary for effective antigen recognition and T-cell triggering to occur [5] and for the induction of a local immune response [6,7]. The correlation of hepatocyte surface expression of accessory molecules with the presence of liver-infiltrating T cells support the notion that locally released T-cell-derived immune mediators (cytokines) are responsible for the modulation of the hepatocyte phenotype. In acute hepatitis, these activators and hepatocellular adhesion molecules are diffusely distributed throughout the inflamed liver parenchyma, whereas in chronic hepatitis, their expression is restricted to periportal and intralobular areas of inflammation [8]. In order to exert their regulatory role, these cytokines interact with specific receptors displayed on the surface of target cells. A de novo expression of the human interferon-γ receptor and tumor necrosis factor (TNF) receptors on hepatocytes is observed in inflammatory liver diseases [9,10], indicating that hepatocytes can serve as target cells of cytokines released by monocyte/macrophages in the early immune response. In later phases of immune responses, interferon-γ release by activated T-lymphocytes may dominate. The expression of the cytokine receptor CD40 on hepatocytes [11], a glycoprotein found on many lymphoid and non-lymphoid cell types, is enhanced by several cytokines, including interferon-γ and interleukin-4 (IL-4). CD40 is a member of a cytokine receptor family that may render hepatocytes more efficient antigen-presenting cells during the immune response.

Thus, it is likely that cytokines or the antigenic material itself are responsible for induction of an activated hepatic phenotype, followed by antigen-independent interactions between hepatocytes and T-lymphocytes that further enable and modulate antigen-specific TCR-mediated recognition.

1.1.2. Sinusoidal endothelial cells

SEC are involved in the clearance of components from the sinusoidal blood. Furthermore, they participate in extracellular matrix biosynthesis [12]. SEC function as a barrier between macromolecules or leukocytes present in the sinusoidal lumen and hepatocytes [13]. Direct contact between passenger leukocytes and hepatocytes is prevented by SEC. The uptake of macromolecules by SEC occurs via pattern recognition receptors, such as the scavenger receptor and the mannose receptor [14–17]. They enable SEC to remove non-enzymatically glycosylated proteins and other potentially harmful substances from the circulation [18] and allow a vectorial transport of macromolecules across SEC as a physiologic mechanism to increase their delivery from the sinusoidal lumen to hepatocytes [19–21].

SEC are efficient antigen-presenting cells and induce proliferation and cytokine expression in $CD4^+$ cells in vitro [22,23]. Similar to dendritic cells [24], SEC use the mannose receptor for efficient uptake of antigen [23]. Whereas effective antigen presentation by macro- and microvascular endothelial cells is present only after prestimulation with exogenous cytokines, microvascular SEC need no activation with proinflammatory stimuli to induce efficient antigen presentation to $CD4^-$ T cells [22,23].

The SEC phenotype has further characteristics (MHC class II, CD80, CD86, and CD40) consistent with an antigen-presenting cell [22,23]. In humans, SEC express CD58 [25], the ligand for CD2 that triggers the alternative pathway of T-cell activation [26]. Moreover, SEC bear the CD4 molecule [27] and low levels of CD11c [28].

1.1.3. Kupffer cells

KC are hepatic macrophages that reside in the lumen of hepatic sinusoids and play a key role in host defense. The main properties of KC are endocytosis, destruction of ingested material, antigen presentation, and secretion of biologically active products [29]. KC have a high phagocytosis capacity but show a low-level synthesis of superoxide [30,31]. Activated KC can release cytokines such as TNF-α, interferons, interleukins, and transforming growth factors α and β, and can activate hepatic natural killer cells. A further important action of KC is clearance and modification of endotoxins and the transport to hepatocytes for further modification and excretion into the bile [32]. On the other hand, endotoxin are crucial for KC in promoting phagocytosis and synthesis of biochemically active products, such as prostaglandins, thromboxanes, leukotrienes, fibronectin, IL-1, interferons, TNF-α, erythropoietin, procoagulants, collagenase, lysozymes, and plasminogen activator [33]. Thus, KC not only play a role in host defense, but also in several pathophysiological processes such as endotoxin-induced liver injury, immune modulation and inflammatory responses, and connective tissue remodeling and fibrosis. The crucial role of KC in immunoregulation is shown by two important experiments: Antigens injected into the portal venous system failed to induce an immune response, but injection into the vena cava did, and portacaval anastomosis or blockade of KC phagocytosis prevented immune tolerance [34,35]. Thus, Kupffer cells are effective scavengers of immunogenic antigens before they reach the peripheral lymphoid tissue.

KC express IL-10 in response to physiological concentrations of lipopolysaccharide [36]. IL-10 expression in KC is regulated by a negative autoregulatory feedback loop [37] and has important immunoregulatory effects on KC and SEC. In particular, IL-10 down-regulates $CD4^+$ T-cell activation by antigen-presenting KC and SEC by suppression of receptor-mediated antigen uptake and down-regulation of MHC class II and the co-stimulatory molecules CD80 and CD86 [23]. The immunoregulatory potential of IL-10 in the liver is restricted to the time of its presence in the sinusoids. Once washed away, IL-10 likely has no further influence on the development and quality of immune response in the liver.

1.1.4. Liver-associated lymphocytes

LAL are considered as a hepatic intrasinusoidal immune cell population. Because liver and gut are derived from the endoderm, both organs can support tissue-specific lymphocyte differentiation as evidenced by expression of genes such as recombinase activation genes 1 and 2 that are otherwise only expressed by immature thymocytes undergoing gene rearrangement [38–41]. Similarly, CD45, CD34, and CD7 expression indicate the presence of hematopoietic stem cells and early lymphoid progenitors in the liver [42], and indeed, hematopoiesis can take place in the fetal liver and in liver grafts [43].

LAL differs considerably from that found in the blood. Specifically, the CD4 : CD8 ratio is reversed, and the $CD8^+$ T-cell population is extremely heterogeneous and contains a large percentage of unconventional lymphocytes that are not frequently found in the peripheral blood [42]. These include $CD4^-CD8^-$ double-negative T cells [65–67], $CD4^+CD8^+$ double-positive T cells [42], T cells that display the $\gamma\delta$ T-cell receptor instead of the $\alpha\beta$ T-cell receptor that characterizes peripheral blood T cells [44], and cells that express both the natural killer (NK) cell marker CD56 and the T-cell marker CD3 [45]. The latter have been termed NKT cells and have distinct functional characteristics, such as the ability to recognize non-peptide antigens presented by non-classical MHC molecules [46].

1.1.5. Stellata cells (fat-storing cells)

Stellata cells (Ito cells, fat-storing cells, peri- or parasinusoidal cells, lipocytes) [47] are located in the space of Dissé under the endothelial cell lining and are in close contact with hepatocytes [48]. Beside many metabolic functions [48], stellata cells contribute to the production of connective tissue and have morphologic characteristics in common with fibroblasts. In a chronically injured liver, stellata cells acquire a new fibroblast-like phenotype and participate in fibrogenesis [49–51]. In liver injury, stellata cells undergo an activation which represents a cascade of cellular events due to all forms of liver damage. The initiation of activation results from paracrine mediators from SEC, KC and hepatocytes. Perpetuation of activation leads to several activation-dependent functional changes [52].

1.1.6. Cytokines and chemokines released by liver cells

The unique microenvironment within the sinusoid is the basis for cell-specific interactions between hepatocytes, sinusoidal endothelial cells, Kupffer cells, liver-associated lymphocytes and stellata cells. Cytokines and chemokines released by these cells are important mediators with physiological and pathological implications [53]. They are crucial for both either immunologic homeostasis and induction of tolerance or local immune cell development and activation, recruitment of immune cells to the liver and induction of immunity. Furthermore, they play a key role in the regulation of hepatic cell growth and regeneration, hepatic fibrogenesis, and acute phase response.

1.2. Tolerance induction

The physiological intestinal and sinusoidal microenvironment of the organism seems to be crucial for the immune system to react well balanced between tolerance and immunity [28,54]. Tolerance induction is part of the physiological functions of the immune systems. With respect to oral tolerance, the gastrointestinal immune system is primarily involved. The liver may function as a second security line to ensure tolerance towards dietary antigens coming via portal vein from the gastrointestinal tract [55]. This notion is evidenced by portal systemic shunting experiments [56,57].

The concept of peripheral tolerance induction in the liver is based on the transfer of tolerance-mediating cells from a tolerized animal to a naive animal [58]. Additional evidence that the liver may be of central importance for peripheral tolerance induction stem from [1] apoptosis research, [2] transplantation immunology and from [3] functional studies of SEC.

The role of apoptosis in peripheral tolerance induction in the liver has not yet been well elucidated. There are no convincing data to show that apoptosis is mediated in the liver and that detection of apoptotic cells in the liver is not only a reflection of accumulation of dying lymphocytes [54]. Antigen specificity of apoptosis induction in the liver is a prerequisite for its involvement in tolerance induction, but there are no convincing data so far [59–63]. Apoptosis may take part in the immune regulatory processes in the liver [64,65], but their role in peripheral tolerance induction remains to be determined.

Induction of donor-specific tolerance is a central aim in transplantation immunology. Important observations support this concept [66–71]. Injection of donor-specific leukocytes via the portal vein, but not via the lateral tail vein results in donor-specific acceptance of skin grafts [72], which seems to be mediated by T cells that preferentially express IL-4 and IL-10, but not IL-2, upon contact with specific antigen in vitro [73]. Adoptive transfer of tolerance by hepatic $\gamma\delta$ T cells suggests that tolerance is not mediated by clonal deletion, but by immune deviation, and that maintenance of tolerance depends on the persistent presence of antigen [74]. Recently, a molecule termed OX-2 has been identified that is involved in the non-MHC-restricted induction of tolerance [75]. It appears that OX-2-expressing dendritic cells are able to inhibit T-cell stimulation by allogeneic dendritic cells.

As mentioned before, KC are critically involved in tolerance induction towards porto-venous injection of allogeneic cells. Thus, it is likely that tolerance induction to allogeneic cells may be different from those operative in tolerance induction to soluble antigens. This is probably due to the different liver cells that are involved in uptake/clearance of entire cells or subcellular components (Kupffer cells) and soluble antigens (SEC) [75–81].

Recently, it has been shown that SEC may have a regulatory influence on peripheral tolerance induction in the liver. SEC stimulate naive $CD4^+$ T cells to become Th-0 cells and to secrete the cytokines IL-4 and IL-10 and not IFN-γ, but fail to differentiate to Th1-phenotypes. IL-4 seems to be essential during the early priming phase of regulatory T cells. Cytokines promoting Th-1 differentiation such as IL-12, IL-2, or IFN-γ show no effect on regulatory T-cell differentiation by SEC [28]. Very recently it was reported that SEC are capable of cross-presenting soluble exogenous antigen to $CD8^+$ T cells. Although SEC use similar molecular mechanisms for cross-presentation as dendritic cells, presentation of soluble antigen by SEC results in antigen-specific $CD8^+$ T-cell tolerance rather than in immunity. Thus it is likely that SEC may play a key role in hepatic immune tolerance induction particularly towards soluble antigens such as food and self proteins [82].

In conclusion, the microenvironment within the sinusoid preferentially tries either to induce peripheral tolerance against antigens or to confine pathogen host interactions locally. SEC, Kupffer cells, liver dendritic cells, and liver-associated lymphocytes are involved in keeping the balance between induction of tolerance and immunity.

2. HOST DEFENSE MECHANISMS

2.1. Innate immune responses

The innate immune system constitutes the early phase of immune defense and interacts with and controls adaptive immune response [83]. Only after recognition by the innate immunity the adaptive immunity is able to respond to pathogens. The effector mechanisms of innate immunity are activated immediately after infection and control rapidly the replication of the infected agent [84,85]. The main differences between the innate and the adaptive immune system are the mechanism and repertoire used for immune recognition. Innate immune recognition is mediated by germ-line encoded receptors and is thereby genetically predetermined. The total number of receptors involved in innate immunity is limited as compared to the large and diverse amount of somatically generated receptors of the adaptive immune response. The innate immune response is directed on few highly conserved structures named pathogen-associated molecular patterns (PAMP) which have common features and are present in large groups of agents [86].

The PAMP receptors differ from other antigen receptors substantially. They are expressed on many effector cells (macrophages, dendritic cells and B-cells), belong to several families of proteins, and are divided into three classes: secreted, endocytic and signaling. The recently identified receptors of the Toll family seem to play a major role in the induction of immune and inflammatory response [87–92]. Innate receptors are specific for structures expressed in pathogens and thereby can quickly signal the presence of infection. Self antigens are not recognized by receptors of the innate immune system. Dysfunctions of components of the innate immune systems, i.e. genetic alterations, may lead to immune abnormalities and diseases, including autoimmune disorders [93].

The role of the innate immune system in liver diseases is not well elucidated so far. The liver is enriched in cells of the innate immune response, i.e. NK cells, NKT cells, $\gamma\delta$-receptor-positive T cells and macrophages [42], indicating that a pathogen-induced activation of the innate immune system may locally lead to an early inhibition of viral replication, viral gene expression and viral protein synthesis. Furthermore, cytokines and chemokines released by cells of the innate immune system may modify the distribution and migration of immune cells [94,95]. IL-15 seems to be one of the most important stimulators of the innate immunity [96] that preferentially supports innate cell development, activation, and homeostasis. The pleiotropic action of IL-15 in the case of viral infections selectively activates NK cells, NK T cells, $\gamma\delta$-receptor-positive cells and $CD8^+$ cells [96].

2.2. Adaptive immune response

The adaptive immune response consists of T- and B-cells that display somatically developed, structurally unique receptors which can react with infectious and harmless environmental antigens as well as autoantigens. Antigen–receptor interactions of individual lymphocytes lead to clonal selection and expansion and to an adequate immune response after several days. This interval is mostly too large to avoid organ and/or host damage. Thus, activation of the adaptive immune response can in principle be dangerous to the host, particularly in case of immune reactions against self or environmental antigens. Therefore, interaction and control of the adaptive immune response by the innate immune system is of crucial importance in determining the origin of antigens (foreign or self), for the maintenance of host integrity and host defense [42,92]. In liver diseases, the adaptive immune response plays an important role in host defense against non-cytopathic agents, but is also responsible for organ damage [85].

2.3. The role of cytokines and chemokines

Cytokines are important proteins that are involved in many physiological and pathological processes of the liver. They are secreted after activation of naive T-helper cells and influence the pattern of T-helper cell differentiation towards pro- (Th1) or anti-inflammatory (Th2) actions [97–100]. The transcription factors T-bet on the one side and $GATA_3$ and C-MAF on the other side are decisive for the final function and action of developing T cells. The molecular mechanisms that direct lineage commitment in the immune system remains to be determined [100]. Factors that may influence the T-cell differentiation program are the TCR–peptide MHC complex itself [101,102], immune response genes, the structure of the MHC class II molecules on the various antigen-presenting cells, the characteristics and the load of the pathogens, and the affinity and alteration of the ligands [103].

Chemotactic cytokines or chemokines are important mediators of the immune system [104]. Based on their structure and target cell specificity, they are divided into two major groups: C–X–C chemokines and C–C chemokines [105,106]. They preferentially function as chemoattractants and activators of leukocytes. Chemokines are produced by monocytes, macrophages, Kupffer cells, liver sinusoidal and vascular endothelial cells, various epithelial cells, and fibroblasts. Important inducers of chemokines are IL-1, TNF-α, bacterial endotoxin, and oxidant stress [105].

Chemokine receptor expression and tissue-specific migration is related to the type and activation status of T cells [104–109]. Liver associated lymphocytes express higher amounts of CXC receptor 3 and the CC-receptor 5 than lymphocytes in the peripheral blood.

The ligands of the CXC receptor 3 and the CC receptor 5 are IFN-γ inducible protein 10 (IP10) and the monokine induced by IFN-γ (MIG). Eotaxin is the ligand of the CC receptor 3 and 4. Of special importance for the induction of periportal inflammation may be the ligands of the CC receptor 5, i.e. the chemokines MIP-1α, MIP-1β and RANTES. They are expressed on vascular endothelial cells within the portal tract in normal and viral infected livers [110–112].

3. IMMUNE MECHANISMS IN LIVER DISEASES

3.1. Autoimmune liver diseases

Acute and chronic liver diseases resulting from autoimmunity are distinct entities in which immune-mediated reactions against self seem to be the major pathogenetic mechanism. This is believed to be true in autoimmune hepatitis (AIH), primary sclerosing cholangitis (PSC), and primary biliary cirrhosis (PBC). Several studies have failed to show any significant associations between infection with hepatitis A, B, C and D viruses and autoimmune liver diseases (AILD) [113,114]. The co-existence of viral hepatitis and AILD is a rare event and appears to be due to chance. Hepatitis A, B, D and C, however, are able to induce autoantibodies in a significant number of patients. [115]. These autoantibodies usually tend to be low in titer in viral infections and mainly have one autoantibody subtype. Interferon-α therapy can induce a transient appearance of autoantibodies in viral liver diseases [116]. A special autoantibody observed in about 50% of patients with chronic hepatitis C, named anti-Gor [117] is a rare finding in AIH or other liver diseases. In hepatitis C anti-Gor correlates with disease-activity [118]. The viral trigger mechanism of autoimmunity is of special interest pathophysiologically. Upregulation of autoimmune reactions against membrane antigens of hepatocytes are observed in all types of hepatic viral infections, but they usually do not run to self-perpetuating autoimmune liver disease. The same seems to be true for non-hepatotropic viruses [119].

3.1.1. Autoimmune hepatitis

Cellular and humoral autoimmune reactions have the capability of causing hepatocellular damage. Direct cytotoxicity of T cells directed against organ-specific antigens expressed on the liver plasma membrane is probably the most important action in the initial phase of autoimmune liver injury. Evidence for this comes from animal models of AIH [120]. The essential role of T-cell recognition of liver antigens has been shown by a passive transfer of the disease by CD4-positive T cells in syngeneic mice. In this model, autoantibodies appear at the time of spontaneous recover from the disease [121,122].

Considering the clinical, experimental and immunological findings, there is increasing evidence that autoimmune diseases are partially regulated by each patient's own immune system [121,122]. AIH usually runs a subacute or chronic course with intermittent phases of acute disease exacerbation and recovery. This clinical pattern can only be explained by an active interplay between disease-promoting factors [genetic predisposition (HLA-D3/Dr4 associations) and/or environmental factors] and counter-regulatory elements of the immune system. The experimental data mentioned above give accumulating evidence that T-cell-mediated cytotoxicity may be the primary event of liver injury in AIH. The quality of downregulation of T-cell response involving antigen-specific and, to a lesser extent, -non-specific suppression may be course-determining. An impaired natural control and early downregulation of liver-specific T-cell response may be decisive for AIH initiation and progression. In the chronic self-perpetuating phase of AIH, both cellular and autoantibody-mediated as well as the patterns of pro- and anti-inflammatory cytokines may shape the clinical pictures.

3.1.2. Primary sclerosing cholangitis

PSC is a chronic cholestatic liver disease of unknown etiology which is characterized by fibro-obliterative inflammation of the intra- and extrahepatic bile ducts [123]. The usually progressive course leads to biliary cirrhosis and in about 20% of the cases to cholangiocarcinoma. Special features are the male predominance (2 : 1) and the association with inflammatory bowel diseases (IBD) in particular with ulcerative colitis (UC) which shows geographical variations between 20 and 90%. Recent studies have implicated genetic and immunological factors as important pathogenetic mechanisms [124].

There is increasing evidence that PSC is mediated by organ-specific autoimmune mechanisms. Susceptibility to PSC is strongly linked to MHC class II molecules particularly HLA-B8 DR3 haplotypes which are associated with other autoimmune disorder and that are believed to be mediated by T cells. T-cell reactivity against bile duct epithelia and several humoral autoimmune epiphenomena support this notion. Finally, an overlap of PSC with autoimmune hepatitis [125,126] and inflammatory bowel diseases [127] is in agreement with the presence of immune-mediated pathogenetic mechanisms. But the question of whether PSC is an autoimmune disorder cannot yet be answered. The main problem is the lack of an organ- and disease-specific autoantigen as targets of T- and B-cell immune responses.

3.1.3. Primary biliary cirrhosis

PBC is a chronic cholastatic liver disease characterized by progressive destruction of biliary epithelial cells lining the small intrahepatic bile ducts. PBC has all the features of a classic autoimmune disorder, particularly a female predominance, disease-specific immune abnormalities, overlapping with AIH, autoimmune cholangitis, and other autoimmune disorders, immunogenetic associations, and no link to viral liver diseases [128].

Cellular and humoral immune reactions specific for PBC are directed against the mitochondrial autoantigen PDC-E2 as immunodominant target structure. The identification of humoral autoepitopes present in nearly all patients with PBC and the characterization of an immunodominant autoreactive T-cell epitope (PDC-E2 163–176 peptide) gives strong evidence that PBC is a T-cell-mediated autoimmune disorder. The autoantigen is highly expressed on the apical surface of biliary epithelial cells in PBC [129,130]. The nature and identity of the tissue-specific autoantigen which cross-reacts with PDC-E2 remains to be defined, but there is strong evidence that mitochondrial autoantigens may be the cause for the induction of a disease-specific autoimmunity. Etiology and disease-promoting factors or agents of the disease-specific autoimmune response have not yet been identified. But the fact that PDC-E2 is evolutionarily highly conserved among various species and is displayed on the cell surface of bacteria supports the notion that cross-reactivity or molecular mimicry at the T-cell level may be a decisive step for the break of tolerance to biliary autoantigens. This disease-promoting factor may mainly be effective in females with a special immunogenetic background.

3.2. Viral liver diseases

The liver is the primary site of viral replication of probably all clinically relevant hepatitis viruses. The early interaction between hepatitis viruses and the host determines the fate of viral infections. Although the relevance of the antigen non-specific (innate) immune response of the host is not well documented, it is likely that an early and strong innate immune reaction which regulates the virus-specific adaptive immune mechanisms is a prerequisite for viral control and clearance. The fact that infected hepatocytes usually display no or little liver damage suggests that the antiviral immune response is not only responsible for viral clearance, but also the most important factor in the pathogenesis of viral liver diseases and the individual clinical pictures and courses [131].

As mentioned before, the normal liver is able to eliminate activated immune cells after pathogen-induced expansion to restore homeostasis of the resident immune cell repertoire. In the case of hepatic viral infection, the intrahepatic induction of specifically primed naive T cells, the release of proinflammatory cytokines and chemokines by resident cells may be the primary and early antiviral response of the host to control the infection locally [132,133]. With respect to the incubation time the local host viral interaction may last about 3 months or more in HBV and about 2 months in HCV infections. The recruitment of specific Th1 cells, CTLs, and monocytes/macrophages from the peripheral blood may in case of an insufficient local control of viral infection lead to intrahepatic inflammation, tissue damage, and clinical disease [134–136].

What is known about the dynamic of immune mechanisms during the usually very long incubation time in hepatitis B and hepatitis C compared with other viral diseases [131]? In a chimpanzee model of HBV infection, a marked reduction of viral load already occurs before clinical disease [137]. Furthermore, it has been shown in a transgenic mouse model of HBV infection that viral clearance or reduction of viral load seems not to be due to viral specific CTL, but other antiviral host defense mechanisms i.e. cytokines. This notion received support through a prospective analysis of cellular immune mechanisms during the incubation time of a single source outbreak of HBV infection [138,139]. Thus, clinical diseases which develop in only one-third of individuals infected with the hepatitis B virus seem to be the result of an insufficient host defense at the sites of viral replication and of an activation of adaptive immune mechanisms. Due to the wide distribution of MHC class I molecule-expression, the adaptive cellular immune response has the ability to recognize viral antigens in infected cells throughout the body. At the site of viral replication, HLA class II-restricted T-helper cell responses are of particular importance for the outcome of infections.

Which factors influence viral persistence in HBV and HCV infections, and what makes the difference between HBV and HCV infections?

In HBV infections, host defense mechanisms are effective in the majority of individuals after HBV inoculation. It is well documented that about 70% of HBV-infected subjects clear the virus without clinical disease. The remaining 30% develop acute hepatitis, but only 5–10% of them become chronic HBV carriers. The majority of individuals with long or life-long HBV persistence stem from vertical HBV transmission or HBV infection during early childhood, thus in individuals with a poorly developed immune system. These HBV-carriers seem to have a status of immune tolerance to HBV as documented by the high rate (90%) of persistent infections, lack of disease activity in the presence of high viral load, and the very low rate of spontaneous or interferon-induced seroconversion from HBE antigen to anti-HBE. However, clinical and immunological studies clearly show that HBV-specific T cells are still present in so-called tolerant HBV carriers as evidenced by the small number of carriers that develop HBV-specific T-cell proliferation and seroconversion [140]. The trigger mechanisms that allow the immune system to overcome tolerance to HBV in patients with perinatally acquired HBV infections are unknown. Persistent HBV infections in adults are mainly related to the male sex, various forms of T-cell immune deficiencies and immunosuppressions. Thus the majority of persistent HBV infections are associated with poor host defense mechanisms which allow the virus to develop immune escape mechanisms [141].

One of the most important features of HCV infections is the high rate of chronicity (70–90%) that follows acute hepatitis C which often shows subclinical courses. Chronic HCV infections resulting from vertical viral transmission is a rare event. In contrast to HBV infection, viral factors seem to be of central importance for HCV persistence and the outcome of the disease [142]. The genetic variability of HCV is very complex. Genotypes, subgenotypes, isolates, and quasi-species are the basis for the development of a large reservoir of biologically different variants and for viral load [142]. Another important factor is the early extrahepatic expression and viral replication in particular in cells of the immune system including the immune-privileged sites of the liver that may lead, like in HIV infections, to an alteration and suppression of the local immune response, particularly in the early phase of infection [143]. Furthermore, extrahepatic manifestations of HCV infections, such as autoimmunity, immune abnormalities and B-cell lympho-proliferative disorders, are very common [144].

From observations in immune-incompetent patients, HCV appears to be non-cytopathic. Thus, as in HBV infections, the antiviral immune response seems to play a critical role for both viral clearance and the pathogenesis of the various courses of HCV-related liver diseases [143]. Self-limited HCV infections are associated with strong and long-lasting HCV-specific $CD4^+$ T-cell response [145–148].

The pathogenesis of the different courses of chronic hepatitis C and hepatocellular injury is not yet fully understood, but there is increasing evidence that a loss of HCV-specific $CD4^+$ and $CD8^+$ T-cell response is one of the central factors of HCV persistence and disease chronicity. With respect to the impaired HCV-specific T-cell function, disease progression and hepatocellular damage seem to be related to non-specific immune reactivity and proinflammatory cytokine production. But not only Th1 cytokines may be course-determining. A switch in the cytokine secretion patterns from Th1 to Th2/Th0 and vice versa — probably different from chronic HBV carriers [149] — is more likely to explain the different clinical pictures and the development of fibrosis and cirrhosis in chronic hepatitis C [150].

REFERENCES

[1] Wisse E, De Zanger RB, Charels K et al. The liver sieve: considerations concerning the structure and function of endothelial fenestrae, the sinusoidal wall and the space Disse. Hepatology 1985; 5: 683–692.

[2] Van den Oord JJ, De Vos R, Desmet VM. HLA expression in liver diseases. In: Popper H, Schaffner F, editors. Progress in Liver Diseases, Vol. IX. Philadelphia, PA, Saunders, 1990; pp. 73–88.

[3] Geppert TD, Lipsky PE. Antigen presentation at the inflammatory site. Crit Rev Immunol 1989; 9: 313–318.
[4] Geppert TD, Davis LS, Gur H et al. Accessory cell signals involved in T-cell activation. Immunol Rev 1990; 117: 5–12.
[5] Springer TA. Adhesion receptors of the immune system. Nature 1990; 346: 425–432.
[6] Volpes R, van den Oord JJ, Desmet VJ. Immunochemical study of adhesion molecules in liver inflammation. Hepatology 1990; 12: 59–66.
[7] Steinhoff G, Behrend M, Wonigkeit K. Expression of adhesion molecules on lymphocytes/monocytes and hepatocytes in human liver grafts. Hum Immunol 1990; 28: 123–131.
[8] Volpes R, van den Oord JJ, Desmet VJ. Hepatic expression of intercellular adhesion molecule 1 (ICAM-1) in viral hepatitis B. Hepatology 1990; 12: 148–155.
[9] Volpes R, van den Oord JJ, De Vos R et al. Expression of interferon gamma receptor in normal and pathological human liver tissue. J Hepatol 1991; 12: 195–203.
[10] Volpes R, van den Oord JJ, De Vos R, Desmet VJ. Hepatic expression of type A and type B receptors for tumor necrosis factor. J Hepatol 1992; 14: 61–69.
[11] Volpes R, van den Oord JJ, Desmet VJ. Expression of B-cell growth factor receptor (CDw40) on hepatocytes in areas of inflammation. J Hepatol 1989; 9 (Suppl): 243–251.
[12] Smedsrød B. Pathobiology of sinusoidal endothelial cells. In: Gresner A, Ramadori G, editors. Molecular and Cell Biology of Liver Fibrogenesis. Dordrecht, Kluwer Academic Press, 1992; pp. 454–467.
[13] Fraser R, Dobbs BR, Rogers GW. Lipoproteins and the liver sieve: the role of the fenestrated sinusoidal endothelium in lipoprotein metabolism, atherosclerosis and cirrhosis. Hepatology 1995; 21: 863–874.
[14] Blomhoff R, Eskild W, Berg T. Endocytosis of formaldehyde treated serum albumin via scavenger pathway in liver endothelial cells. Biochem J 1984; 218: 81–86.
[15] Laurent TC. Scavenger functions of the liver endothelial cell. Biochem J 1990; 266: 313–327.
[16] Magnusson S, Berg T. Extremely rapid endocytosis mediated by the mannose receptor of sinusoidal endothelial rat liver cells. Biochem J 1989; 257: 651–656.
[17] Melkko J, Hellevik T, Risteli L et al. Clearance of NH2-terminal propeptides of types I and III procollagen is a physiological function of the scavenger receptor in liver endothelial cells. J Exp Med 1994; 1879: 405–412.
[18] Horiuchi S. Advanced glycation end products are eliminated by scavenger-receptor-mediated endocytosis in hepatic sinusoidal Kupffer and endothelial cells. Biochem J 1997; 322: 567–573.
[19] Tavassoli M, Kishimoto T, Soda R et al. Liver endothelium mediates the uptake of iron-transferrin complex by hepatocytes. Exp Cell Res 1986; 165: 369–379.
[20] Tavassoli M, Kishimoto T, Kataoka M. Liver endothelium mediates the hepatocyte's uptake of ceruloplasmin. J Cell Biol 1986; 102: 1298–1303.
[21] Irie S, Kishimoto T, Tavassoli M. Desialation of transferrin by rat liver endothelium. J Clin Invest 1988; 82: 508–513.
[22] Lohse AW, Knolle PA, Bilo K et al. Antigen-presenting function and B7 expression of murine sinusoidal endothelial cells and Kupffer cells. Gastroenterology 1996; 110: 1175–1181.
[23] Knolle PA, Uhrig A, Hegenbarth S et al. IL-10 down-regulates T cell activation by antigen-presenting liver sinusoidal endothelial cells through decreased antigen uptake via the mannose receptor and lowered surface expression of accessory molecules. Clin Exp Immunol 1998; 114: 427–433.

[24] Sallusto F, Cella M, Danieli C, Lanzavecchia A. Dendritic cells use macropinocytosis and the mannose receptor to concentrate macromolecules in the major histocompatibility complex class II compartment: downregulation by cytokines and bacterial products. J Exp Med 1995; 182: 389–400.
[25] Autschbach F, Meuer S, Moebius U et al. Hepatocellular expression of lymphocyte function-associated antigen 3 in chronic hepatitis. Hepatology 1991; 14: 223–230.
[26] Meuer SC, Hussey RE, Fabbi M et al. An alternative pathway of T-cell activation: a functional role for the 50 kd TI 1 sheep erythrocyte receptor protein. Cell 1984; 36: 897–906.
[27] Scoazec JY, Feldmann G. Both macrophages and endothelial cells of the human hepatic sinusoid express the CD4 molecule, a receptor for the human immunodeficiency virus. Hepatology 1990; 12: 505–510.
[28] Knolle P, Schmitt E, Jin S et al. Induction of cytokine production in naive $CD4^+$ T cells by antigen-presenting murine liver sinusoidal endothelial cells but failure to induce differentiation toward Th1 cells. Gastroenterology 1999; 116: 1428–1440.
[29] Winwood PJ, Arthur MJP. Kupffer cells: their activation and role in animal models of liver injury and human liver disease. Semin Liver Dis 1993; 13: 50–58.
[30] Laskin DL, Sirak AA, Pilaro AM. Functional and biochemical properties of rat Kupffer cells and peritoneal macrophages. J Leukocyte Biol 1988; 44: 71–76.
[31] Lepay DA, Nathan CF, Steinmann RM. Murine Kupffer cells: mononuclear phagocytes deficient in the generation of reactive oxygen intermediates. J Exp Med 1985; 161: 1079–1087.
[32] Van Vossuyt H, Zahger RB, Wisse E. Cellular and subcellular distribution of injected lipopolysaccharide in rat liver and its inactivation by bile salt. J Hepatol 1988; 7: 325–331.
[33] McCuskey RS, McCuskey PA, Urbaschek R, Urbaschek B. Kupffer cell function in host defense. Rev Infect Dis 1987; 9: 616–622.
[34] Rogoff TM, Lipsky PE. Role of the Kupffer cells in local and systemic immune response. Gastroenterology 1981; 80: 854–863.
[35] Callery MP, Kamei T, Flye MW. Kupffer cell blockade inhibits induction of tolerance by the portal venous route. Transplantation 1989; 47: 1092–1098.
[36] Knolle P, Schlaak J, Uhrig A et al. Human Kupffer cells secrete IL-10 in response to lipopolysaccharide (LPS) challenge. J Hepatol 1995; 22: 226–229.
[37] Knolle PA, Uhrig A, Protzer U et al. Interleukin-10 expression is autoregulated at the transcriptional level in human and murine Kupffer cells. Hepatology 1998; 27: 93–99.
[38] Collins C, Norris S, McEntee G et al. RAG1, RAG2 and pre-T cell receptor alpha chain expression by adult human hepatic T cells; evidence for extrathymic T cell maturation. Eur J Immunol 1996; 26: 3114–3118.
[39] Lynch S, Kelleher D, McManus R, O'Farrelly C. RAG1 and RAG2 expression in human intestinal epithelium: evidence of extrathymic T cell differentiation. Eur J Immunol 1995; 25: 1143–1447.
[40] Guy-Grand D, Vanden Broecke C, Briottet C et al. Different expression of the recombination activity gene RAG-1 in various populations of thymocytes, peripheral T cells and gut thymus-independent intraepithelial lymphocytes suggests two pathways of T cell receptor rearrangement. Eur J Immunol 1992; 22: 505–510.
[41] Lundqvist C, Varanov V, Hammarstrom S et al. Intra-epithelial lymphocytes. Evidence for regional specialization and extrathymic T cell maturation in the human gut epithelium. Int Immunol 1995; 7: 1473–1487.
[42] O'Farrelly C, Crispe IN. Prometheus through the looking glass: reflections on the hepatic immune system. Immunol Today 1999; 20: 394–398.

[43] Schlitt HJ, Schafers S, Deiwick A et al. Extramedullary erythropoiesis in human liver grafts. Hepatology 1995; 21: 689–696.
[44] Bandeira A, Itohara S, Bonneville M et al. Extrathymic origin of intestinal intraepithelial lymphocytes bearing T-cell antigen receptor gamma delta. Proc Natl Acad Sci USA 1991; 88: 43–47.
[45] MacDonald HR. NK1.1+ T cell receptor-alpha/beta+ cells: New clues to their origin, specificity, and function. J Exp Med 1995; 182: 633–638.
[46] Bendelac A, Lantz O, Quimby ME et al. CD1 recognition by mouse NK1+ T lymphocytes. Science 1995; 268: 863–865.
[47] Wake K. 'Sternzellen' in the liver: perisinusoidal cells with special reference to storage of vitamin A. Am J Anat 1971; 132: 429–436.
[48] Hendriks HFJ, Verfoofstad WA, Brouwer A et al. Perisinusoidal fat-storing cells are the main vitamin A storage sites in rat liver. Exp Cell Res 1985; 160: 138–144.
[49] Ramadori G. Kupffer cells and fibrogenesis. In: Clement A, Guillozo EDS, editors. Cellular and Molecular Aspects of Cirrhosis. Paris: John Libbey Eurotext, 1992; 215: 169–177.
[50] Knittel T, Kobold D, Salle B et al. Rat liver myofibroblasts and hepatic stellate cells: different cell populations of the fibroblast lineage with fibrogenic potential. Gastroenterology 1999; 117: 1205–1221.
[51] Friedman SL. The virtuosity of hepatic stellata cells. Gastroenterology 1999; 117: 1244–1246.
[52] Friedman SL. Hepatic stellata cells. Progress in Liver Disease 1996; 14: 101–130.
[53] Maher JJ. Cytokines: Overview. Semin Liver Dis 1999; 19(2): 109–115.
[54] Knolle PA, Gerken G, Local control of the immune response in the liver. Immunol Rev 2000; 174: 21–34.
[55] Weiner HL, Mayer LF. Oral tolerance: mechanisms and application. Ann New York Acad Sci 1996; 778–792.
[56] Yang R, Liu Q, Grosfeld JL, Pescovitz MD. Intestinal venous drainage through the liver is a prerequisite for oral tolerance induction. J Pediatr Surg 1994; 29: 1145–1148.
[57] Callery MP, Kamei T, Flye MW. The effect of portacaval shunt on delayed-hypersensitivity responses following antigen feeding J Surg Res 1989; 46: 391–394.
[58] Gorczynski RM. Adoptive transfer of unresponsiveness to allogeneic skin grafts with hepatic $\gamma\delta^-$ T cells. Immunology 1994; 81: 27–35.
[59] Dini I, Caral EC. Hepatic sinusoidal endothelium heterogeneity with respect to the recognition of apoptotic cells. Exp Cell Res 1998; 240: 388–398.
[60] Müschen M, Warskulat U, Douillard P et al. Regulation of CD95 (APO-1/Fas) receptor and ligand expression by lipopolysaccharide and dexamethasone in parenchymal and nonparenchymal rat liver cells. Hepatology 1998; 27: 200–208.
[61] Müschen M, Warskulat U, Peters-Regehr T et al. Involvement of CD95 (APO-1/Fas) ligand expressed by rat Kupffer cells in hepatic immunoregulation. Gastroenterology 1999; 116: 666–667.
[62] Bertolino P, Trescol-Biemont MC, Rabourdin-Combe C. Hepatocytes induce functional activation of naive $CD8^+$ T lymphocytes but fail to promote survival. Eur J Immunol 1998; 28: 221–236.
[63] Galle PR, Hofmann WJ, Walczak M et al. Involvement of the CD95 (APO-1/Fas) receptor and ligand in liver damage. J Exp Med 1995; 182: 1223–1230.
[64] Cooper S, Erickson AL, Adams EJ et al. Analysis of a successful immune response against hepatitis C virus. Immunity 1999; 10: 439–449.

[65] Crispe IN, Mehal WZ. Strange brew: T cells in the liver. Immunol Today 1996; 17: 522–525.
[66] Kamada N, Wight DG. Antigen-specific immunosuppression induced by liver transplantation in the rat. Transplantation 1984; 38: 217–221.
[67] May AG, Bauer S, Leddy JP et al. Survival of allografts after hepatic portal venous administration of specific transplantation antigen. Ann Surg 1969; 170: 824–832.
[68] Gorczynski RM. Immunosuppression induced by hepatic portal venous immunization spares reactivity in IL-4 producing T lymphocytes. Immunol Lett 1992; 33: 67–77.
[69] Barker CF, Corrier JN Jr. Canine renal homotransplantation with venous drainage via the portal vein. Ann Surg 1967; 165: 279–282.
[70] Boeckx W, Sobis H, Lacqzet A et al. Prolongation of allogeneic heart graft survival by pretransplant transfusion and/or by varying the route of allograft venous drainage. Transplantation 1975; 19: 145–149.
[71] Gorczynski RM, Chan Z, Chung S et al. Prolongation of rat small bowel or renal allograft survival by pretransplant transfusion and/or by varying the route of allograft venous drainage. Transplantation 1994; 58: 816–820.
[72] Rossi-Bergman B. A subset of $\gamma\delta$ T-cell receptor-positive cells produce T-helper type-2 cytokines and regulate mouse skin graft rejection following portal venous pretransplant preimmunization. Immunology 1996; 87: 381–389.
[73] Gorczynski RM, Hozumi N, Wolf S, Chen Z. Interleukin 12 in combination with anti-interleukin 10 reverses graft prolongation after portal venous immunization. Transplantation 1995; 60: 1337–1341.
[74] Gorczynski RM. Regulation of IFN-γ and IL-10 synthesis in vivo as well as continuous antigen exposure, is associated with tolerance to murine skin allografts. Cell Immunol 1995; 160: 224–231.
[75] Gorczynski L, Chen Z, Hu, J et al. Evidence that an OX-2-positive cell can inhibit the stimulation of type 1 cytokine production by bone marrow-derived B7-1 and B7-2-positive dendritic cells. J Immunol 1999; 162: 774-781.
[76] Cosse L. Electron microscopy of Kupffer cells in the orthotopic porcine liver homograft during the late stage after transplantation (phagocytosis of host cells by Kupffer cells). Exp Pathol (Jena) 1975; 11: 168–181.
[77] Falsca L, Bergamini A, Serafino A et al. Human Kupffer cell recognition and phagocytosis of apoptotic peripheral blood lymphocytes. Exp Cell Res 1996; 224: 152–162.
[78] Caliery MP, Kamei T, Flye MW. Kupffer cell blockade inhibits induction of tolerance by the portal venous route. Transplantation 1989; 47: 1091–1094.
[79] Kamei T, Callery MP, Flye MW. Kupffer cell blockade prevents induction of portal venous tolerance in rat cardiac allograft transplantation. J Surg Res 1990; 48: 393–396.
[80] Roland CR, Mangino MJ, Duffy BF, Flye MW. Lymphocyte suppression by Kupffer cells prevents portal venous tolerance induction: a study of macrophage function after intravenous gadolinium. Transplantation 1993; 55: 1151–1158.
[81] Steinbrink K, Wolf M, Jonuleit H et al. Induction of tolerance by IL 10–treated dendritic cells. J Immunol 1997; 159: 4772–4780.
[82] Limmer A, Ohl J, Kurts Ch et al. Efficient presentation of exogenous antigen by liver endothelial cells to $CD8^{+}$ T cells results in antigen-specific T–cell tolerance. Nat Med 2999; 6(12): 1348–1355.
[83] Fearon DT, Locksley RM. The instructive role of innate immunity in the acquired immune response. Science 1996; 272: 50–53.
[84] Epstein J, Eichbaum Q, Sheriff S, Ezekowitz RA. The collectins in innate immunity. Curr Opin Immunol 1996; 8: 29–35.

[85] Biron CA. Role of early cytokines, including alpha and beta interferons (IFN-alpha/beta), in innate and adaptive immune responses to viral infections. Semin Immunol 1998; 10: 383–390.
[86] Medzhitov R, Janeway CA Jr. Innate immunity: impact on the adaptive immune response. Curr Opin Immunol 1997; 9: 4–9.
[87] Fraser IP, Koziel H, Ezekowitz RA. The serum mannose-binding protein and the macrophage mannose receptor are pattern recognition molecules that link innate and adaptive immunity. Semin Immunol 1998; 10: 363–372.
[88] Suzuki H, Kurihara Y, Takeya M et al. A role for macrophage scavenger receptors in atherosclerosis and susceptibility to infection. Nature 1997; 386: 292–156.
[89] Thomas CA, Li Y, Kodama T et al. Protection from lethal Gram-positive infection by macrophage scavenger receptor-dependent phagocytosis. J Exp Med 2000; 191: 147–156.
[90] Hashimoto C, Hudson KL, Anderson KV. The Toll gene of Drosophila, required for dorsal-ventral embryonic polarity, appears to encode a transmembrane protein. Cell 1988; 52: 269–279.
[91] Hoffmann JA, Kafatos FC, Janeway CA, Ezekowitz RA. Phylogenetic perspectives in innate immunity. Science 1999; 284: 1313–1318.
[92] Takeuchi O, Kaufmann A, Grote K et al. Cutting edge: preferentially the R stereoisomer of the mycoplasmal lipopeptide macrophage-activating lipopeptide-2 activates immune cells through a Toll-like receptor 2- and MyD88-dependent signaling pathway. J Immunol 2000; 164: 554–557.
[93] Medzhitov R, Janeway CA. Innate Immunity. New Engl J Med 2000; 343(5): 338–344.
[94] Ishikawa R, Biron CA. IFN induction and associated changes in splenic leukocyte distribution. J Immunol 1993; 150: 3713–3727.
[95] Salazar-Mather TP, Ishikawa R, Biron CA. NK cell trafficking and cytokine expression in splenic compartments after IFN induction and viral infection. J Immunol 1996; 157: 3054–3064.
[96] Ma A. Pleiotropic functions of IL 15 in innate and adoptive immunity. Mod Asp Immunobiol 2000; 1(3): 102–104.
[97] Ihle JN. Cytokine receptor signaling. Nature 1995; 377: 591–601.
[98] Scabo SJ, Kim ST, Costa GL et al. A novel transcription factor, T-bet, directs Th1 lineage commitment. Cell 2000; 100: 655–669.
[99] Ouyang W, Löhming M, Gao Z et al. Stat6-independent Gata-3 autoactivation directs IL4-independent Th2 development and commitment. Immunity 2000; 12: 27–37.
[100] O'Garra A. Commit ye helpers. Nature 2000; 404: 719–720.
[101] Leitenberg D, Boutin Y, Lu DD, Bottomly K. Biochemical association of CD45 with the T cell receptor complex: regulation by CD45 isoform and during T cell activation. Immunity 1999; 10(6): 701–711.
[102] Tao X, Constant S, Jorritsma P, Bottomly K. Strength of TCR signal determines the costimulatory requirements for Th1 and Th2 $CD4^+$ T cell differentiation. J Immunol 1997; 159: 5956–5964.
[103] Hsieh CS, Macatonia SE, O'Garra A, Murphy KM. Pathogen-induced Th1 phenotype development in $CD4^+$ $\alpha\beta$-TCR transgenic T cells is macrophage dependent. Int Immunol 1993; 5: 371–382.
[104] Springer TA. Traffic signals for lymphocyte recirculation and leukocyte emigration: the multiple paradigma. Cell 1994; 76: 304–314.
[105] Shields PL, Morland CM, Salmon M et al. Chemokine and chemokine receptor interactions provide a mechanism for selective T cell recruitment to specific liver compartments within hepatitis C-infected liver. J Immunol 1999; 163: 6236–6243.

[106] Zlotnik A, Yoshic O. Chemokines: a new classification system and their role in immunity. Immunity 2000; 12: 121–127.
[107] Jung S, Littman DR. Chemokine receptors in lymphoid organ homeostasis. Curr Opin Immunol 1999; 11: 319–325.
[108] Sallusto F, Lenig D, Mackay CR, Lanzavecchia A. Flexible programs of chemokine receptor expression on human polarized T helper 1 and 2 lymphocytes. J Exp Med 1998; 187: 875–883.
[109] Bonechhi R, Bianchi G, Bordignon PP et al. Differential expression of chemokine receptors and chemotactic responsiveness of type 1 T helper cells (Th1s) and Th2s. J Exp Med 1998; 187: 129–134.
[110] Murai M, Yoneyama H, Harada A et al. Active participation of CCR5(+) T lymphocytes in the pathogenesis of liver injury in graft-versus-host disease. J Clin Invest 1999; 104: 49–57.
[111] Mehal WZ, Juedes AE, Crispe IN. Selective retention of activated $CD8^+$ T cells by the normal liver. J Immunol 1999; 163: 3202–3210.
[112] Cocchi F, DeVico AL, Garzino-Demo A et al. Identification of RANTES, MIP-1 alpha, and MIP-1 beta as the major HIV-suppressive factors produced by $CD8^+$ T cells. Science 1995; 270: 1811–1815.
[113] Mitchel LS, Jeffers LJ, Reddy KR et al. Detection of hepatitis C virus antibody by first and second generation assays and polymerase chain reaction in patients with autoimmune chronic active hepatitis types I, II, and III. Am J Gastroenterol 1993; 88: 1027–1034.
[114] Lohse AW, Gerken G, Mohr H et al. Relation between autoimmune liver diseases and viral hepatitis: clinical and serological characteristics in 859 patients. Ger J Gastroenterol 1995; 33: 527–533.
[115] Philipp J, Durrazo M, Trautwein CH et al. Recognition of uridine diphosphate glucuronosyl transferase by LKM_3 antibodies in chronic hepatitis D. Lancet 1994; 344: 578–581.
[116] Mayet WH, Hess G, Gerken G et al. Treatment of chronic type B hepatitis with recombinant alpha interferon induces autoantibodies not specific for autoimmune chronic hepatitis. Hepatology 1989; 10: 24–28.
[117] Michel G, Ritter A, Gerken G et al. Anti-GOR and hepatitis C virus in autoimmune liver diseases. Lancet 1992; 339: 267–269.
[118] Löhr HF, Gerken G, Michel G et al. In vitro secretion of anti-GOR protein and anti-hepatitis C virus antibodies in patients with chronic hepatitis C. Gastroenterology 1994; 107: 1443–1448.
[119] McFarlane IG. Autoimmunity and hepatotropic viruses. Semin Liver Dis 1991; 11: 221–223.
[120] Lohse AW, Manns M, Dienes HP et al. Experimental autoimmune hepatitis: disease induction, time course and T-cell reactivity. Hepatology 1990; 11: 24–30.
[121] Lohse AW, Kögel M, Meyer zum Büschenfelde KH. Evidence for spontaneous immunosuppression in autoimmune hepatitis. Hepatology 1995; 22: 381–388.
[122] Cohen IR, Miller A. Autoimmune disease models. New York, London: Academic Press, 1994.
[123] Thorpe ME, Scheuer PJ, Sherlock S. Primary sclerosing cholangitis, the biliary tree and ulcerative colitis. Gut 1967; 8: 435–448.
[124] Chapman RW, Marborgh BA, Rhodes JM et al. Primary sclerosing cholangitis: A review of its clinical features, cholangiography, and hepatic histology. Gut 1980; 21: 870–877.
[125] Gohlke F, Lohse AW, Dienes HP et al. Evidence for an overlap of autoimmune hepatitis and primary sclerosing cholangitis. J Hepatol 1996; 24: 699–705.
[126] Van Bauren HR, von Hoogstraten HJF, Terkivatan T et al. High prevalence of autoimmune

hepatitis among patients with primary sclerosing cholangitis. J Hepatol 2000; 33: 543–548.

[127] Duerr RH, Targan SR, Landers CJ et al. Neutrophilic cytoplasmic antibodies: a link between primary sclerosing cholangitis and ulcerative colitis. Gastroenterology 1991; 100: 1385–1391.

[128] Mackay JR, Gershwin ME. The nature of autoimmune disease. Semin Liver Dis 1997; 17: 3–11.

[129] Tsuneyama K, Van de Water J, Leung PSC et al. Abnormal expression of the E2 component of the pyruvate dehydrogenase complex on the luminal surface of biliary epithelium occurs before major histocompatibility complex class II and BB1/B7 expression. Hepatology 1995; 21: 1031–1937.

[130] Joplin R, Gershwin ME. Ductular expression of autoantigens in primary biliary cirrhosis. Semin Liver Dis 1997; 17: 97–103.

[131] Zuckermann AJ, Zuckermann JN. Hepatitis viruses. In: Weatherall DJ, Ledingham JGG, Warrell DA, editors. Oxford Textbook of Medicine, 2nd ed. Oxford: Oxford University Press, 1996; pp. 452–460.

[132] Biron CA, Nguyen KB, Pien GC et al. Natural killer cells in antiviral defense: function and regulation by innate cytokines. Annu Rev Immunol 1999; 17: 189–220.

[133] Welsh RM, Brubaker JO, Vargas-Cortes M, O'Donnell CL. Natural killer (NK) cell response to virus infections in mice with severe combined immunodeficiency. The stimulation of NK cells and the NK cell-dependent control of virus infections occur dependently of T and B cell function. J Exp Med 1991; 173: 1053–1063.

[134] Guidotti LG, Chisari FV. To kill or cure: options in host defense against viral infection. Curr Opin Immunol 1996; 8: 478–483.

[135] Maini MK, Boni C, Ogg GS et al. Direct ex vivo analysis of hepatitis B virus-specific CD8(+) T cells associated with the control of infection. Gastroenterology 1999; 117: 1386–1396.

[136] Maini MK, Boni C, Lee CK et al. The role of virus-specific $CD8^+$ cells in liver damage and viral control during persistent hepatitis B virus (HBV) infection. J Exp Med 2000; 191: 1269–1280.

[137] Guidotti LG, Rochford R, Chung J et al. Viral clearance without destruction of infected cells during acute HBV infection. Science 1999; 284: 825–829.

[138] Webster GJM, Hallett R, Whalley SA et al. Molecular epidemiology of a large outbreak of hepatitis B linked to 'autohaemotherapy'. Lancet 2000; 356: 379–384.

[139] Webster GJM, Reignat S, Maini MK et al. Incubation phase of acute hepatitis B in man: dynamics of cellular immune mechanisms. Hepatology 2000; 32: 117–124.

[140] Hsu HY, Chang MH, Lee CY et al. Spontaneous loss of HBsAg in children with chronic hepatitis B virus infection. Hepatology 1992; 15: 382–386.

[141] Protzer U, Schaller H. Immune escape by hepatic B viruses. Virus Genes 2000; 21: 27–37.

[142] Farci P, Purcall RH. Clinical significance of hepatitis C virus. Genotypes and quasispecies. Semin Liver Dis 2000; 20: 103–126.

[143] Rehermann B. Interaction between the hepatitis C virus and the immune system. Semin Liver Dis 2000; 20: 127–141.

[144] Rammacco F, Sansonno D, Piccoli C et al. The lymphoid system in hepatitis C infection: Autoimmunity, mixcoyoglobulinemia, and overt B cell malignancy. Semin Liver Dis 2000; 20: 143–157.

[145] Diepolder H, Zachoval R, Hoffmann R et al. Possible mechanism involving T-lymphocyte response to non-structural protein 3 in viral clearance in acute hepatitis C virus infection. Lancet 1995; 346: 1006–1007.

[146] Missale G, Bertoni R, Lamonaca V et al. Different clinical behaviors of acute hepatitis C infection are associated with different vigor of the anti-viral cell-mediated immune response. J Clin Invest 1996; 98: 706–714.
[147] Cramp ME, Carucci P, Rossol S et al. Hepatitis C virus (HCV) specific immune responses in anti-HCV positive patients with hepatitis C viraemia. Gut 1999; 44: 424–429.
[148] Gerlach JT, Diepolder HM, Jung MC et al. Recurrence of hepatitis C virus after loss of virus-specific $CD4^+$ T-cell response in acute hepatitis C. Gastroenterology 1999; 117: 933–941.
[149] Bertoletti A, D'Elios MM, Boni C et al. Different cytokine profiles of intrahepatic T cells in chronic hepatitis B and hepatitis C virus infections. Gastroentrology 1997; 112: 193–199.
[150] Poynard T, Ratzin V, Bermanov Y et al. Fibrosis in patients with chronic hepatitis C: Detection and significance. Semin Liver Dis 2000; 20: 47–55.

Viral Hepatitis

Edited by T. Tsuji, T. Higashi, M. Zeniya and K.-H. Meyer zum Büschenfelde

CHAPTER 2

The Mechanisms of Liver Injury in Hepatitis B Virus Infection

Tetsuya Ishikawa and Shinichi Kakumu

First Department of Internal Medicine, Research Center for Infectious Disease, Aichi Medical University School of Medicine, Aichi, Japan

INTRODUCTION

HBV (hepatitis B virus) is a noncytopathic virus with a circular double stranded DNA genome. It causes acute and chronic necroinflammatory liver disease and hepatocellular carcinoma [1]. Since the disease spectrum associated with HBV is extraordinarily variable, it is believed that the host immune response plays a critical role in the pathogenesis of the associated liver disease. In fact, a great deal of evidence suggests that the several mechanisms of the immune system deal with free extracellular HBV and HBV-infected cells and that they relate to the pathogenesis of type B hepatitis [1]. However, it has been difficult to examine the roles of immune responses in detail because of the limited host range of this virus and the lack of an in vitro culture system to propagate it. Until recently, most studies of HBV pathogenesis were limited to the analysis of HBV-infected patients and chimpanzees or of HBV-related hepadonavirus infections in the woodchuck, ground squirrel, and Peking duck, outbred species whose immune systems have not been characterized and have limited value for analysis of the antiviral immune response.

Just recently, it became evident that many questions relating to HBV immunobiology and pathogenesis might be directly examined by introducing partial or complete copies of the HBV genome into transgenic mice. For example, a model for acute and fulminant hepatitis initiated by HBsAg-specific CTL (cytotoxic T lymphocyte) response has been developed [2,3]. In the same model system, the clearance of the virus also initiated by HBsAg-specific CTL response without the destruction of antigen- or virus-loaded cells has been observed [4,5]. Also the disease pathogenesis induced by HBsAg-specific helper T cell (Th) response was studied in the same mice [6]. Using this model, we tried to elucidate the detailed mechanisms of liver injury and viral clearance, and the relationship of both events to the strength of immune response, using the variety of CTLs that showed different characteristics in vitro. The results indicated that the viral clearance was highly dependent on the amount of cytokines produced by CTLs, being consistent with the previous. On the other hand, it was shown that the disease magnitude was dependent on the unknown characteristics of CTLs but on cytokine profiles of CTLs.

1. HBV IMMUNOPATHOGENESIS AND FULMINANT HEPATITIS IN HUMAN

The immune responses to HBV encoded antigens are responsible for viral clearance and for disease pathogenesis during this infection. While the humoral antibody response to viral envelope antigens contribute to the clearance of circulating virus particles, the cellular immune responses to the envelope, nucleocapsid, and polymerase antigens eliminated infected cells, thus directly contribute to the disease pathogenesis. The class I- and class II-restricted T cell responses to the viral antigens are detected in the infected patients, and are vigorous, polyclonal, and multispecific in acutely infected patients who successfully clear the virus [1]. These responses are thought to play central roles in the development of hepatic injury, and it may be reasonable to think that their strength determines the extent of the disease. The relationship of mutant HBV to development of fulminant hepatitis has been discussed in the literature. It is reported that severe hepatitis such as fulminant hepatitis is caused by the mutant HBV lacking HBeAg production [7,8]. On the other hand, the wild type HBV without such mutations is also reported to cause fulminant hepatitis [9,10]. In consideration of this unsolved subject, we tried to examine the roles of immune responses, especially cellular immune responses in disease exacerbation using the hepatitis model with HBV transgenic mice as described below.

2. CTL-MEDIATED IMMUNOPATHOGENESIS

Fig. 1 illustrates the system that was developed to study the pathogenesis of immune-mediated hepatitis. HBsAg-specific CTLs were derived from B10.D2 (H-2^d) non-transgenic mice. Briefly, the mice were immunized two to three times weekly with recombinant vaccinia virus harboring HBs gene. One week after the last immunization, their spleen cells were recovered, stimulated in vitro with HBsAg-expressing tumor cells, and cloned by limiting dilution. The obtained CTL clones were all $CD8^+$, MHC class I (L^d)-restricted, recognized a twelve-mer peptide within HBsAg (HBsAg aa28–39) as a minimal optimal motif, and secreted IFN-γ (interferon-γ) and TNF-α (tumor necrosis factor-α) after antigen stimulation in vitro [5,6]. After expansion in vitro, CTL clones were injected intravenously to transgenic mice that have same background (H-2^d) as the source of CTLs (B10.D2) and express HBsAg in the liver. The extent of disease severity was assessed by serum ALT levels and by the histology of the liver. HBV proteins, mRNA, and DNA level in the liver were also analyzed to assess the antiviral effect of CTLs.

The transgenic lineages that are used in this work are reviewed in Table 1.

3. PATHOGENETIC POTENTIAL OF THE CTL RESPONSE TO HBV

If the CTLs are injected into these transgenic mice, they develop hepatitis, but the severity of the disease is lineage-specific [2–5]. In the lineage designated as 107-5D, which retains HBsAg in hepatocytes, severe and sometimes fatal liver disease,

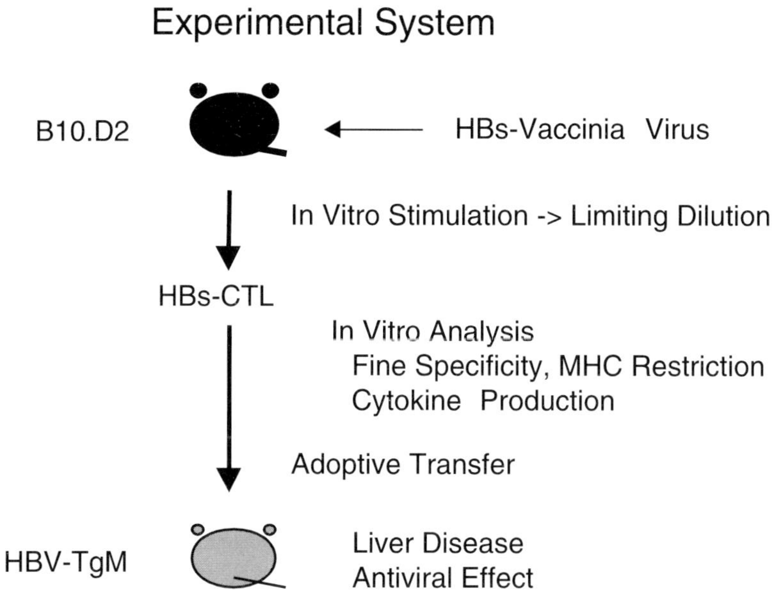

Fig. 1. The strategy to construct the hepatitis model with HBV-transgenic mice. See the text for details.

with higher ALT elevation that reaches around 10,000 IU/l, was observed by the adoptive transfer of 1×10^7 CTLs (6C2, most of the experiments were done using this representative clone). On the other hand, in the lineage designated as 1.3.32, which replicates HBV in the liver and secretes HBsAg from the hepatocytes, less severe disease, with moderate ALT elevation around 3000 IU/l, was observed by the same procedure. In both these mice, the disease was self-limited and ALT levels went back to normal in 7 to 10 days after CTL injection.

The difference in the manifestation and the process of the liver disease between two transgenic mouse lineages is summarized in Fig. 2 [2]. As shown in Fig. 2, the disease process consists of three steps.

The first step is 'apoptosis' caused by the direct attack of the CTLs against HBsAg-positive hepatocytes. This step occurs immediately after the transfer of CTLs to mice, and is a critical initiating event. The direct CTL–target cell interaction

TABLE 1

Hepatitis B virus transgenic mice

Lineage	Background	Gene product expressed	Characteristics	Model for
107-5D	H-2^d	Large S and Small S	Retain HBsAg	Fulminant hepatitis
1.3.32, 1.3.46	H-2^d	All HBV ORFs	Secrete HBsAg Replicate virus	Acute hepatitis Viral clearance

HBV: Hepatitis B virus, ORF: open reading frame.

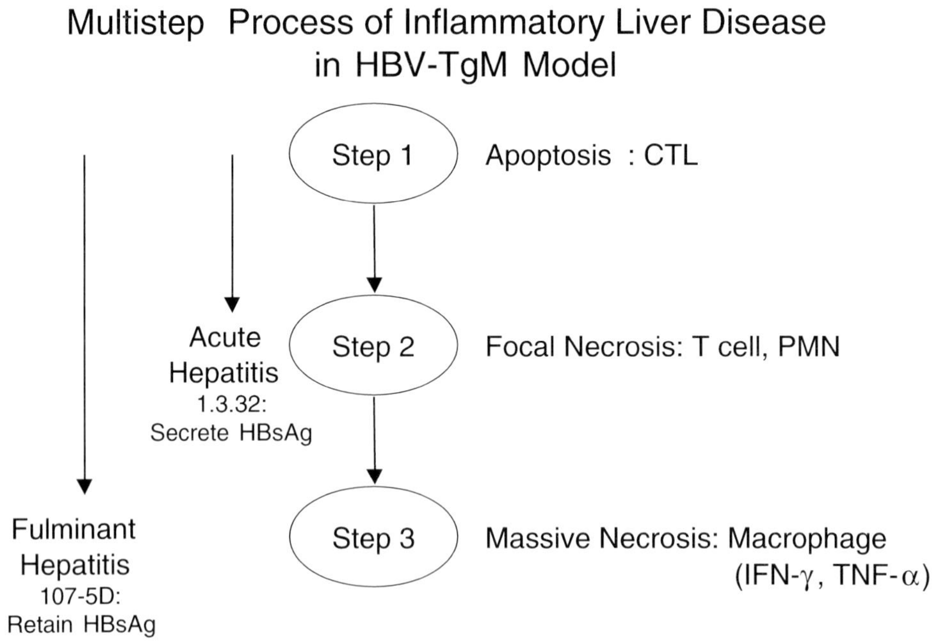

Fig. 2. Class I-restricted immunopathology is a multistep process in HBV-transgenic mice. The ability of HBV-specific CTLs to induce the HBV hepatocytes to undergo apoptosis (step 1) represents a critical initiating event, but most of the liver cell injury is caused by the antigen-nonspecific inflammatory cells that the CTLs recruit. The CTLs induce a stereotypic response in which polymorphonuclear cells and nonspecific lymphonuclear cells amplify the effects of the CTLs locally, forming discrete necroinflammatory foci (step 2) surrounding each CTL. The CTLs also release inflammatory cytokines such as IFN-γ and TNF-α (step 3) that activate intrahepatic macrophages and destroy a subset of HBsAg-positive hepatocytes that retain the large HBsAg polypeptide in their endoplasmic reticulum ('ground glass' hepatocytes). If the process proceeds to step 3, the histological features in those mice resemble that of fulminant hepatitis in man. In the transgenic mice that do not retain but secrete HBsAg, the disease process stops at step 2, thereby resembling acute hepatitis in man.

results in the appearance of widely scattered, acidophilic, Councilman bodies (apoptotic hepatocytes) that are characteristic of acute viral hepatitis in humans.

The second step is 'focal necrosis', which is also known as a feature of acute hepatitis in human. The factors or signals that cause this process are unknown. However, from the histology and other additional experiments, it has been shown that this process is characterized by the migration of host-derived, antigen-nonspecific inflammatory cells, like T cells and polymorphomononuclear cells, into the immediate vicinity of the lesion of apoptosis caused by the CTLs. In this step, hepatocellular necrosis extends well beyond the CTLs, indicating that most of hepatocytes are killed by host-derived cells infiltrating to the inflammatory locus. These two steps are common in the two transgenic lines. However, in 1.3.32, the liver disease does not progress beyond this point, in contrast to most cases of acute hepatitis in humans.

The third step is 'massive necrosis', which happens only in 107-5D. This step is characterized by the widespread necrosis of HBsAg-laden hepatocytes with marked diffuse lymphomononuclear inflammatory cell infiltration and Kupffer cell hyperplasia, thereby resembling the histological features of HBV-induced fulminant hepatitis in humans. Deleting macrophages by carrageenan or blocking IFN-γ by neutralizing antibody can block about 90% of ALT elevation. This suggest that most of the destruction is caused by the inflammatory cells that the CTLs recruit or activate and not by the CTLs themselves. It has been shown that the hepatocytes retaining HBsAg are sensitive to these cytokines, even though the detailed mechanism or the final mediators that cause massive necrosis to hepatocytes are not clarified yet.

4. NONCYTOPATHIC ANTIVIRAL POTENTIAL OF THE IMMUNE RESPONSE TO HBV

CTL injection develops acute or fulminant hepatitis in HBV transgenic mice depending upon the nature of HBsAg produced in the hepatocytes as described above. More importantly, CTL injection also causes the downregulation of the HBV antigens, HBV mRNA and even HBV DNA, not only by the direct killing of the HBV antigen-expressing targets but also by the indirect pathway, which is mediated by cytokines, like TNF-α and IFN-γ [4,5].

Fig. 3 summarizes the process of disease progression and the mechanisms of viral clearance caused by CTL administration. HBV-specific CTLs initiate a complex antiviral response within the liver, but that viral clearance is attributable primarily to the effects of inflammatory cytokines, especially IFN-γ and TNF-α, that are released by the CTLs when they recognize their viral target antigen on the hepatocyte. These cytokines activate the Kupffer cells to produce additional TNF-α, which activates the hepatocytes to an anti-viral state that is destructive for the virus while being compatible with survival of the cell [4,5]. In the transgenic mouse lineage designated as 1.3.32, which replicates the HBV genome, it was shown that all of the viral gene products, including the intrahepatic nucleocapsid and the viral replicative intermediates, were eliminated by the CTL administration [5]. The observation suggests that, in addition to destroying HBV-infected hepatocytes, a strong intrahepatic immune response to HBV might be able to suppress viral replication and perhaps even cure the infected hepatocytes without killing them. In support of this hypothesis, it has been shown that the woodchuck hepatitis virus is cleared from all of the hepatocytes in the acutely infected woodchuck liver without massive hepatic necrosis [11], suggesting that a noncytolytic clearance mechanism may be also operative in that model.

5. TH1-MEDIATED IMMUNOPATHOGENESIS

Using the same HBV-transgenic mouse lineages (107-5, 1.3.46), Franco et al. demonstrated that disease pathogenesis caused by HBsAg-specific Th was similar to that caused by HBs-CTLs. They established I-A^d-restricted Th1 clone specific to HBs 182–196 peptide, that produced IFN-γ and TNF-α, but IL-4 after antigen stimulation [6]. Adoptive transfer of this Th1 clone to 107-5 caused acute necroinflammatory liver disease, which resembled CTL-mediated disease with regard to the magnitude of

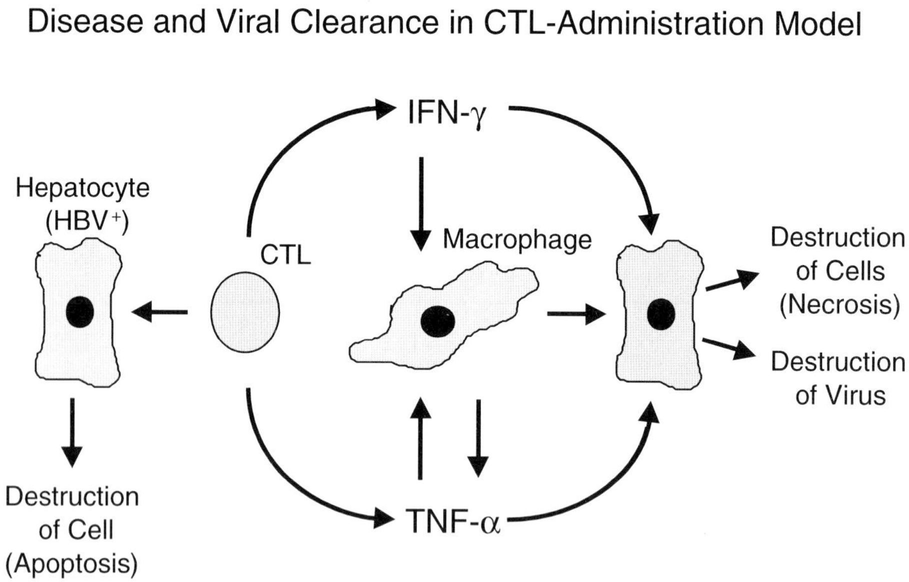

Fig. 3. The disease and the viral clearance pathways. HBV-specific CTLs initiate a complex antiviral response within the liver, but that viral clearance is attributable primarily to the effects of inflammatory cytokines, especially IFN-γ and TNF-α, that are released by the CTLs when they recognize their viral target antigen on the hepatocyte. These cytokines activate the Kupffer cells to produce additional TNF-α, which activates the hepatocyte to an antiviral state that is destructive to the virus while being compatible with the survival of the cell. This pathway is responsible for the noncytopathic clearance of virus from 10 to 100 times as many cells as the CTLs kill by apoptosis at the time that they are activated by antigen and secrete their antiviral cytokines (as seen in the transgenic mice lineage, 1.3.32). On the other hand, these cytokines induce massive necrosis in the HBsAg-retaining hepatocytes that are sensitive to the cytokines (as seen in the transgenic mice lineage, 107-5).

disease and the lineage specificity. When 1×10^7 HBs-Th were injected to 107-5, sALT elevation reached a peak of more than 4000 U/l in 48 to 72 hr and returned to normal in 5 to 7 days. Histologically, at the peak of the disease initiated by the clone, they observed diffuse mixed inflammatory infiltrates throughout the hepatic lobule, consisting of hyperplastic sinusoidal lining cells, polymorphomononuclear cells, macrophages, and lymphocytes. In addition, several dead and degenerating (apoptotic) hepatocytes were present. Importantly, inflammation was almost completely blocked by the administration of antibodies for IFN-γ and TNF-α. Since there were marked similarities between CTL- and Th-mediated disease, analysis for the factors that determined disease severity was done in the CTL-administration model.

6. FACTORS RESPONSIBLE FOR THE DISEASE EXACERBATION

In order to analyze the relationship between the characteristics of CTLs and the disease severity or the efficacy of viral clearance, eight CTL clones with different cytokine profiles were applied in the same system.

TABLE 2

T cell receptor β gene usage of HBsAg-specific CTLs

Clone	Vβ	Dβ	Jβ
6C2	1	2.1	2.5
11B5	1	2.1	2.5
11B10	8.2	2.1	2.2
13F6	8.2	1.1	2.6
14F7	8.2	1.1	2.6
SWB1	16	2.1	2.6
SWD10	6	1.1	2.1
B6D	2	1.1	1.1

Through the in vitro analysis of HBsAg-specific CTL clones, it was found that all the clones recognized exactly the same peptide (aa 28 to aa 39 of HBsAg) as the minimal optimal motif and that they recognized it in combination with L^d. In spite of the variety of TCRβ (T cell receptor β) gene usage as shown in Table 2, they showed the similar specificity and affinity to the antigenic peptide [12]. The cytokine profiles tested in vitro with antigen-specific stimulation indicated that they all produced IFN-γ and TNF-α. However, the amount of each cytokine produced by these clones was extremely variable (in the typical case more than a hundred-fold difference was observed among the clones, when 1×10^6 CTLs were stimulated in vitro and the amount of the cytokine in the culture supernatant was tested by ELISA). When the individual CTL clones were injected into 1.3.32, the extent of viral gene downregulation was variable, reflecting the ability to produce cytokines in vitro. This finding is consistent with the observation described above, that IFN-γ and/or TNF-α was important for the antiviral effect of CTLs. At first, it was also expected that the disease magnitude was regulated by the amount of cytokines produced by the CTLs, since IFN-γ and TNF-α were shown to be necessary for the progression of the hepatitis in 107-5D. However, opposed to the expectation, the disease magnitude did not correlate to the amount of cytokines produced by the CTLs. Even though CTL administration simultaneously causes two events, the liver disease and the viral downregulation, the factors responsible for the individual events are suggested to be different. From these results, by further analysis of the exacerbation factors of the hepatitis, it may be possible to design a therapeutic approach that specifically blocks the disease exacerbation without disturbing the viral clearance. More detailed analysis of the relationship between the disease severity and the immunological factors, especially the extent of CTL activation, are necessary and currently under investigation.

In conclusion, CTLs initiate the cascade of immune response that is responsible for the progression of the disease and for the eradication of the virus. While the latter event is controlled by the amount of inflammatory cytokines produced by CTLs, the exact factor responsible for the former event remains to be elucidated. The study of that factor may make possible a therapeutic approach that reduces the disease severity without affecting the process of viral clearance.

ACKNOWLEDGEMENTS

The authors thank Drs. Francis V. Chisari and Kazuki Ando for the encouragement and helpful suggestion for the preparation of the manuscript.

REFERENCES

[1] Chisari FV, Ferrari C. Hepatitis B virus immunopathogenesis. Annu Rev Immunol 1995; 13: 29–60.
[2] Ando K, Moriyama T, Guidotti LG, Wirth S, Schreiber RD, Schlicht HJ, Huang S, Chisari FV. Mechanisms of class I restricted immunopathology: a transgenic mouse model of fulminant hepatitis. J Exp Med 1993; 178: 1541–1554.
[3] Ando K, Guidotti LG, Wirth S, Ishikawa T, Missale G, Moriyama T, Schreiber RD, Schlicht HJ, Huang S, Chisari FV. Class I restricted cytotoxic T lymphocytes are directly cytopathic for their target cells in vivo. J Immunol 1994; 152: 3245–3253.
[4] Guidotti LG, Ando K, Hobbs MV, Ishikawa T, Runkel RD, Schreiber RD, Chisari FV. Cytotoxic T lymphocytes inhibit hepatitis B virus gene expression by a noncytolytic mechanism in transgenic mice. Proc Natl Acad Sci USA 1994; 91: 3764–3768.
[5] Guidotti LG, Ishikawa T, Hobbs MV, Matzke B, Schreiber RD, Chisari FV. Intracellular inactivation of the hepatitis B virus by cytotoxic T lymphocytes. Immunity 1996; 4: 25–36.
[6] Franco A, Guidotti, LG, Hobbs MV, Pasquetto V, Chisari FV. Pathogenetic effector function of CD4-positive T helper 1 cells In heptitis B virus transgenic mice. J Immunol 1997; 159: 2001–2008.
[7] Omata M, Ehata T, Yokosuka O, Hosoda K, Ohto M. Mutations in the precore region of hepatitis B virus DNA In patients with fulminant and severe hepatitis. N Engl J Med 1991; 324: 1699–1704.
[8] Yotsumoto S, Kojima M, Shoji I, Yamamoto K, Okamoto H, Mishiro S. Fulminant hepatitis related to transmission of hepatitis B variants with precore mutations between spouses. Hepatology 1992; 16: 31–35.
[9] Laskus T, Persing DH, Nowicki MJ, Mosley JW, Rakela J. Nucleotide sequence analysis of the precore region In patients with fulminant hepatitis B in the United States. Gastroenterology 1993; 105: 1173–1178.
[10] Liang TJ, Hasegawa K, Munoz SJ, Shapiro CN, Yoffe B, McMahon BJ, Feng C, Bei H, Alter MJ, Dienstag JL. Hepatitis B virus precore mutation and fulminant hepatitis in the United States. A polymerase chain reaction-based assay for the detection of specific mutation. J Clin Invest 1994; 93: 550–555.
[11] Jilbert AR, Wu T-T, England JM, De La M Hall P, Carp NZ, O'Connell AP, Manson WS. Rapid resolution of duck hepatitis B virus infections occurs after massive hepatocellular involvement. J Virol 1992; 66: 1377–1388.
[12] Ishikawa T, Kono D, Chung J, Fowler P, Theofilopoulos A, Kakumu S, Chisari FV. Polyclonality and multispecificity of the CTL response to a single viral epitope. J Immunol 1998; 161: 5842–5850.

Edited by T. Tsuji, T. Higashi, M. Zeniya and K.-H. Meyer zum Büschenfelde

CHAPTER 3

Genetic Diversity and Pathophysiology of Hepatitis B Virus

Hiroshi Yatsuhashi and Michitami Yano

Institute for Clinical Research, National Nagasaki Medical Center, and WHO Collaborating Center for Reference and Research on Viral Hepatitis, Nagasaki, Japan

INTRODUCTION

The hepatitis B virus (HBV), discovered in 1966, infects more than 350 million people worldwide. One third of the global population has been acutely infected with HBV. Hepatitis B is a leading cause of chronic hepatitis, cirrhosis, and hepatocellular carcinoma, accounting for 1 million deaths annually. Viral and host factors, such as age, immunosuppression, and sex contribute to the patient outcome [1]. Recent advances in polymerase chain reaction (PCR) and DNA sequencing technique made it possible to identify various HBV mutations. So far, increasing attention focused on the contribution of variant HBV strains to the clinical course of acute or chronic infection has been reported and discussed widely. Mutant HBV might display enhanced virulence with increased levels of HBV replication, resistance to antiviral therapies, facilitated cell attachment/penetration, or alteration of epitopes important in the host immune response [2]. This review addresses clinical aspects of genetic diversity and pathophysiology of HBV, including our data.

1. HBV-DNA

HBV belongs to a family of closely related DNA viruses called the hepadnaviruses. The viral genome of HBV is a partially double-stranded circular DNA of approximately 3200 base pairs that encodes four overlapping open reading frames. The four genes are core, surface, X, and polymerase. The core gene encodes the core nucleocapsid protein (important in viral packaging) and hepatitis B e antigen (HBeAg). The surface gene encodes pre-S1, pre-S2, and S protein (yielding large, middle, and small surface proteins, respectively). The X gene encodes the X protein, which has transactivating properties and may be important in hepatic carcinogenesis. The polymerase gene encodes a large protein with functions critical for packaging and DNA replication (including priming, RNA- and DNA-dependent DNA polymerase) [1,2] (Fig. 1).

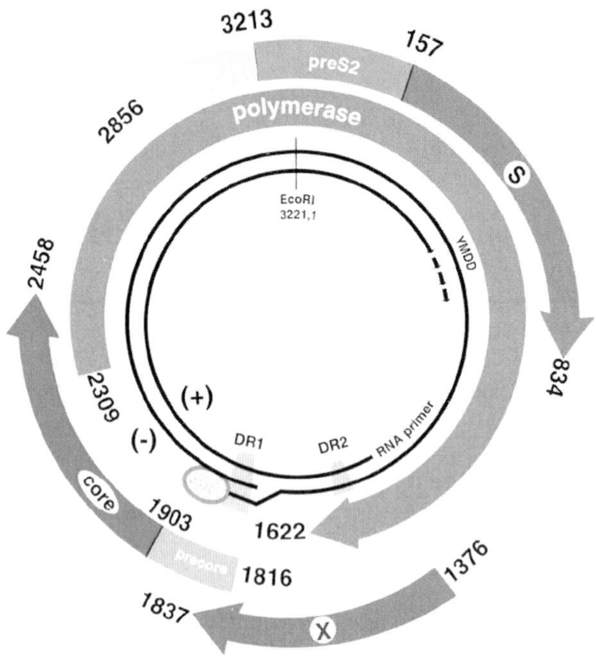

Fig. 1. Genome of HBV (genotype A). The inner circles represent the minus (−) and (+) DNA strands of the viral genome. The HBV polymerase is shown as an circle covalently bound to the 5′-end of the (−) DNA strand. The different open reading frames encoded by the genome, designated as S, core, polymerase, and X, are indicated by arrows. Nucleotide numbers designate the boundaries of each open reading frame with position 1 mapped at the *Eco*RI site. S, surface antigen; Y, tyrosine; M, methionine; D, aspartate; DR, direct repeat segment, used in viral replication

It is known that HBV replication cycle requires a reverse transcription step. HBV undergoes a higher rate of mutations than other DNA viruses, because the HBV P protein, like the reverse transcriptase of other viruses, lacks proofreading functions. Therefore, HBV exhibits a mutation rate more than 10-fold higher than other DNA viruses, the estimated mutation rate is approximately 1 nucleotide/10,000 bases/infection year [3].

2. MUTATIONS IN THE PRECORE/CORE REGION

The X open reading frame encodes the X protein that has transactivating activity and contains the basic core promoter (BCP). The BCP, mapping between nucleotides 1744 and 1804, controls the transcription of both precore messenger RNA (mRNA), which codes for the protein that is the precursor of the e antigen, and pregenomic RNA (pgRNA), which controls HBV replication. A variety of precore/core mutants have been described. The two well-defined precore mutations include a stop codon mutation at nucleotide (nt) 1896 and mutations in the basal core promoter (BCP) at nt 1762 and nt 1764.

2.1. Precore stop mutation

Mutations in the precore region of the HBV genome have been reported in many HBeAg-negative patients with chronic HBV infection. The predominant mutation involves a G-to-A change at nucleotide 1896 (A1896), which creates a premature stop codon at codon 28. This mutation prevents the translation of the precore protein and completely abolishes the production of HBeAg. Longitudinal studies found that A1896 emerges or is selected around the time of HBeAg seroconversion. These findings suggest that A1896 plays an important role in HBeAg clearance [4].

However, not all patients develop A1896 after HBeAg seroconversion; some patients retain wild-type precore sequence, while others have undetectable HBV DNA in serum by PCR. Furthermore, marked geographic differences in the prevalence of these precore stop mutant viruses have been noted. Only 10% of HBV isolates from US patients with fulminant hepatitis and 12–27% of isolates from US and European patients with chronic active hepatitis exhibit these precore stop mutations, whereas 47–60% of isolates from patients with chronic active hepatitis in Asia, Africa, Southern Europe, and the Middle East exhibit these stop mutations [5,6].

Recently, seven genotypes of HBV are recognized that are distinguished by differences of more than 8% in the entire nucleotide sequence of approximately 3,200 nt, and they are designated by capital letters from A to G [7]. HBV genotypes have distinct geographical distributions [8]. Overall, genotypes B and C are frequent in Asia, whereas genotypes A and D prevail in Western countries. Genotype E is restricted to Africa, and genotype F prevails in Central America. Genotype G was added to the alphabet list very recently, and its distribution is yet to be determined. It is now recognized that the occurrence of A1896 is restricted to HBV genotypes with T at nucleotide 1858. A change from G to A at nucleotide 1896 increases the stability of the stem–loop structure of the pregenome encapsidation sequence (e) when the opposite nucleotide at 1858 is a T (T1858), but this change disrupts a pre-existing C–G pair when the nucleotide at 1858 is a C (C1858) [9]. The restriction of A1896 to specific HBV genotypes accounts for its high prevalence in Asia and the Mediterranean basin, where the predominant HBV genotypes (B, C, and D) frequently have T1858, and its low prevalence in North America and Europe, where the predominant HBV genotype (A) almost always has C1858.

2.2. BCP mutations (X-ORF region)

The core promoter controls the transcription of the two core gene products: core and precore RNA. The core RNA is essential for viral replication because it encodes the major capsid protein and the viral polymerase; it also serves as the pregenomic RNA. The nonessential precore RNA encodes the precore protein, which is processed in the endoplasmic reticulum to produce the secreted HBeAg.

A pair of mutations in the BCP that is associated with a reduced level of HBeAg expression was first described in Japanese patients; an adenine (A) to thymine (T) transversion at position 1762 together with a guanine (G) to A transition at 1764 in the second AT-rich region of the BCP are often present in patients with chronic hepatitis B and fulminant hepatitis B, and less often in asymptomatic carriers, immunosuppressed patients, and carriers without serological HBV markers [10,11].

In some patients, the TA changes were not associated with A1896, suggesting that mutations in the core promoter region alone may play a role in HBeAg clearance. This is supported by in vitro observations that the TA changes decrease transcription of precore mRNA and secretion of HBeAg [12]. However, TA changes have also been found in some HBeAg-positive patients, especially those with chronic hepatitis.

Recently, Orito et al. [13] have reported the BCP double mutation was significantly associated with genotype C, more severe disease (liver cirrhosis with or without hepatocellular carcinoma) and old age (more than 35 years), but it was not associated with sex, HBeAg, HBV-DNA,or the precore mutation (A1896) in a case-control study. Their study indicated that the occurrence of BCP double mutation was associated with genotype C and a longer duration of infection in aggravation of chronic hepatitis B. They also indicated that BCP double mutation was not associated with the HBeAg/anti-HBe status,unlike the preC mutation that was closely associated with anti-HBe.

From these considerations, all discussion on preC and BCP double mutation in patients with chronic HBV infection should carried out with regard to the association with HBV genotypes. The study of HBV genotypes is required to define the clinical significance of these mutations.

3. MUTATIONS IN PATIENTS WITH HBV-RELATED FULMINANT HEPATITIS

Approximately 1% of patients with acute HBV infection develop fulminant hepatitis. Fulminant hepatitis B is widely thought to be caused by a well-described HBeAg-negative mutant of HBV, which has a point mutation (G to A at nucleotide (nt) 1896) in the precore region that blocks synthesis of HBeAg. Omata et al. [14] found precore mutations in all of seven Japanese patients with fulminant hepatitis B. Similarly, Liang et al. [15] found precore mutations in all five patients with fulminant hepatitis in an outbreak of hepatitis B in Israel. However, subsequent studies in patients from the United States and France have indicated that these mutations are neither necessary nor sufficient for fulminant hepatitis B [16–18]. Sato et al. [11] reported an association between core promoter mutations (especially an A-to-T substitution at nt 1762 and a G-to-A transition at nt 1764) and fulminant hepatitis B in Japan. These mutations were uniformly present in patients with fulminant hepatitis without, as well as in a majority of patients with, the classic nt 1896 mutation.

In order to investigate the association of mutations in the precore and core promoter region of HBV with fulminant and severe acute hepatitis, we demonstrated our study results in Japanese patients with acute HBV infection, including 12 patients with fulminant hepatitis, 23 with severe acute hepatitis and 98 with acute self-limited hepatitis (Fig. 2). They were all admitted to five hospitals (National Nagasaki Medical Center, Osaka National Hospital, Shinsyu Medical University Hospital, Miyazaki Medical University Hospital and Kurume Medical University Hospital). We used the following diagnostic criteria for fulminant hepatitis as described by Trey et al. [19]: (1) the development of stage II–IV hepatic encephalopathy within 8 weeks of the onset of illness; (2) prothrombin time less than 40%; and (3) no known history of liver disease

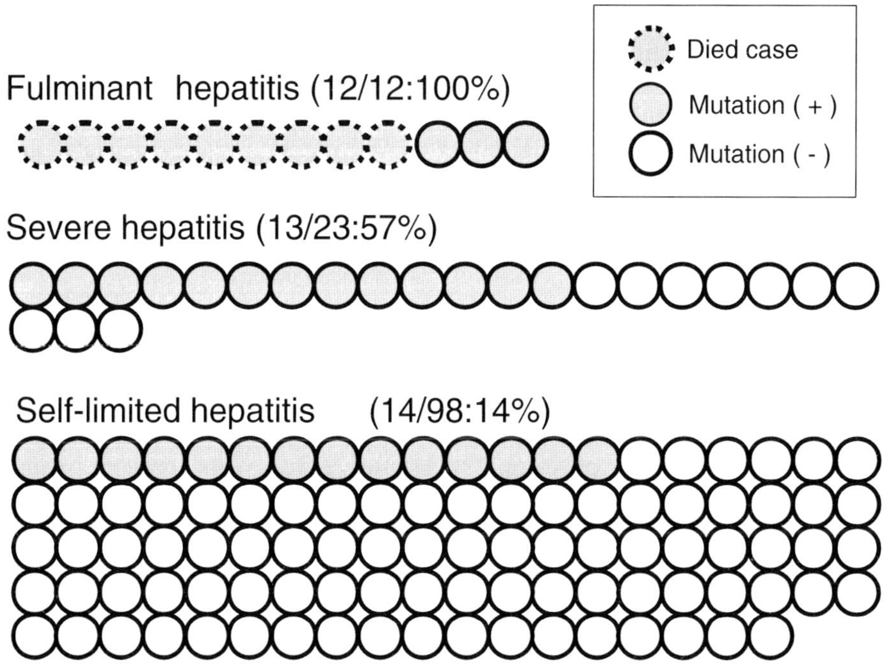

Fig. 2. Association of mutations in the precore and core promoter region of HBV with fulminant and severe acute hepatitis in Japanese patients with acute HBV infection, including 12 patients with fulminant hepatitis, 23 with severe acute hepatitis and 98 with acute self-limited hepatitis. Among 12 patients with fulminant hepatitis, nine patients died due to acute hepatic failure. The presence of HBV mutants was examined by using a point mutation assay (PMA) to detect a G-to-A transition at position 1896 in the precore region and an A-to-T transition at position 1762 and a G-to-A transition at position 1764 in the core promoter region.

(to rule out the possibility of chronic liver failure). The diagnostic criteria for severe hepatitis were: (1) stage I hepatic encephalopathy; and (2) prothrombin time less than 40%. The diagnosis of acute HBV infection was based on detection of high titers of IgM antibody to hepatitis B core antigen (anti-HBc) in the absence of any evidence of acute infection with other hepatitis viruses. Among 12 patients with fulminant hepatitis, nine died due to acute hepatic failure. All patients who survived were clear of hepatitis B surface antigen (HBsAg) after the episode of acute hepatitis. The presence of HBV mutants was examined by using a point mutation assay (PMA) to detect a G-to-A transition at position 1896 in the precore region and an A-to-T transition at position 1762 and a G-to-A transition at position 1764 in the core promoter region. PMA was HBV-DNA mutations detection PCR kit whose sensitivity was 100 copies/ml [20].

Mutations were detected in either the precore or core promoter region in all 12 patients (100%) with fulminant hepatitis B including nine patients who died. Among 23 patients with severe hepatitis, 13 (57%) had mutations of HBV. Among 98 patients with self-limited acute hepatitis B, 14 (14%) had mutations in either the precore or core promoter regions. Significant differences in the proportion of mutations in the precore or core promoter region were present between patients with fulminant hepatitis and self-limited acute hepatitis [12/12 (100%) vs. 14/98 (14%), $P < 0.01$] and between severe acute hepatitis and self-limited acute hepatitis [13/23 (57%) vs. 14/98 (14%), $P < 0.01$]. The frequency of mutation increased proportionately with the severity of disease in patients with acute HBV infection. Our results indicate that mutations in the core promoter and precore regions, together or independently, are associated with fulminant or severe acute hepatitis and that HBV strains with such mutations cannot direct the production of HBeAg. A low prevalence of HBeAg or anti-HBe in patients with fulminant and severe acute hepatitis B has also been noted.

As we had described previously, the G-to-A switch at nt 1896 of the precore region of HBV gene results in a translational stop codon which causes a lack of secretion of HBeAg, and mutations within the core promoter region down-regulate HBeAg expression at the transcriptional level. It is generally believed that immunoelimination of HBV-infected cells occurs following specific targeting of HBeAg on the membrane of liver cells by activated T-lymphocytes [21]. Secretory HBeAg may distract the immune system from eliminating infected hepatocytes, possibly by down-regulation of cellular factors important in recognition by the immune system [21,22]. Therefore, the presence of replicating HBV associated with a lack of circulating HBeAg may result in a higher degree of inflammatory activity and determine an unfavorable clinical outcome.

Baumert et al. [23] demonstrated that two adjacent mutations in the HBV core promoter region were responsible for enhanced replication of the viral genome of a HBV strain associated with an outbreak of fulminant hepatitis (strain FH). Moriyama et al. [24] also demonstrated that mutations at nt 1762 and 1764 in the core promoter were responsible for reduced HBeAg production as well as enhanced replication and core production. Buckwold et al. [25] proved experimentally that HBeAg production was decreased, as a liver-specific transcription factor which normally binds to the basal core promoter was prevented from binding by the mutations and that this mutation did not affect the transcription of the core RNA and protein. This mutation appeared to increase the packaging efficiency of pregenomic RNA and, therefore, increase viral replication. However, there is no direct evidence that the enhanced replication of strain FH HBV contributes to the development of fulminant hepatitis. Studies in an animal model are necessary to demonstrate the biological significance of these mutations in the pathogenesis of HBV infection.

We must discuss the relationship between HBV genotype and precore mutation again. Lindh et al. [26] have demonstrated how the regional differences in precore mutation prevalence have occurred. In patients with genotype A HBV infection, which is a predominant genotype in North America and Europe, a dCTP is at nt 1858. Impaired base-pairing of the pregenomic RNA results when the C1858 tries to pair with a U1858 in the RNA genome. In contrast, among chronic HBV carriers from Asia, Africa or the Middle East, U1858 permits stable basepair formation with a G-to-A mutation at nt 1896 which forms a TAG stop codon. Other studies [27,28] also demonstrated a high prevalence of precore mutation in HBV sequences with genotype D and a low prevalence in sequences with genotype A. Such differences may explain why mutation at nt 1896 is not common in patients with fulminant hepatitis in France or the United States, where HBV of genotype A predominates.

There is still a lack of reliable clinical markers that predict the outcome of acute hepatitis. The most important clinical implication of our findings is that we may be able to predict the outcome of liver disease in patients with acute HBV infection by using PMA for HBV precore and core promoter analysis in patients without HBV genotype A [20].

REFERENCES

[1] Lee WM. Hepatitis B virus infection. New Engl J Med 1997; 337: 1733–1745.

[2] Hunt CM, McGill JM, Allen MI, Condreay LD. Clinical relevance of hepatitis B viral mutations. Hepatology 2000; 31: 1037–1044.

[3] Blum HE. Variants of hepatitis B, C, and D viruses: molecular biology and clinical significance. Digestion 1995; 56: 85–95.

[4] Carman WF, Jacyna MR, Hadziyannis S, Karayiannis P, McGarvey MJ, Makris A, Thomas HC. Mutation preventing formation of hepatitis B e antigen in patients with chronic hepatitis B infection. Lancct 1989; 2: 588–591.

[5] Laskus T, Rakela J, Nowicki MJ, Persing DH. Hepatitis B virus core promoter sequence analysis in fulminant and chronic hepatitis B. Gastroenterology 1995; 109: 1618–1623.

[6] Lindh M, Horal P, Dhillon AP, Furuta Y, Norkrans G. Hepatitis B virus carriers without precore mutations in hepatitis B e antigen-negative stage show more severe liver damage. Hepatology 1996; 24: 494–501.

[7] Okamoto H, Tsuda F, Sakugawa H, Sastrosoewignjo RI, Imai M, Miyakawa Y et al. Typing hepatitis B virus by homology in nucleotide sequence: comparison of surface antigen subtypes. J Gen Virol 1988; 69: 2575–2583.

[8] Mizokami M, Nakano T, Orito E, Tanaka Y, Sakugawa H, Mukaide M, Robertson BH. Hepatitis B virus genotype assignment using restriction fragment length polymorphism patterns. FEBS Lett 1999; 450: 66–71.

[9] Lok AS, Akarca U, Greene S. Mutations in the pre-core region of hepatitis B virus serve to enhance the stability of the secondary structure of the pre-genome encapsidation signal. Proc Natl Acad Sci USA 1994; 91: 4077–4081.

[10] Okamoto H, Tsuda F, Akahane Y, Sugai Y, Yoshiba M, Moriyama K, Tanaka T et al. Hepatitis B virus with mutations in the core promoter for an e antigen-negative phenotype in carriers with antibody to e antigen. J Virol 1994; 68: 8102–8110.

[11] Sato S, Suzuki K, Akahane Y et al. Hepatitis B virus strains with mutations in the core promoter in patients with fulminant hepatitis. Ann Intern Med 1995; 122: 241–248.

[12] Buckwold VE, Xu Z, Chen M, Yen TSB, Ou JH. Effects of a naturally occurring mutation in the hepatitis B virus basal core promoter on precore gene expression and viral replication. J Virol 1996; 70: 5845–5851.

[13] Orito Orito E, Mizokami M, Sakugawa H, Michitaka K, Ishikawa K, Ichida T, Okanoue T, Yotsuyanagi H, Iino S. A case-control study for clinical and molecular biological differences between hepatitis B viruses of genotypes B and C. Hepatology 2001; 33: 218–123.

[14] Omata M, Ehata T, Yokosuka O, Hosoda K, Ohto M. Mutations in the precore region of hepatitis B virus DNA in patients with fulminant and severe hepatitis. New Engl J Med 1991; 324: 1699–1704.

[15] Liang TJ, Hasegawa K, Rimon N, Wands J, Ben-Porath E. A hepatitis B virus mutant associated with an epidemic of fulminant hepatitis. New Engl J Med 1991; 324: 1705–1709.

[16] Laskus T, Persing DH, Nowicki MJ, Mosley MJ, Rakela J. Nucleotide sequence analysis of the precore region in patients with fulminant hepatitis B in the United States. Gastroenterology 1993; 105: 1173–1178.

[17] Liang TJ, Hasegawa K, Munoz SJ et al. Hepatitis B virus precore mutation and fulminant hepatitis in the United States. J Clin Invest 1994; 93: 550–555.
[18] Feray C, Gigou M, Samuel D, Bernuau J, Bismuth H, Brechot C. Low prevalence of precore mutations in hepatitis B virus DNA in fulminant hepatitis B in France. J Hepatol 1993; 18: 119–122.
[19] Trey C, Lipworth L, Chalmers TC et al. Fulminant hepatic failure. Presumable contribution of halothane. New Engl J Med 1968; 279: 798–801.
[20] Aritomi T, Yatsuhashi H, Fujino T, Yamasaki K, Inoue O, Koga M, Kato Y et al. Association of mutations in the core promoter and precore region of hepatitis virus with fulminant and severe acute hepatitis in Japan. J Gastroenterol Hepatol 1998; 13: 1125–1132.
[21] Yamada G, Takaguchi K, Matsuda K et al. Immunoelectron microscopic observation of intrahepatic HBeAg in patients with chronic hepatitis B. Hepatology 1990; 12: 133–140.
[22] Milich DR, Jones JE, Hughes JL, Price J, Raney AK, McLanchen A. Is a function of the secreted hepatitis B e antigen to induce immunologic tolerance in utero. Proc Natl Acad Sci USA 1990; 87: 6599–6603.
[23] Baumert T, Rogers SA, Hasegawa K, Liang TJ. Two core promoter mutations identified in a hepatitis B virus strain associated with fulminant hepatitis result in enhanced viral replication. J Clin Invest 1996; 98: 2268–2276.
[24] Moriyama K, Okamoto H, Tsuda F, Mayumi M. Reduced precore transcription and enhanced core-pregenome transcription of hepatitis B virus DNA after replacement of the precore–core promoter with sequences associated with e antigen-seronegative persistent infections. Virology 1996; 226: 269–280.
[25] Buckwold VE, Xu Z, Chen M, Yen TS, Ou JH. Effects of a naturally occurring mutation in the hepatitis B virus basal core promoter on precore gene expression and viral replication. J Virol 1996; 70: 5845–5851.
[26] Lindh M, Horal P, Dhillon AP, Furuta Y, Norkrans G. Hepatitis B virus carriers without precore mutations in hepatitis B e antigen-negative stage show more severe liver damage. Hepatology 1996; 24: 494–501.
[27] Rodriguez-Frais F, Buti M, Jardi R et al. Hepatitis B virus infection; precore mutants and its relation to viral genotypes and core mutations. Hepatology 1995; 22: 1641–1647.
[28] McMillan JS, Bowden DS, Angus PW, McCaughan GW, Locarnini SA. Mutations in the hepatitis B virus precore/core gene and core promoter in patients with severe recurrent disease following liver transplantation. Hepatology 1996; 24: 1371–1378.

Molecular Biology and Immunology in Hepatology
Edited by T. Tsuji, T. Higashi, M. Zeniya and K.-H. Meyer zum Büschenfelde

CHAPTER 4

Immunopathogenesis of Hepatitis C

Margaret James Koziel

Department of Infectious Diseases, Beth Israel Deaconess Medical Center, and Harvard Medical School, Boston, MA 02215, USA

INTRODUCTION

Following the cloning of hepatitis C virus (HCV) in 1989, it was recognised as a common cause of chronic liver disease, cirrhosis, and hepatocellular carcinoma [1]. More than 170 million people are estimated to be infected worldwide with an estimated 2.8 million persistently infected in the US. Acute HCV infection is typically mild and often subclinical, yet 85% of healthy adults will develop persistent infection, with at least 50–70% of those infected developing chronic elevations in transaminases [2]. Individuals may present later in the course of infection with a range of symptoms and signs, ranging from minimal elevations in liver function tests to frank cirrhosis. Some individuals with persistent viraemia have normal transaminases, which might suggest complete recovery; however, more than half of these individuals will have abnormal liver biopsies, including the presence of cirrhosis [3]. In immunocompetent individuals, chronic active hepatitis, cirrhosis, and HCC typically develop approximately 10, 21, and 29 years after infection, respectively [4]. However, the natural history is highly variable, with rates of cirrhosis after known exposures ranging from 2 to 32% of affected individuals [5–9].

HCV is approximately 9400 nucleotides in length, and consists of a single open reading frame encoding a polyprotein of 3011 amino acids. Although functional characterisation of the proteins is largely through analogy with corresponding sequences of other members of the flaviviridae family, a few functions have been identified (reviewed in ref. [10]). The structural proteins include a core protein, as well as two envelope proteins, which likely form a heterodimer in vivo. The NS3 region of the virus is important for post-translational processing of the polyprotein into individual proteins, and the NS5 region is probably an RNA-dependent RNA polymerase. The primary site of replication is the hepatocyte, although cells of the macrophage/monocyte lineage in bone marrow and peripheral blood mononuclear cells (PBMC) also appear to support viral replication in vivo [11]. Macrophage and hepatocellular cell lines cannot be infected with HCV, however; the only tissue culture system reported utilises retrovirus-transformed cells or

Daudi cells, neither of which support high levels of viral production [12,13]. The only species known to be susceptible to HCV infection are humans and chimpanzees, which has limited hypothesis-driven studies of immunopathogenesis.

1. HOST IMMUNE DEFENSES

1.1. Innate immunity

An effective host response against a viral infection requires a coordinated effort of both non-specific and antigen-specific immune responses (Fig. 1). Immediately after viral infection, there are several antigen-non-specific effector mechanisms which are activated. The innate immune responses which constitute the first line of defence are generally antigen-non-specific and include the production of interferons (IFN) and activation of natural killer (NK) cells, macrophages and natural killer T cells (NK T) which are capable of recognising viral antigens in the absence of antigen presenting cells (APCs). IFNs are a family of related proteins that act against many phases of

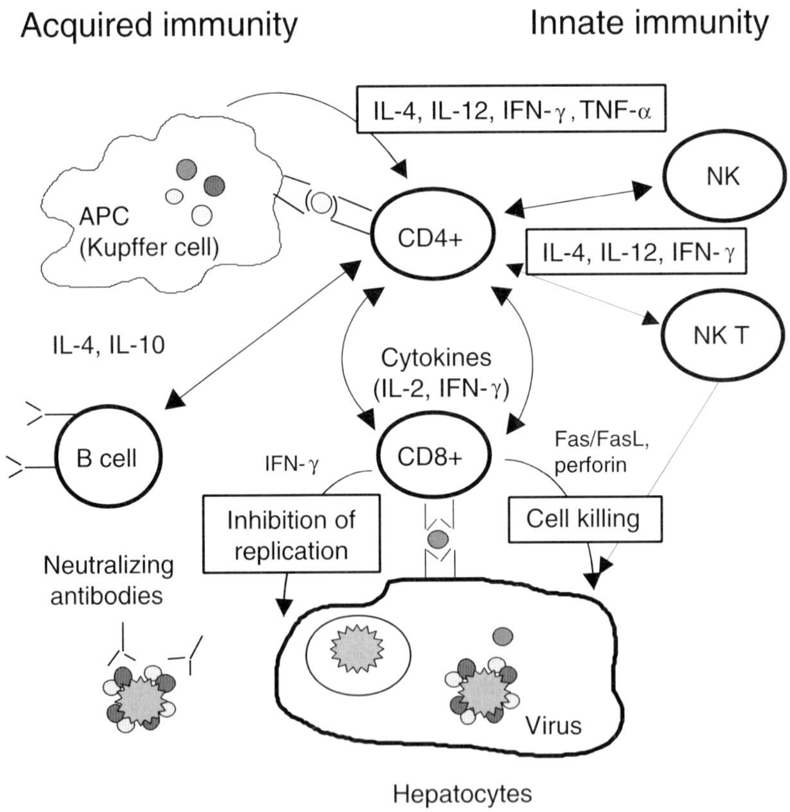

Fig. 1. Innate and acquired immunity.

the viral life cycle [14]. The two principal types of IFN are the type 1 interferons, IFNα, -β, and -ω, which have antiproliferative and antiviral effects, and type 2 IFN, or IFNγ, which principally acts as an immunomodulatory cytokine. The type 1 IFNs activate transcription of a wide number of cellular genes, at least some of which, such as Mx protein, 2-5 oligo-adenylate synthetase (2-5′OAS) and the IFN-induced protein kinase (PKR), have antiviral activity. PKR is a serine/threonine-specific protein kinase which phosphorylates the protein synthesis initiation factor eIF-2, resulting in a global inhibition of protein synthesis and thus viral replication [15]. These interferons also increase the expression of major histocompatibility (MHC) class I antigens, thereby enhancing the presentation of viral antigens to $CD8^+$ cytotoxic T lymphocytes (CTLs). Some of these effects are both virus- and species-specific. For example, in murine cells Mx protein protects against influenza but not vesicular stomatitis virus, whereas in human cells Mx protects against both viruses in vitro [16]. In addition to these direct effects on viral replication, IFNs also increase the susceptibility of infected cells to immune mediated destruction by increasing HLA class I expression on the cell surface.

Large numbers of NK cells, γδ T cells and NK T cells are demonstrated in both the normal and inflamed adult human liver [17–19]. NK cells are very primitive cells that non-specifically lead to lysis of infected cells [20]. The induction, activation of cytotoxicity, and proliferation of NK cells is dependent upon interferons and IL-12 [21]. NK cells are also critical mediators of cytokine production by other, antigen-specific cells, through the production of IFNγ, which helps promote cellular immune responses. Although the precise role of NK cells in viral hepatitis in humans is not known, on the basis of animal models of infection it is likely that these cells play a critical role in the resolution of acute viral hepatitis [20,22,23]. Limited studies suggest that NK cells are functionally impaired in chronic HCV infection [24,25]. However, little is known about other components of the innate immune system in the normal or HCV-infected liver.

1.2. Acquired immunity

The adaptive or acquired immune system is comprised of $CD8^+$ cytotoxic T-cell responses (CTLs), $CD4^+$ helper T-cell responses, and antibody responses, which typically become armed several days after a viral infection. Antibodies typically are thought to prevent infection of cells via neutralisation. Once a virus has achieved entry into the cell, the cellular immune system is the dominant means of limitation of viral spread. Both $CD8^+$ and $CD4^+$ T cells function as a result of the specific interaction of T-cell receptor (TCR) with a complex consisting of processed viral protein and a HLA class I or class II molecule. After engagement of the TCR with the appropriate molecular complex, T cells are activated and display a number of effector functions, including cytolysis and cytokine production.

$CD4^+$ T cells recognise exogenous antigen taken up, processed by antigen presenting cells and presented in the context of MHC class II molecules with co-stimulatory molecules required for activation. $CD4^+$ cells, by virtue of their capacity to produce cytokines, play a central role in control of immune responses. Recently, the characterisation of distinct patterns of cytokines produced by $CD4^+$ T cells had led to the adoption of the Th1/Th2 paradigm [26]; since $CD8^+$ cells can also produce cytokines, this is more accurately termed the type 1 and 2 paradigm. Precursor cells initially acquire the capacity to produce both interleukin (IL)-4 and IFNγ, termed the type 0 pattern, but then differentiate into either type 1 or type 2 cells. Type 1 responses are characterised by production of IL-2 and IFNγ responses, which prime and maintain antigen-specific cellular immunity and type I IFNs, and thus are important in the defense against intracellular pathogens such as viruses. Type 2 responses are characterised by IL-4, -5, and -10, which promote humoral immune responses and defense against helminthic infections. The cytokines driving the initial commitment of the type 0 cell are produced by non-T cells; for example, IL-12 is made by macrophages and NK cells, whereas IL-4 may be produced by mast cells and NK T cells [27,28]. Later, cytokines produced by antigen-specific cells, such as IL-2, tumour necrosis factor alpha (TNFα), and IL-6 can activate naive ($CD45RA^+$) and memory ($CD45RO^+$) resting $CD4^+$ T cells to proliferate; this novel Ag-independent pathway of T-cell activation may play an important role in vivo in recruiting effector T cells at the site of immune response and in maintaining the clonal size of memory T cells in the absence of antigenic stimulation [29].

In certain murine and human infections, a particular pattern of cytokine production by $CD4^+$ cells is associated with differential outcome from infection [30,31]. The prototypic example of this polarisation of immune responses is found in experimental *Leishmania major* infection. C57/BL6 mice, which mount a strong type 1 response, are resistant to *L. major* infection, whereas Balb/C mice, which mount a type 2 response, are susceptible to this infection [32]. In vivo, therapy with IL-4, which promotes a type 2 response, is associated with a switch from a resistant to a sensitive phenotype. Experiments in a wide variety of bacterial, fungal, and helminthic infections have confirmed this finding [33–37]. In viral infections, a type 1 response is often viewed as a correlate of strong cellular immunity, and thus as 'protective'.

Generally, CTLs characteristically recognise endogenous antigen presented in the context of the MHC class I antigen and β-2 microglobulin by the target cells. Historically, CTL have been thought to control viruses principally through their ability to recognise infected cells and kill them, either through direct cytolysis or induction of apoptosis [38]. The mechanisms by which the CTLs kill target cells are by release of preformed secretory granules, which contain perforin and granzymes, or by Fas or TNFα mediated induction of apoptosis. Fas ligand (FasL) expression is induced in cytotoxic T cells and is capable of ligating the molecule Fas expressed on the surface of target cells. Fas is expressed on many cells, including hepatocytes, and ligation of Fas induces hepatocyte apoptosis [39,40]. In chronic HCV infection, areas of active inflammation are composed of cytotoxic T cells surrounding areas of Fas expressing hepatocytes with acidophilic bodies, indicating that CTLs may be inducing hepatocyte apoptosis. A third potential effector molecule used by CTL to induce cell death is TNFα. TNFα belongs to a family of nine ligands known as the TNF receptor superfamily produced by activated macrophages and lymphocytes and is an important mediator of apoptosis. Following sensitisation, hepatocytes can undergo apoptosis as a result of TNF stimulation [41,42].

CTLs can also contribute to host defence by the production of cytokines that are capable of non-cytopathic viral elimination. CTLs are capable of producing multiple cytokines, including IFNγ, TNFα, IL-8 and multiple chemokines [43,44]. Of these, the role of IFNγ in inhibiting viral replication has been characterised the best. In HBV-transgenic mice, IFNγ has been shown to contribute to the non-cytopathic reduction in viral gene expression and replication; super-infection of these mice with another pathogen such as LCMV, which results in IFNγ, leads to a reduction in viral replication [43,45,46]. The importance of cytokines in the control of viral replication has also been shown in a number of other systems including vaccinia virus, herpes simplex virus, measles, Semliki Forest virus, and Theiler's virus [47]. However, not all viruses are controlled by IFNγ: for example, after influenza challenge, IFNγ receptor knockout mice have the same susceptibility to influenza as wild type mice [48]. Depending on the kinetics of viral replication, either cytotoxicity or cytokine production may be the more important factor in control of a given viral infection. Recent experiments with perforin-deficient mice have shown that T-cell-mediated cytotoxicity is crucial for the resolution of infection by non-cytopathic viruses, such as most strains of lymphocytic choriomeningitis virus, but not for the resolution of infection with cytopathic viruses such as vaccinia, vesicular stomatitis, Semliki Forest or influenza virus [49]. In addition, IFNγ production by CTL is required to clear infections where the CTL does not have a high affinity for its target [50].

2. ACUTE HCV

The natural history of the infection is such that only about 15% of infected individuals successfully clear the infection and the remainder develop chronic disease of varying severity. The host and viral factors that are responsible for viral persistence and those that are associated with successful spontaneous eradication have not been clearly elucidated as of yet. This is mainly because the vast majority of acute HCV infections are sub-clinical with only 20% presenting with jaundice, therefore making it difficult to identify and study individuals during the critical period that is thought to dictate eventual disease outcome [51]. For the most part, patients with HCV infection present with chronic infection rather than the acute illness and because of this, the vast majority of studies on HCV-specific immune responses have focused on chronic rather than acute/resolving infection. Furthermore, our understanding of the immune responses during the acute phase of HCV infection is also limited by the absence of a small animal model. The only available animal model of HCV infection is the chimpanzee, which, because of the limited number of animals, reagents, and expense has hampered our understanding of acute HCV [52].

2.1. Antibody responses

After HCV was cloned in 1989, screening of overlapping cDNA clones against sera from individuals with post-transfusion NANB hepatitis resulted in the identification of reactive peptides, which encoded for B-cell epitopes. Subsequently the development of multiple generations of antibody testing to detect HCV antigens provided clear evidence that HCV infection is associated with the development of antibodies against both structural and non-structural antigens. After exposure to HCV, the majority of immunocompetent individuals will seroconvert within a 4-week period [53]. Both the order and pattern of antibody response is variable but the first antibody responses to develop are usually those against the NS3 (anti-c33) and core (anti-c22) with anti-NS4 and anti-E1/E2 developing later. Unlike the development of antibodies in HBV infection, the development of anti-HCV antibodies does not herald resolution of the disease process and lasting immunity. Similarly, IgM responses to core have been described in HCV infection, but they do not necessarily represent acute infection as the appearance of these antibodies may post-date the development of IgG response, are usually associated with the presence of viraemia, and do not occur in all individuals [54]. In the face of continuing viraemia, antibody responses are directed against multiple epitopes, while acute self-limiting infection is generally associated with a transient antibody response that gradually declines or one that does not develop at all [55–57]. Numerous studies have proposed associations between the pattern of antibody response and disease outcome, but have given conflicting results about the nature of this response and outcome [58,59].

Studies in the chimpanzee have demonstrated that repetitive re-challenge of convalescent animals with homologous or heterologous strains of HCV results in reappearance of viraemia in spite of the presence of antibodies to HCV indicating that they have no protective value [60]. However, more recent animal studies have shown that neutralising antibodies can be raised by repeated immunisation that are protective against infection with homologous virus; and plasma infectivity can be neutralised by serum from the same animal after 2 years but not after 11 years, indicating development of escape mutants over time [61,62]. Thus, it appears that while weak neutralising antibody responses are formed, escape mutation allows evasion of the humoral immune response. Furthermore, antibody responses to the envelope proteins develop slowly, achieve only modest titres and tend to be short lived, suggesting that neutralising antibodies may emerge too late or may not be strong enough to prevent chronic infection [63].

2.2. CD4 responses in acute HCV

$CD4^+$ responses are critical to both the generation and maintenance of anti-viral immune responses, since they secrete cytokines that augment antibody production by B cells and prime $CD8^+$ cells specific for virus-infected cells. Without $CD4^+$ cells, induction of new immune responses is impaired and CTL memory cannot be maintained in vivo [64]. The importance of vigorous $CD4^+$ responses in clearance of HCV is found in several lines of evidence. First, individuals who mount a polyclonal HCV-specific $CD4^+$ are more likely to clear HCV, whereas individuals who do not are more likely to become persistently infected [65–68]. Second, loss of HCV-specific $CD4^+$ is associated with relapse of infection [69]. Third, increased HCV-specific $CD4^+$ T cells are associated with an increase likelihood of sustained response after treatment [70]. Finally, in a cross-sectional analysis vigorous HCV-specific $CD4^+$ responses are associated with less aggressive disease recurrence following orthotopic liver transplantation [71]. Furthermore, these cellular responses can persist for long periods as suggested by the strong Th1 responses directed against both structural and non-structural HCV antigens persisting in individuals up to 17 years after spontaneous clearance [57,72]. Among patients who clear hepatitis C infections, there are higher levels of IL-12 than in chronic carriers and their peripheral $CD4^+$ T-cell responses preferentially produce IFNγ and IL-2 [68,73,74]. The reasons for an ineffective immune response in the majority (80–85%) of acutely infected individuals is not known and remains an important area of research. However, it would appear that the vigour, epitope specificity, and cytokine profile of the initial $CD4^+$ response have an important bearing on the outcome of acute HCV infection.

2.3. CD8 responses in acute HCV

CTL-mediated lysis of virally infected cells may result in clearance of the infection or, if incomplete, persistence of the infection and eventual tissue damage. Based on this, it would appear that a successful CTL response is crucial in preventing liver damage. Analysis of CTL responses is limited because of the small numbers of patients presenting with acute HCV and because of the inherent technical difficulties in working with these cells. Moreover, it is not ethical to perform liver biopsies on patients with acute viral hepatitis and so all human studies examining HCV-specific CTL responses have been performed on peripheral blood samples. Many of the studies on HCV-specific CTLs have used predicted epitopes based on known HLA class I binding motifs, such as HLA A2.1, which limits one's scope to those predicted peptides and HLA class I responses for which sufficient data are available. Similarly, the use of techniques such as chromium release cytotoxicity assays to enumerate antigen specific cells may result in underestimation of these cells because of apoptosis during repeated rounds of stimulation.

Despite this we know from chimpanzee studies that elimination of HCV infection in the acute phase is associated with the development of a multispecific intra-hepatic CTL response, while the persistence of infection is associated with a delayed and weaker intrahepatic response against fewer epitopes [75]. In humans, a similar early and polyclonal response is seen in those with self-limiting disease [76–78]. The development of newer techniques such as class I tetramers and ELISPOT assays, which can detect antigen-specific cells by virtue of their secreted cytokines in response to specific antigen, have provided further tools with which we can more efficiently measure the effectiveness of the early CTL responses [79,80]. Gruener et al. have demonstrated using ELISPOT techniques, a significant $CD8^+$ T-cell response directed against multiple class I-restricted HCV epitopes of structural and non-structural regions of the HCV polyprotein, which correlates with elimination of the virus. The frequency reported by Gruener in the peripheral blood of individuals with acute HCV was 0.2% of total $CD8^+$ cells. Significant proliferative responses of $CD4^+$ T cells to NS3 and NS4 proteins accompanied the CTL responses and were maintained in those patients with resolving infection [78]. Lechner et al. using a combination of class I tetramer staining and ELISPOT techniques have also demonstrated that the successful eradication of HCV is associated with a peripheral blood CTL frequency of greater than 7% at the peak of clinical illness, which is similar to that noted for infectious mononucleosis, and that this CTL response was simultaneously directed against eight different epitopes. This frequency of CTL contrasts with the low levels (0.07%) found in the peripheral blood of those individuals with chronic infection [81]. Several studies have demonstrated the persistence of HCV-specific CTL responses in the absence of serological or molecular evidence of HCV infection indicating the presence of CTL memory, possible persisting undetectable virus, or cross reactive responses against heterologous proteins [82–84]. Whether these 'memory' CTL responses can protect against future exposure remains to be seen. Therefore, acute self-limiting HCV infection is characterised by vigorous multispecific $CD4^+$ Th1 and CTL response.

3. CHRONIC HCV

Circumstantial evidence suggests that HCV replication is limited by cellular immune responses, but this hypothesis is still unproven. As discussed above, in chronic infection, peripheral HCV-specific $CD4^+$ T cells are present, but at much lower frequency than is found in acute clearance [65–68]. Several recent studies have demonstrated an association between strong $CD4^+$ T-cell responses and the absence of histological progression in immunocompetent hosts and in determining disease progression in recurrence of disease following liver transplantation [71,85,86]. Several groups, including our own, have published reports of HCV-specific CTL in the PBMC and liver infiltrating lymphocytes of persons with chronic HCV [44,87–98]. These CTL target multiple epitopes within the viral polyprotein, even within a single patient [44,88,91,96,99]. Certainly the HCV-specific CTL response is ineffective at completely controlling viral replication, as it coexists with robust viral replication. The relative weakness of virus-specific T-cell responses is reflected in the unusually low frequency of HCV-specific T cells in patients with chronic HCV infection as compared with other viral infections including hepatitis B. In rhesus monkeys that are chronically infected with simian immunodeficiency virus (SIV), at least 1.3–6.0% of peripheral blood lymphocytes and 7.0–28.8% of intrahepatic lymphocytes are SIV-specific, as revealed by staining with a tetrameric MHC/peptide complex that detects T cells specific for one epitope in the Gag protein [100]. In contrast, the frequency of HCV-specific $CD8^+$ T cells detected by the same techniques is much lower in chronic HCV infection. In one study, He et al. showed that the frequency of HCV-specific $CD8^+$ T cells, as revealed by staining with two MHC/HCV peptide tetrameters that detect $CD8^+$ T cells specific for two epitopes in the NS3 protein, was only 1–2% of intrahepatic $CD8^+$ T cells [97].

Recent reports suggest that the presence or absence of HCV core-specific CTL correlates with viral titre, indicating that HCV core-specific CTL serve to limit viral replication [94,101]. However, when more detailed examinations are performed analysing multiple CTL epitopes, there is no clear-cut correlation between the presence or absence of any CTL response and viral titre [91,102]. Although our bias is that cellular immune responses are beneficial, large and long-term trials are addressing the relationship of the immune response and natural history of HCV. Part of the difficulty in assessing such relationships is the prolonged and highly variable natural history of HCV, which makes it difficult to accumulate sufficient numbers of patients in these studies.

4. MECHANISMS OF LIVER INJURY

The absence of a robust tissue culture system limits our understanding of the effect of HCV upon cell survival, but at least two lines of evidence support the fact that HCV is not directly cytopathic in the classic sense. First, transgenic animals expressing HCV proteins do not develop cytopathic changes or liver inflammation [103,104]. Second, cell lines expressing HCV under the control of inducible promoters do not develop cytopathic changes once HCV expression is turned on, although the cells do have delayed growth kinetics [105]. Some other lineages of transgenic animals do develop hepatic steatosis and HCC, presumably in the setting of T-cell tolerance, which suggests that HCV proteins or RNA may interfere with host cell function [106–108].

The role of antigen-specific CTLs in mediating hepatocyte toxicity is well established in murine models of viral hepatitis. The classic model of liver injury in viral hepatitis is the adoptive transfer of syngeneic HBV-specific CTL clones into HBV transgenic mice, which results in the development of acute hepatitis [109,110]. Both of these experiments suggest that the liver injury occurs as a direct consequence of the CTLs. There is some direct evidence for this in hepatitis C. Animals who only express HCV under the control of an inducible promoter develop inflammation of the liver, whereas those animals who are constitutively tolerant to HCV proteins do not develop inflammation [111]. Similarly, treatment of an HCV-infected patient with anti-CD8 monoclonal antibodies resulted in improvement of serum transaminases, suggesting that the $CD8^+$ T cells were the cause of liver damage. However, HCV-specific cellular immune responses may not be the sole explanation, as evidenced by multiple clinical observations that describe an accelerated natural history of HCV-related liver damage in patients with immunosuppression, whether that is exogenously induced after liver transplantation or subsequent to human immunodeficiency virus (HIV)-induced loss of $CD4^+$ T cells [112,113].

Production of cytokines may also contribute to liver injury as well as mediate viral clearance. In animal models of Concanavalin A-induced hepatitis, the absence of $CD4^+$ T cells or IFNγ is associated with failure to develop liver injury [114], which is likely related to NK T-cell activation [115]. Similarly, transgenic mice constitutively producing IFNγ develop liver injury independent of any pathogen [116]. This illustrates a key paradox in understanding viral hepatitis, as one of the same molecules, IFNγ, involved in recovery is also implicated in liver injury; the result may be a matter of local kinetics of release. The vigour of the inflammatory response as measured by cytokine production within the liver is also correlated with the extent of liver injury [117,118]. Understanding to what extent cellular immune responses limit viral replication and liver injury and to what extent they induce liver injury remains a paradox that awaits resolution.

5. MECHANISMS OF HCV PERSISTENCE

Viruses have evolved a number of potential mechanisms to evade host immune responses, including replication in immunologically privileged sites, latent infections, induction of immunosuppression, alterations in cytokine patterns, viral variation, and alterations in antigen presentation (reviewed in ref. [119]). It is not clear why, in the majority of cases, HCV fails to induce an effective immune response. For example, the failure of most acutely infected individuals to develop an adequate $CD4^+$ response has not been linked to a class II allele, as many such studies of class I and II alleles provide contradictory results [120]. The intensity of the initial immune response is generally dependent on the cytopathic effects of virus, viral load, co-stimulatory signals, and type of APC. There is little information about the interaction of innate immunity with HCV, although HCV may interfere with the dimerisation of PKR, which is a key molecule induced by IFN, thus inhibiting the normal antiviral response of endogenous IFN [121,122]. Dendritic cell function also appears to be impaired, at least as measured by the capacity of these cells to induce reactions against alloantigens [123–125]. Failure of these professional antigen presenting cells early in infection would enhance the possibility of chronicity.

HCV exhibits extensive genetic variation among sequenced isolates with a degree of sequence variation analogous to that observed with HIV-1 [126]. At least six related but distinct families of isolates are known, and multiple closely related viral variants, the so-called quasispecies, can be identified within individual patients. Given the high degree of variability in the viral quasispecies within infected individuals, the emergence of viral escape mutants in antibody-recognising sites and CTL epitopes is a potential mechanism of persistence. During the acute infection there is relative stasis of the quasispecies population in those who have acute self-limited infection, but significant variation in the quasispecies of those that develop progressive infection [127]. Furthermore, complex quasispecies with sequence change variation in the HVR1 have been shown to correlate with disease persistence [128]. Mutations in the hypervariable region 1 (HVR1) of the envelope are less numerous in immunocompromised individuals than they are in immunocompetent individuals suggesting that antibody pressure may result in viral escape mutants; however, it has also been noted that persistent infection in chimpanzees can occur without variation in the HVR1 [129,130]. Similarly, CTL escape mutants have been reported in chimpanzees and chronically infected humans [92,128,131]. A recent report demonstrated that mutant epitopes in HVR1 can function as TCR antagonists capable of inhibiting HVR1-specific CTL activity, consistent with the notion that early CTL escape promotes chronicity [95]. However, the concept of CTL escape was recently challenged in a longitudinal study of virus mutations [132]. Over a 2-year period there were mutations in the envelope region of HCV which are not associated with known B-cell or CTL epitopes, and no mutations in the core region despite CTL recognition of this region. Since HCV infection may coexist with multispecific $CD4^+$ T-cell and CTL responses to both the conserved and variable epitopes [92,132], this argues that immune selection of escape mutants is not a complete explanation of virus persistence. Other mechanisms for viral persistence include alterations in cytokine secretion pattern induced by variation within cellular epitopes [133,134], which might reduce the functional capacity of these cells.

5.1. Compartmentalisation of immune responses in the liver

The hepatotropic nature of HCV may also contribute to persistence, as the liver is a site of relative immune privilege. An immune response is characterised by activation and massive expansion of antigen-specific T cells. To maintain lymphocyte homeostasis, the majority of these activated T cells, with the exception of a few long-lived memory T cells, will need to be eliminated after successful elimination of the invading pathogen.

In vivo, the major site of depletion of activated T cells appears to be the liver, especially for activated $CD8^+$ T cells [135]. Following activation, T cells appear in the periphery and spleen initially. As these T cells disappear from the lymph nodes and spleen, they accumulate in the liver, where they undergo apoptosis [136,137]. This apoptosis of activated T cells has been shown in two different systems, namely autoreactive cells in $H\text{-}2^k$ transgenic mice [138] and T cells isolated from TCR transgenic mice injected with peptide [137,139]. This is specific for activated cells, as activated but not resting cells are selectively retained by the normal liver [137]. In a more physiologic model, during influenza infection in the mouse, where the infection is limited to the respiratory tract, the resolution phase of the infection is associated with accumulation of abundant, apoptotic, virus-specific $CD8^+$ T cells in the liver, not in the lymph node or lung [140]. This deletion of activated $CD8^+$ T cells has been postulated to play a significant role not only in T-cell homeostasis, but also in the relative tolerance of liver allografts [141]. For example, in a B10 ($H\text{-}2^b$) to C3H ($H\text{-}2^k$) transplant model, manipulation of the model to decrease apoptosis of infiltrating T cells in the liver led to an increase in rejection.

Multiple lines of evidence support the compartmentalisation of immune responses in chronic HCV. Minutello et al. demonstrated that there is sequestration of virus-specific T cells in the liver during chronic HCV infection, as indicated by a different pattern of epitope specificity and T-cell receptor usage [142]. Schirren et al. have also demonstrated that the $CD4^+$ T-cell responses are compartmentalised to the liver as opposed to the peripheral blood, where they secrete a Th1 cytokine profile (IFNγ) which theoretically could continually stimulate the CTL and result in chronic liver disease [143]. Similarly, epitopes recognised by CTL isolated from PBMC and liver infiltrating lymphocytes appear to be of markedly different specificity (ref. [144] and M. Koziel, D. Wong and B. Walker, unpublished results). This suggests that the physiologic role of the liver in immune modulation may actually play a role in chronicity of hepatitis C. However, this needs to be confirmed in animal studies of acute infection.

CONCLUSION

In acute resolving infections, a co-ordinated and well-orchestrated innate immune response resulting in non-cytopathic viral elimination, mediated predominantly by the production of Th1 cytokines followed by vigourous $CD4^+$ Th1 responses which serve a critically important regulatory function by secreting cytokines that can facilitate B-cell maturation, expansion and antibody secretion or that foster the development of a strong CTL response. In spite of all the progress in determining the mechanism of cell injury and many pieces of experimental evidence reported on viral chronicity, we still lack the knowledge to explain adequately why and how viral persistence occurs in the case of HCV. It may result because of an inefficient immune response, evasion by the virus, escape mutations, or virus-induced apoptosis of antigen-specific CTLs. It would appear that some or all of these mechanisms play some role to a greater or lesser degree depending on the virus involved. Understanding the kinetics of the immune response and the balance between effective control and liver damage remains an important challenge for the future.

REFERENCES

[1] Cheney CP, Chopra S, Graham C. Hepatitis C. Infect Dis Clin N Am 2000; 14: 633–667.
[2] Alter MJ, Margolis HS, Krawczynski K, Judson F, Mares A, Alexander W et al. The natural history of community-acquired hepatitis C in the United States. New Engl J Med 1992; 327: 1899–1905.
[3] Alberti A, Morsica G, Chemello L, Cavalletto D, Noventa F, Pontisso P et al. Hepatitis C viraemia and liver disease in symptom-free individuals with anti-HCV. Lancet 1992; 340: 697–698.
[4] Iwarson S, Norkrans G, Wejstal R. Hepatitis C: natural history of a unique infection [review]. Clin Infect Dis 1995; 20: 1361–1370.
[5] Seeff LB, Buskell-Bales Z, Wright EC, Durako SJ, Alter HJ, Iber FL et al. Long-term mortality after transfusion-associated non-A, non-B hepatitis. The National Heart, Lung, and Blood Institute Study Group. New Engl J Med 1992; 327: 1906–1911.
[6] Di Bisceglie AM, Goodman ZD, Ishak KG, Hoofnagle JH, Melpolder JJ, Alter HJ. Long-term clinical and histopathological follow-up of chronic posttransfusion hepatitis. Hepatology 1991; 14: 969–974.
[7] Tong MJ, el-Farra NS, Reikes AR, Co RL. Clinical outcomes after transfusion-associated hepatitis C. N Engl J Med 1995; 332: 1463–1466.
[8] Kenny-Walsh E. Clinical outcomes after hepatitis C infection from contaminated anti-D immune globulin. Irish Hepatology Research Group. N Engl J Med 1999; 340: 1228–1233.
[9] Seeff LB. Natural history of hepatitis C. Am J Med 1999; 107: 10S–5S.
[10] Brechot C. Hepatitis C virus: molecular biology and genetic variability. Dig Dis Sci 1996; 41: 6S–21S.
[11] Lerat H, Berby F, Trabaud MA, Vidalin O, Major M, Trepo C et al. Specific detection of hepatitis C virus minus strand RNA in hematopoietic cells. J Clin Invest 1996; 97: 845–851.
[12] Shimizu Y, Imawoto A, Hijikata M, Purcell R, Yoshikura H. Evidence for in vitro replication of hepatitis C virus genome in a human T-cell line. Proc Natl Acad Sci USA 1992; 89: 5477–5481.
[13] Shimizu YK, Purcell RH, Yoshikura H. Correlation between the infectivity of hepatitis C virus in vivo and its infectivity in vitro. Proc Natl Acad Sci USA 1993; 90: 6037–6041.
[14] Koziel MJ, Walker BD. Viruses, chemotherapy and immunity. Parasitology 1992; 105 Suppl: S85–92.
[15] Clemens MJ, Elia A. The double-stranded RNA-dependent protein kinase PKR: structure and function. J Interferon Cytokine Res 1997; 17: 503–524.
[16] Samuel CE. Antiviral actions of interferon. Interferon-regulated cellular proteins and their surprisingly selective antiviral activities. Virology 1991; 183: 1–11.
[17] Doherty DG, Norris S, Madrigal-Estebas L, McEntee G, Traynor O, Hegarty JE et al. The human liver contains multiple populations of NK cells, T cells, and $CD3^+CD56^+$ natural T cells with distinct cytotoxic activities and Th1, Th2, and Th0 cytokine secretion patterns. J Immunol 1999; 163: 2314–2321.
[18] Doherty DG, O'Farrelly C. Innate and adaptive lymphoid cells in the human liver. Immunol Rev 2000; 174: 5–20.
[19] Nuti S, Rosa D, Valiante NM, Saletti G, Caratozzolo M, Dellabona P et al. Dynamics of intra-hepatic lymphocytes in chronic hepatitis C: enrichment for Valpha24+ T cells and rapid elimination of effector cells by apoptosis. Eur J Immunol 1998; 28: 3448–3455.
[20] Bukowski JF, Woda BA, Habu S, Okumura K, Welsh RM. Natural killer cell depletion enhances virus synthesis and virus-induced hepatitis in vivo. J Immunol 1983; 131: 1531–1538.

[21] Trinchieri G. Biological properties and therapeutic applications of interleukin-12. Eur Cytokine Netw 1997; 8: 305–307.
[22] Kakimi K, Guidotti LG, Koezuka Y, Chisari FV. Natural killer T cell activation inhibits hepatitis B virus replication in vivo. J Exp Med 2000; 192: 921–930.
[23] Liu ZX, Govindarajan S, Okamoto S, Dennert G. NK cells cause liver injury and facilitate the induction of T cell-mediated immunity to a viral liver infection. J Immunol 2000; 164: 6480–6486.
[24] Corado J, Toro F, Rivera H, Bianco NE, Deibis L, De Sanctis JB. Impairment of natural killer (NK) cytotoxic activity in hepatitis C virus (HCV) infection. Clin Exp Immunol 1997; 109: 451–457.
[25] Kawarabayashi N, Seki S, Hatsuse K, Ohkawa T, Koike Y, Aihara T et al. Decrease of CD56(+)T cells and natural killer cells in cirrhotic livers with hepatitis C may be involved in their susceptibility to hepatocellular carcinoma. Hepatology 2000; 32: 962–969.
[26] Spellberg B, Edwards JE Jr. Type 1/Type 2 immunity in infectious diseases. Clin Infect Dis 2001; 32: 76–102.
[27] Croft M, Carter L, Swain SL, Dutton RW. Generation of polarized antigen-specific CD8 effector populations: reciprocal action of interleukin (IL)-4 and IL-12 in promoting type 2 versus type 1 cytokine profiles. J Exp Med 1994; 180: 1715–1728.
[28] Spada FM, Koezuka Y, Porcelli SA. CD1d-restricted recognition of synthetic glycolipid antigens by human natural killer T cells. J Exp Med 1998; 188: 1529–1534.
[29] Unutmaz D, Pileri P, Abrignani S. Antigen-independent activation of naive and memory resting T cells by a cytokine combination. J Exp Med 1994; 180: 1159–1164.
[30] Guidotti LG, Chisari FV. Noncytolytic control of viral infections by the innate and adaptive immune response. Annu Rev Immunol 2001; 19: 65–91.
[31] Koziel MJ. Cytokines in viral hepatitis. Semin Liver Dis 1999; 19: 157–169.
[32] Scott P, Pearce E, Cheever AW, Coffman RL, Sher A. Role of cytokines and $CD4^+$ T-cell subsets in the regulation of parasite immunity and disease. Immunol Rev 1989; 112: 161–182.
[33] Cenci E, Mencacci A, Del Sero G, Bistoni F, Romani L. Induction of protective Th1 responses to *Candida albicans* by antifungal therapy alone or in combination with an interleukin-4 antagonist. J Infect Dis 1997; 176: 217–226.
[34] Daugelat S, Kaufmann SH. Role of Th1 and Th2 cells in bacterial infections. Chem Immunol 1996; 63: 66–97.
[35] Matyniak JE, Reiner SL. T helper phenotype and genetic susceptibility in experimental Lyme disease. J Exp Med 1995; 181: 1251–1254.
[36] Spaccapelo R, Del Sero G, Mosci P, Bistoni F, Romani L. Early T cell unresponsiveness in mice with candidiasis and reversal by IL-2: effect on T helper cell development. J Immunol 1997; 158: 2294–2302.
[37] Urban JF Jr, Katona IM, Paul WE, Finkelman FD. Interleukin 4 is important in protective immunity to a gastrointestinal nematode infection in mice. Proc Natl Acad Sci USA 1991; 88: 5513–5517.
[38] Berke G. Killing mechanisms of cytotoxic lymphocytes. Curr Opin Hematol 1997; 4: 32–40.
[39] Ogasawara J, Watanabe-Fukunaga R, Adachi M, Matsuzawa A, Kasugai T, Kitamura Y et al. Lethal effect of the anti-Fas antibody in mice. Nature 1993; 364: 806–809.
[40] Nagata S, Golstein P. The Fas death factor. Science 1995; 267: 1449–1456.
[41] Nagaki M, Sugiyama A, Osawa Y, Naiki T, Nakashima S, Nozawa Y et al. Lethal hepatic apoptosis mediated by tumor necrosis factor receptor, unlike Fas-mediated apoptosis, requires hepatocyte sensitization in mice. J Hepatol 1999; 31: 997–1005.

[42] Diehl AM. Cytokine regulation of liver injury and repair. Immunol Rev 2000; 174: 160–171.
[43] Guidotti LG, Ando K, Hobbs MV, Ishikawa T, Runkel L, Schreiber RD et al. Cytotoxic T lymphocytes inhibit hepatitis B virus gene expression by a noncytolytic mechanism in transgenic mice. Proc Natl Acad Sci USA 1994; 91: 3764–3768.
[44] Koziel MJ, Dudley D, Afdhal N, Grakoui A, Rice CM, Choo QL et al. HLA class I-restricted cytotoxic T lymphocytes specific for hepatitis C virus. Identification of multiple epitopes and characterization of patterns of cytokine release. J Clin Invest 1995; 96: 2311–2321.
[45] Guidotti LG, Borrow P, Hobbs MV, Matzke B, Gresser I, Oldstone MB et al. Viral cross talk: intracellular inactivation of the hepatitis B virus during an unrelated viral infection of the liver. Proc Natl Acad Sci USA 1996; 93: 4589–4594.
[46] Guidotti LG, Ishikawa T, Hobbs MV, Matzke B, Schreiber R, Chisari FV. Intracellular inactivation of the hepatitis B virus by cytotoxic T lymphocytes. Immunity 1996; 4: 25–36.
[47] Ramshaw IA, Ramsay AJ, Karupiah G, Rolph MS, Mahalingam S, Ruby JC. Cytokines and immunity to viral infections. Immunol Rev 1997; 159: 119–135.
[48] Graham MB, Dalton DK, Giltinan D, Braciale VL, Stewart TA, Braciale TJ. Response to influenza infection in mice with a targeted disruption in the interferon gamma gene. J Exp Med 1993; 178: 1725–1732.
[49] Kagi D, Hengartner H. Different roles for cytotoxic T cells in the control of infections with cytopathic versus noncytopathic viruses. Curr Opin Immunol 1996; 8: 472–477.
[50] Von Herrath MG, Coon B, Oldstone MB. Low-affinity cytotoxic T-lymphocytes require IFN-gamma to clear an acute viral infection. Virology 1997; 229: 349–359.
[51] Borrow P. Mechanisms of viral clearance and persistence. J Viral Hepat 1997; 4: 16–24.
[52] Grakoui A, Hanson HL, Rice CM. Bad time for Bonzo? Experimental models of hepatitis C virus infection, replication, and pathogenesis. Hepatology 2001; 33: 489–495.
[53] Rubin R, Falestiny M, Malet P. Chronic hepatitis C: advances in diagnostic testing and therapy. Arch Int Med 1994; 154: 387–392.
[54] Quinti I, Hassan NF, El Salman D, Shalaby H, El Zimatty D, Monier MK et al. Hepatitis C virus-specific B cell activation: IgG and IgM detection in acute and chronic hepatitis C. J Hepatol 1995; 23: 640–647.
[55] Beld M, Penning M, van Putten M, Lukashov V, van den Hoek A, McMorrow M et al. Quantitative antibody responses to structural (Core) and nonstructural (NS3, NS4, and NS5) hepatitis C virus proteins among seroconverting injecting drug users: impact of epitope variation and relationship to detection of HCV RNA in blood. Hepatology 1999; 29: 1288–1298.
[56] Chien DY, Choo QL, Tabrizi A, Kuo C, McFarland J, Berger K et al. Diagnosis of hepatitis C virus (HCV) infection using an immunodominant chimeric polyprotein to capture circulating antibodies: reevaluation of the role of HCV in liver disease. Proc Natl Acad Sci USA 1992; 89: 10011–10015.
[57] Takaki A, Wiese M, Maertens G, Depla E, Seifert U, Liebetrau A et al. Cellular immune responses persist and humoral responses decrease two decades after recovery from a single-source outbreak of hepatitis C. Nat Med 2000; 6: 578–582.
[58] Kobayashi M, Chayama K, Arase Y, Tsubota A, Saitoh S, Suzuki Y et al. Predictive value of different hepatitis C serological assays in the treatment of chronic hepatitis C with interferon alpha. J Gastroenterol 1999; 34: 94–99.
[59] Lesniewski RR, Watanabe S, Devare SG. Expression of HCV envelope proteins and the serological utility of the anti-E2 immune response. Princess Takamatsu Symp 1995; 25: 129–137.

[60] Farci P, Alter H, Govindarajan S, Wong D, Engle R, Lesniewski R et al. Lack of protective immunity against reinfection with hepatitis C virus. Science 1992; 258: 135–140.
[61] Choo QL, Kuo G, Ralston R, Weiner A, Chien D, Van Nest G et al. Vaccination of chimpanzees against infection by the hepatitis C virus. Proc Natl Acad Sci USA 1994; 91: 1294–1298.
[62] Farci P, Alter HJ, Wong DC, Miller RH, Govindarajan S, Engle R et al. Prevention of hepatitis C virus infection in chimpanzees after antibody-mediated in vitro neutralization. Proc Natl Acad Sci USA 1994; 91: 7792–7796.
[63] Chen M, Sallberg M, Sonnerborg A, Weiland O, Mattsson L, Jin L et al. Limited humoral immunity in hepatitis C virus infection. Gastroenterology 1999; 116: 135–143.
[64] Matloubian M, Concepcion RJ, Ahmed R. $CD4^+$ T cells are required to sustain $CD8^+$ cytotoxic T-cell responses during chronic viral infection. J Virol 1994; 68: 8056–8063.
[65] Diepolder HM, Zachoval R, Hoffmann RM, Wierenga EA, Santantonio T, Jung MC et al. Possible mechanism involving T-lymphocyte response to non-structural protein 3 in viral clearance in acute hepatitis C virus infection. Lancet 1995; 346: 1006–1007.
[66] Lechmann M, Ihlenfeldt HG, Braunschweiger I, Giers G, Jung G, Matz B et al. T- and B-cell responses to different hepatitis C virus antigens in patients with chronic hepatitis C virus infection and in healthy anti-hepatitis C virus-positive blood donors without viremia. Hepatology 1996; 24: 790–795.
[67] Missale G, Bertoni R, Lamonaca V, Valli A, Massari M, Mori C et al. Different clinical behaviors of acute hepatitis C virus infection are associated with different vigor of the anti-viral cell-mediated immune response. J Clin Invest 1996; 98: 706–714.
[68] Tsai SL, Liaw YF, Chen MH, Huang CY, Kuo GC. Detection of type 2-like T-helper cells in hepatitis C virus infection: implications for hepatitis C virus chronicity. Hepatology 1997; 25: 449–458.
[69] Gerlach JT, Diepolder HM, Jung MC, Gruener NH, Schraut WW, Zachoval R et al. Recurrence of hepatitis C virus after loss of virus-specific CD4(+) T-cell response in acute hepatitis C. Gastroenterology 1999; 117: 933–941.
[70] Cramp ME, Rossol S, Chokshi S, Carucci P, Williams R, Naoumov NV. Hepatitis C virus-specific T-cell reactivity during interferon and ribavirin treatment in chronic hepatitis C. Gastroenterology 2000; 118: 346–355.
[71] Rosen HR, Hinrichs DJ, Gretch DR, Koziel MJ, Chou S, Houghton M et al. Association of multispecific CD4(+) response to hepatitis C and severity of recurrence after liver transplantation. Gastroenterology 1999; 117: 926–932.
[72] Cramp ME, Carucci P, Rossol S, Chokshi S, Maertens G, Williams R et al. Hepatitis C virus (HCV) specific immune responses in anti-HCV positive patients without hepatitis C viraemia. Gut 1999; 44: 424–429.
[73] Penna A, Del Prete G, Cavalli A, Bertoletti A, D'Elios MM, Sorrentino R et al. Predominant T-helper 1 cytokine profile of hepatitis B virus nucleocapsid-specific T cells in acute self-limited hepatitis B. Hepatology 1997; 25: 1022–1027.
[74] Rossol S, Marinos G, Carucci P, Singer MV, Williams R, Naoumov NV. Interleukin-12 induction of Th1 cytokines is important for viral clearance in chronic hepatitis B. J Clin Invest 1997; 99: 3025–3033.
[75] Cooper S, Erickson AL, Adams EJ, Kansopon J, Weiner AJ, Chien DY et al. Analysis of a successful immune response against hepatitis C virus. Immunity 1999; 10: 439–449.
[76] Lechner F, Wong DK, Dunbar PR, Chapman R, Chung RT, Dohrenwend P et al. Analysis of successful immune responses in persons infected with hepatitis C virus. J Exp Med 2000; 191: 1499–1512.

[77] Takaki A, Wiese M, Maertens G, Depla E, Seifert U, Liebetrau A et al. Cellular immune responses persist and humoral responses decrease two decades after recovery from a single-source outbreak of hepatitis C. Nat Med 2000; 6: 578–582.
[78] Gruener NH, Lechner F, Jung MC, Diepolder H, Gerlach T, Lauer G et al. Sustained dysfunction of antiviral CD8$^+$ T lymphocytes after infection with hepatitis C virus. J Virol 2001; 75: 5550–5558.
[79] Gallimore A, Glithero A, Godkin A, Tissot AC, Pluckthun A, Elliott T et al. Induction and exhaustion of lymphocytic choriomeningitis virus-specific cytotoxic T lymphocytes visualized using soluble tetrameric major histocompatibility complex class I-peptide complexes. J Exp Med 1998; 187: 1383–1393.
[80] Murali-Krishna K, Altman JD, Suresh M, Sourdive DJ, Zajac AJ, Miller JD et al. Counting antigen-specific CD8 T cells: a reevaluation of bystander activation during viral infection. Immunity 1998; 8: 177–187.
[81] Lechner F, Gruener NH, Urbani S, Uggeri J, Santantonio T, Kammer AR et al. CD8$^+$ T lymphocyte responses are induced during acute hepatitis C virus infection but are not sustained. Eur J Immunol 2000; 30: 2479–2487.
[82] Koziel MJ, Wong DK, Dudley D, Houghton M, Walker BD. Hepatitis C virus-specific cytolytic T lymphocyte and T helper cell responses in seronegative persons. J Infect Dis 1997; 176: 859–866.
[83] Resti M, Azzari C, Lega L, Rossi ME, Zammarchi E, Novembre E et al. Mother-to-infant transmission of hepatitis C virus. Acta Paediatr 1995; 84: 251–255.
[84] Scognamiglio P, Accapezzato D, Casciaro MA, Cacciani A, Artini M, Bruno G et al. Presence of effector CD8$^+$ T cells in hepatitis C virus-exposed healthy seronegative donors. J Immunol 1999; 162: 6681–6689.
[85] Chang KM, Thimme R, Melpolder JJ, Oldach D, Pemberton J, Moorhead-Loudis J et al. Differential CD4 and CD8 T-cell responsiveness in hepatitis C virus infection. Hepatology 2001; 33: 267–276.
[86] Kamal S, Rasenack J, Bianchi L, Taweel A, Khalifa K, Peters T et al. A prospective study of the outcome of acute hepatitis C with and without schistosomiasis: correlation with hepatitis C specific CD4$^+$ T cell and cytokine responses. Gastroenterology 2001; 121: 646–656.
[87] Koziel MJ, Dudley D, Wong JT, Dienstag J, Houghton M, Ralston R et al. Intrahepatic cytotoxic T lymphocytes specific for hepatitis C virus in persons with chronic hepatitis. J Immunol 1992; 149: 3339–3344.
[88] Koziel MJ, Dudley D, Afdhal N, Choo QL, Houghton M, Ralston R et al. Hepatitis C virus (HCV)-specific cytotoxic T lymphocytes recognize epitopes in the core and envelope proteins of HCV. J Virol 1993; 67: 7522–7532.
[89] Battegay M, Fikes J, Di Bisceglie AM, Wentworth PA, Sette A, Celis E et al. Patients with chronic hepatitis C have circulating cytotoxic T cells which recognize hepatitis C virus-encoded peptides binding to HLA-A2.1 molecules. J Virol 1995; 69: 2462–2470.
[90] Kaneko T, Nakamura I, Kita H, Hiroishi K, Moriyama T, Imawari M. Three new cytotoxic T cell epitopes identified within the hepatitis C virus nucleoprotein. J Gen Virol 1996; 77: 1305–1309.
[91] Rehermann B, Chang K-M, McHutchinson J, Kokka R, Houghton M, Chisari F. Quantitative analysis of the peripheral blood cytotoxic T lymphocyte response in patients with chronic hepatitis C virus infection. J Clin Invest 1996; 98: 1431–1440.
[92] Chang KM, Rehermann B, McHutchison JG, Pasquinelli C, Southwood S, Sette A et al. Immunological significance of cytotoxic T lymphocyte epitope variants in patients chronically infected by the hepatitis C virus. J Clin Invest 1997; 100: 2376–2385.

[93] Giuggio VM, Bonkovsky HL, Smith J, Rothman AL. Inefficient recognition of autologous viral sequences by intrahepatic hepatitis C virus-specific cytotoxic T lymphocytes in chronically infected subjects. Virology 1998; 251: 132–140.
[94] Nelson DR, Marousis CG, Ohno T, Davis GL, Lau JY. Intrahepatic hepatitis C virus-specific cytotoxic T lymphocyte activity and response to interferon alfa therapy in chronic hepatitis C. Hepatology 1998; 28: 225–230.
[95] Tsai SL, Chen YM, Chen MH, Huang CY, Sheen IS, Yeh CT et al. Hepatitis C virus variants circumventing cytotoxic T lymphocyte activity as a mechanism of chronicity. Gastroenterology 1998; 115: 954–965.
[96] Chang KM, Gruener NH, Southwood S, Sidney J, Pape GR, Chisari FV et al. Identification of HLA-A3 and -B7-restricted CTL response to hepatitis C virus in patients with acute and chronic hepatitis C. J Immunol 1999; 162: 1156–1164.
[97] He XS, Rehermann B, Lopez-Labrador FX, Boisvert J, Cheung R, Mumm J et al. Quantitative analysis of hepatitis C virus-specific CD8(+) T cells in peripheral blood and liver using peptide-MHC tetramers. Proc Natl Acad Sci USA 1999; 96: 5692–5697.
[98] Urbani S, Uggeri J, Matsuura Y, Miyamura T, Penna A, Boni C et al. Identification of immunodominant hepatitis C virus (HCV)-specific cytotoxic T-cell epitopes by stimulation with endogenously synthesized HCV antigens. Hepatology 2001; 33: 1533–1543.
[99] Rehermann B, Chang K-M, McHutchinson J, Kokka R, Houghton M, Rice CM et al. Differential cytotoxic T-lymphocyte responsiveness to hepatitis B and C viruses in chronically infected patients. J Virol 1996; 70: 7092–7102.
[100] Schmitz JE, Kuroda MJ, Veazey RS, Seth A, Taylor WM, Nickerson CE et al. Simian immunodeficiency virus (SIV)-specific CTL are present in large numbers in livers of SIV-infected rhesus monkeys. J Immunol 2000; 164: 6015–6019.
[101] Nelson DR, Marousis CG, Davis GL, Rice CM, Wong J, Houghton M et al. The role of hepatitis C virus-specific cytotoxic T lymphocytes in chronic hepatitis C. J Immunol 1997; 158: 1473–1481.
[102] Wong DK, Dudley DD, Afdhal NH, Dienstag J, Rice CM, Wang L et al. Liver-derived CTL in hepatitis C virus infection: breadth and specificity of responses in a cohort of persons with chronic infection. J Immunol 1998; 160: 1479–1488.
[103] Kawamura T, Furusaka A, Koziel MJ, Chung RT, Wang TC, Schmidt EV et al. Transgenic expression of hepatitis C virus structural proteins in the mouse. Hepatology 1997; 25: 1014–1021.
[104] Pasquinelli C, Shoenberger JM, Chung J, Chang KM, Guidotti LG, Selby M et al. Hepatitis C virus core and E2 protein expression in transgenic mice. Hepatology 1997; 25: 719–727.
[105] Moradpour D, Kary P, Rice CM, Blum HE. Continuous human cell lines inducibly expressing hepatitis C virus structural and nonstructural proteins. Hepatology 1998; 28: 192–201.
[106] Lemon SM, Lerat H, Weinman SA, Honda M. A transgenic mouse model of steatosis and hepatocellular carcinoma associated with chronic hepatitis C virus infection in humans. Trans Am Clin Climatol Assoc 2000; 111: 146–156.
[107] Moriya K, Yotsuyanagi H, Shintani Y, Fujie H, Ishibashi K, Matsuura Y et al. Hepatitis C virus core protein induces hepatic steatosis in transgenic mice. J Gen Virol 1997; 78: 1527–1731.
[108] Moriya K, Fujie H, Shintani Y, Yotsuyanagi H, Tsutsumi T, Ishibashi K et al. The core protein of hepatitis C virus induces hepatocellular carcinoma in transgenic mice. Nat Med 1998; 4: 1065–1067.
[109] Moriyama T, Guilhot S, Klopchin K, Moss B, Pinkert CA, Palmiter RD et al. Immunobiology and pathogenesis of hepatocellular injury in hepatitis B virus transgenic mice. Science 1990; 248: 361–364.

[110] Zinkernagel RM, Haenseler E, Leist T, Cerny A, Hengartner H, Althage A. T cell-mediated hepatitis in mice infected with lymphocytic choriomeningitis virus. Liver cell destruction by H-2 class I-restricted virus-specific cytotoxic T cells as a physiological correlate of the 51Cr-release assay? J Exp Med 1986; 164: 1075–1092.
[111] Wakita T, Katsume A, Kato J, Taya C, Yonekawa H, Kanegae Y et al. Possible role of cytotoxic T cells in acute liver injury in hepatitis C virus cDNA transgenic mice mediated by Cre/loxP system. J Med Virol 2000; 62: 308–317.
[112] Graham CS, Herren T, Baden L, Mrus J, Yu E, Koziel MJ. Influence of human immunodeficiency virus (HIV) infection on the course of hepatitis C virus (HCV) infection: a meta-analysis. Clin Infec Dis 2001; 33: 562–569.
[113] Rosen HR, Martin P. Viral hepatitis in the liver transplant recipient. Infect Dis Clin N Am 2000; 14: 761–784.
[114] Kusters S, Gantner F, Kunstle G, Tiegs G. Interferon gamma plays a critical role in T cell-dependent liver injury in mice initiated by concanavalin A. Gastroenterology 1996; 111: 462–471.
[115] Takeda K, Hayakawa Y, Van Kaer L, Matsuda H, Yagita H, Okumura K. Critical contribution of liver natural killer T cells to a murine model of hepatitis. Proc Natl Acad Sci USA 2000; 97: 5498–5503.
[116] Toyonaga T, Hino O, Sugai S, Wakasugi S, Abe K, Shichiri M et al. Chronic active hepatitis in transgenic mice expressing interferon-γ in the liver. Proc Natl Acad Sci USA 1994; 91: 614–618.
[117] Napoli J, Bishop GA, McCaughan GW. Increased intrahepatic messenger RNA expression of interleukins 2, 6, and 8 in human cirrhosis. Gastroenterology 1994; 107: 789–798.
[118] Napoli J, Bishop GA, McGuinness PH, Painter DM, McCaughan GW. Progressive liver injury in chronic hepatitis C infection correlates with increased intrahepatic expression of Th1-associated cytokines. Hepatology 1996; 24: 759–765.
[119] Tortorella D, Gewurz BE, Furman MH, Schust DJ, Ploegh HL. Viral subversion of the immune system. Annu Rev Immunol 2000; 18: 861–926.
[120] Thio CL, Thomas DL, Carrington M. Chronic viral hepatitis and the human genome. Hepatology 2000; 31: 819–827.
[121] Gale MJ Jr, Korth MJ, Tang NM, Tan SL, Hopkins DA, Dever TE et al. Evidence that hepatitis C virus resistance to interferon is mediated through repression of the PKR protein kinase by the nonstructural 5A protein. Virology 1997; 230: 217–127.
[122] Taylor DR, Shi ST, Romano PR, Barber GN, Lai MM. Inhibition of the interferon-inducible protein kinase PKR by HCV E2 protein. Science 1999; 285: 107–110.
[123] Auffermann-Gretzinger S, Keeffe EB, Levy S. Impaired dendritic cell maturation in patients with chronic, but not resolved, hepatitis C virus infection. Blood 2001; 97: 3171–3176.
[124] Bain C, Fatmi A, Zoulim F, Zarski JP, Trepo C, Inchauspe G. Impaired allostimulatory function of dendritic cells in chronic hepatitis C infection. Gastroenterology 2001; 120: 512–524.
[125] Kanto T, Hayashi N, Takehara T, Tatsumi T, Kuzushita N, Ito A et al. Impaired allostimulatory capacity of peripheral blood dendritic cells recovered from hepatitis C virus-infected individuals. J Immunol 1999; 162: 5584–5591.
[126] Pawlotsky JM. Hepatitis C virus infection: virus/host interactions. J Viral Hepat 1998; 5(Suppl 1): 3–8.
[127] Farci P, Shimoda A, Coiana A, Diaz G, Peddis G, Melpolder JC et al. The outcome of acute hepatitis C predicted by the evolution of the viral quasispecies. Science 2000; 288: 339–344.

[128] Weiner A, Erickson AL, Kansopon J, Crawford K, Muchmore E, Hughes AL et al. Persistent hepatitis C virus infection in a chimpanzee is associated with emergence of a cytotoxic T lymphocyte escape variant. Proc Natl Acad Sci USA 1995; 92: 2755–2759.
[129] Bassett SE, Guerra B, Brasky K, Miskovsky E, Houghton M, Klimpel GR et al. Protective immune response to hepatitis C virus in chimpanzees rechallenged following clearance of primary infection. Hepatology 2001; 33: 1479–1487.
[130] Odeberg J, Yun Z, Sonnerborg A, Uhlen M, Lundeberg J. Dynamic analysis of heterogeneous hepatitis C virus populations by direct solid-phase sequencing. J Clin Microbiol 1995; 33: 1870–1874.
[131] Kaneko T, Moriyama T, Udaka K, Hiroishi K, Kita H, Okamoto H et al. Impaired induction of cytotoxic T lymphocytes by antagonism of a weak agonist borne by a variant hepatitis C virus epitope. Eur J Immunol 1997; 27: 1782–1787.
[132] Christie JM, Chapel H, Chapman RW, Rosenberg WM. Immune selection and genetic sequence variation in core and envelope regions of hepatitis C virus. Hepatology 1999; 30: 1037–1044.
[133] Eckels DD, Tabatabail N, Bian TH, Wang H, Muheisen SS, Rice CM et al. In vitro human Th-cell responses to a recombinant hepatitis C virus antigen: failure in IL-2 production despite proliferation. Hum Immunol 1999; 60: 187–199.
[134] Wang H, Eckels DD. Mutations in immunodominant T cell epitopes derived from the nonstructural 3 protein of hepatitis C virus have the potential for generating escape variants that may have important consequences for T cell recognition. J Immunol 1999; 162: 4177–4183.
[135] Mehal WZ, Azzaroli F, Crispe IN. Immunology of the healthy liver: old questions and new insights. Gastroenterology 2001; 120: 250–260.
[136] Huang L, Soldevila G, Leeker M, Flavell R, Crispe IN. The liver eliminates T cells undergoing antigen-triggered apoptosis in vivo. Immunity 1994; 1: 741–749.
[137] Mehal WZ, Juedes AE, Crispe IN. Selective retention of activated $CD8^+$ T cells by the normal liver. J Immunol 1999; 163: 3202–3210.
[138] Bertolino P, Heath WR, Hardy CL, Morahan G, Miller JF. Peripheral deletion of autoreactive $CD8^+$ T cells in transgenic mice expressing H-2Kb in the liver. Eur J Immunol 1995; 25: 1932–1942.
[139] Wack A, Corbella P, Harker N, Crispe IN, Kioussis D. Multiple sites of post-activation $CD8^+$ T cell disposal. Eur J Immunol 1997; 27: 577–583.
[140] Belz GT, Altman JD, Doherty PC. Characteristics of virus-specific CD8(+) T cells in the liver during the control and resolution phases of influenza pneumonia. Proc Natl Acad Sci USA 1998; 95: 13812–13817.
[141] Qian S, Lu L, Fu F, Li Y, Li W, Starzl TE et al. Apoptosis within spontaneously accepted mouse liver allografts: evidence for deletion of cytotoxic T cells and implications for tolerance induction. J Immunol 1997; 158: 4654–4661.
[142] Minutello MA, Pileri P, Unutmaz D, Censini S, Kuo G, Houghton M et al. Compartmentalization of T lymphocytes to the site of disease: intrahepatic $CD4^+$ T cells specific for the protein NS4 of hepatitis C virus in patients with chronic hepatitis C. J Exp Med 1993; 178: 17–25.
[143] Schirren CA, Jung MC, Gerlach JT, Worzfeld T, Baretton G, Mamin M et al. Liver-derived hepatitis C virus (HCV)-specific CD4(+) T cells recognize multiple HCV epitopes and produce interferon gamma. Hepatology 2000; 32: 597–603.
[144] Koziel MJ, Walker BD. Characteristics of the intrahepatic cytotoxic T lymphocyte response in chronic hepatitis C virus infection. Springer Semin Immunopathol 1997; 19: 69–83.

Molecular Biology and Immunology in Hepatology
Edited by T. Tsuji, T. Higashi, M. Zeniya and K.-H. Meyer zum Büschenfelde

CHAPTER 5

Recent Advancement in Interferon Therapy for Hepatitis C Treatment

Janos Feher and Gabriella Lengyel

Second Department of Internal Medicine, Semmelweis University, Budapest, Hungary

INTRODUCTION

Viral hepatitis is an infectious disease, where the infecting agent — the virus — elicits mainly the illness of the liver. There are two known forms, acute and chronic hepatitis. As pathogens, mainly hepatotropic viruses are to be counted on, but viruses inducing systemic infections can also cause hepatitis, where the disease of the liver represents only a part of the clinical picture.

According to the current nomenclature so-called hepatotropic viruses are classified as hepatitis A virus (HAV), hepatitis B virus (HBV), hepatitis C virus (HCV), hepatitis D (delta) virus (HDV), hepatitis E virus (HEV), and hepatitis G virus (HGV, HGB-V). Research data suggest that there should be other — not yet identified — primarily hepatotropic non-A–E viruses (e.g. HFV), as well as viruses that are primarily not hepatotropic, but are capable of eliciting an inflammatory reaction in the liver as part of a systemic infection.

HAV and HEV infections cause acute hepatitis accompanied by jaundice in most cases. There is no known chronic form of these infections. On the contrary, HBV, HCV, and HDV, as well as the recently identified HGV, frequently cause chronic hepatitis that can potentially lead to hepatic cirrhosis and to the development of hepatocellular cancer (HCC) during its progression.

The classification of hepatitis viruses is based on their biological and molecular properties. It has been demonstrated that DNA and especially RNA genome of the virus can frequently vary as a consequence of mutations, thus genetic variants (mutants, genotypes) can emerge during each viral infection. These mutants have a significant role in eliciting complications of viral diseases; they have to be taken in consideration in order to diagnose and treat the illness, and to prevent the infection.

The number of people with chronic hepatitis is an estimated half billion worldwide, including about 300 million cases of HBV, and about 170 million cases of HCV origin.

Infection with HCV varies according to continents. In Western Europe and North America anti-HCV can be demonstrated only in less than 1% of the population. In Middle-Eastern Europe the incidence is 1–3%, while in Middle Africa and in Egypt even 10–20% of the population can be infected.

The infection spreads mostly by parenteral route, and it constitutes the main cause of post-transfusion hepatitis since the introduction of HBsAg screening. The disease can be also transmitted by intimate, sexual contact, and from mother to infant. It also resembles HBV infection regarding its most important propagators, the symptom-free carriers.

HCV infection can be transmitted most frequently by blood and blood products. An inadvertent injury by a contaminated needle may be a common source of infection, especially in health care personnel. A known possibility is the concordant infection with both HCV and HIV. Most cases occur in intravenous drug users, people regularly receiving transfusions or blood products (e.g. haemophiliacs), dialysis patients, health care providers as occupational disease (e.g. at surgery, dentistry, and dialysis unit), patients undergoing renal transplantation, and those in close contact with a person infected with HCV (newborn of a virus-positive mother, sexual partner). Screening of the donors also for HCV has reduced the incidence in transfused patients.

Sequential analysis of the HCV genome suggests that HCV isolates from different geographical regions show a significant genetic heterogeneity. There are at least six different known genotypes. HCV-RNA sequence homology is less than 72% among the various genotypes. Subtypes showing 72–80% sequence homology can be separated within each genotype. Comparative sequential analysis demonstrated 12 different HCV variants relating the E1 gene. Mutations can be shown in every part of the HCV genome, especially E1 and E2 genes are characterized by variability. The mutation rate of HCV genome is about ten times greater than that of HBV [1].

The incidence of HCV genotypes varies according to geographical areas, with genotype 1 being characteristic in the USA and Europe, genotypes 1 and 2 in Japan, genotype 3 in the Island of Sardinia, type 4 in Zaire, type 5 in South Africa, and type 6 in Hong Kong (Table 1). HCV genotypes or mutants and clinical symptoms cannot be connected in every respect. Development of more serious chronic hepatitis occurs with a significantly greater frequency in type 1 [2]. The importance of HCV variants in relation to clinical course and efficacy of antiviral treatment has not yet been clearly established. Analytic studies with molecular biologic methods are waited for demonstrating the role of HCV genotypes in the epidemiology, clinical picture, and therapy of the infection, as well as in the prevention of the disease.

Hepatitis C virus (HCV) causes primarily the disease of hepatic cells. The way as HCV attaches to and the process when it enters the cells — as the first step of HCV infection — have not yet been clearly determined. Under natural circumstances HCV infects only humans; however, under experimental circumstances infection can be induced in chimpanzees as well [3].

In case of an HCV infection the amount of virus particles in the serum can reach 10^6/ml both in the patients and in infected chimpanzees. However, in chronic inflammatory processes the serum virus concentrations can be considerably lower. It is characteristic to the dynamics of the HCV virus that it is reproduced in the human organism in a magnitude of 6×10^{11} daily, and the treatment can eliminate it only in a

TABLE 1

Occurrence of HCV genotypes related to geographical location

Country	Genotype					
	1	2	3	4	5	6
Australia	+	+	+		+	
Brasilia, Finland, Japan, Libya, United Kingdom	+	+	+			
Cyprus, Portugal, Turkey	+					
Egypt, Italy, Netherlands, USA, Yemen	+	+	+	+		
France, Saudi-Arabia, Hong Kong	+	+				+
Greece	+	+		+		
China, Taiwan	+	+				
Hungary	+			+		

Note: These genotypes have been found in these countries, so far. That does not necessarily mean exclusion of the other possibilities.

magnitude of millions (10^6). The half-life of a virus particle is about 1/3 of a day (7–8 h) [4]. The pathologic progress of HCV infection is demonstrated in Fig. 1. The acute phase of infection is anicteric in 80% of the cases. Only 20% of patients has icteric syndromes and other symptoms of acute hepatitis. After 6 months the chronic infection causes chronic hepatitis in about 50–90% of the cases and in 10–30 years it leads to liver cirrhosis or hepatocellular cancer.

HCV can injure not only hepatic cells, but also other cells and tissues of the organism. The infected state of these cells is of special importance in case of a re-infection within the organism, including relapse after a lasting remission induced by interferon therapy, as well as hepatitis C developing in the graft following liver transplantation [5].

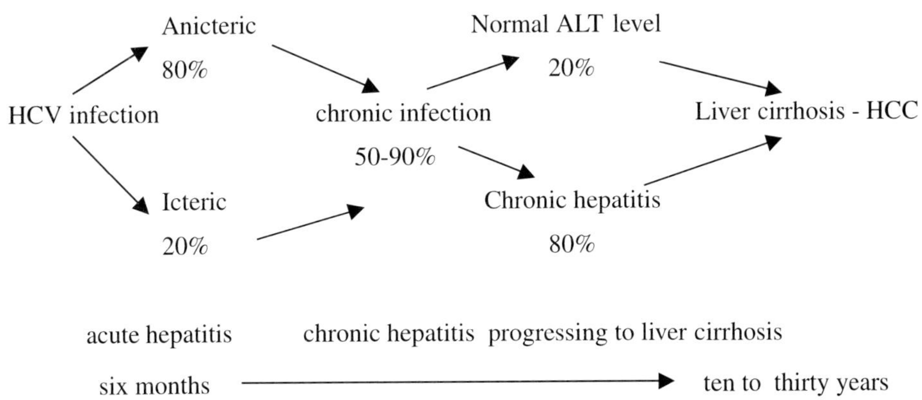

Fig. 1. Pathologic process of HCV infection.

1. THERAPEUTIC POSSIBILITIES IN ACUTE HEPATITIS C

The therapy of clinically obvious acute hepatitis C is supportive. There is no specific drug that could eliminate the virus. In the acute phase hospital admission is needed to make a rest possible, to isolate the patient, to protect people living in the environment, and to provide intensive therapy in case of the rare fulminant forms. The first studies performed with interferon-α reported promising results in acute hepatitis C.

However, no single study on the treatment of acute hepatitis C reported so far has enroled enough patients to demonstrate a significant effect. Some data show that interferon treatment is effective in preventing chronicity in acute hepatitis C with symptoms. A dose greater than 3 MU increasing to a total dose of more than 200 MU is probably more effective in achieving complete response in acute hepatitis C. This rate is about 40% [6].

2. INTERFERON TREATMENT IN CHRONIC HEPATITIS C

The history of interferon therapy in chronic hepatitis C is summarized in the Table 2. The first experiences were the results of interferon monotherapy found after half a year treatment in chronic hepatitis C.

2.1. Interferon monotherapy

At first Hoofnagle and co-workers [7] reported normalization of the alaninamino-transferase (ALT) levels in chronic hepatitis C patients following interferon-α treatment. Since then numerous randomized, controlled trials have been published, confirming that about 45–60% of patients react to interferon-α therapy, when administering 3–6 million units of IFN-α three times a week, for 6–12 months [8]. However, the rate of sustained response to interferon monotherapy is much lower in patients with chronic hepatitis C. Approximately 40% of the patients can reach remission, 50% of the patients reacting to treatment show a relapse after cessation of treatment. Thus, a lasting remission can

TABLE 2

History of treatment modalities with interferon for chronic hepatitis C

Interferon monotherapy (3 MU three times in a week)
6 months
12 months
High-dose induction therapy with interferon (>3 MU up to 10 MU, daily)
Interferon + ribavirin (1000–1200 mg daily) combined therapy
6 months
12 months
Pegylated interferon (once a week) for 12 months
Pegylated interferon + ribavirin combined therapy
Triple combinations (interferon, ribavirin, amantadine)

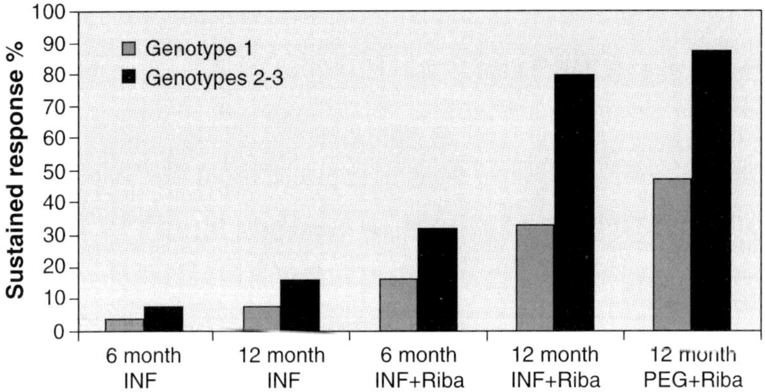

Fig. 2. Long-term sustained response of patients with chronic hepatitis C after interferon or interferon plus ribavirin therapy.

be established in only 18–20% of the cases according to the earlier data. If a relapse occurs, the therapy can be repeated. Liver histology can show clear improvement, and a decrease of the inflammatory process can be obvious also in cases when serum transaminase values have not fully normalized. There have also been data in the literature on the effect of interferon capable of reducing fibrogenesis [9].

The newest data show that there are more relapses after interferon monotherapy than was found in the early trials. Sustained response after several years can be found only in 4% of the cases with genotype 1 and 8% of the cases with genotypes 2–3 after half a year interferon monotherapy [10]. These numbers are doubled after 1 year interferon treatment, that is 8% in genotype 1 and 16% in genotypes 2–3 (Fig. 2).

It is generally accepted that the recommended therapy in chronic hepatitis C is 3–5 million units IFN-α three times a week, for 6–12 months. If there is no result after 2–3 months of treatment, continuation of interferon therapy is not advisable. In case of a partial response, the dose of interferon should be elevated to 5 million units three times a week. For monitoring the effectiveness of therapy determination of serum ALT level and examination of the C virus by PCR technique are recommended. As the latter is not feasible everywhere, anti-HCV IgM test can play an important role in the control of the treatment.

Among predisposing factors of reaction to interferon therapy, the genotype of the C virus is becoming more and more important. A good therapeutic result can be expected in the presence of low pretreatment viraemia, genotypes 2–3, short history, younger age, female gender, and not too high ALT levels (Table 3).

In Hungary we conducted a prospective, multicentre, clinical-pharmacological study [11] on the effect of long-term interferon-α treatment in chronic hepatitis C patients with respect to lasting remission, and to determine how much influence the age of the patients, as well as the time span between hepatitis C virus infection and introduction of treatment exert on the success of interferon therapy. We concluded, similarly to the international data, that interferon therapy for 1 year resulted in a remission of greater

TABLE 3

Characteristics of patients showing the most response to interferon therapy of chronic hepatitis C

Absence of cirrhosis
Age under 50 years
Female gender
γGT normal
Low level of iron in the serum
Low concentration of ferritin
HCV-RNA titre low
HCV genotype 2a, 2b, 3

extent (in 37 of the 91 patients, 40.6%) than the shorter (3–6 months treatments) therapeutic modalities known from the literature. We would like to emphasize that better results are to be expected when interferon treatment is started at a younger age, and as early as possible after the infection.

Recently, interferon monotherapy has been started with a so-called inductive treatment of great dose (10 MU daily) for 10 or 21 days, followed by a maintenance dose of daily 3–5 MU for 6–12 months. The high-dose inductive treatment seems to increase the number of patients reacting to therapy. The induction therapy with high-dose interferon monotherapy resulted in long-term sustained response in 47% of the cases of the trial carried out by Nakamura et al. [12].

During the interferon treatment side effects can be found about in one third of the patients treated. These are mostly flue-like syndromes, joint and myalgia, haematological alterations (leucocytopenia, thrombocytopenia), fatigue, transient alopecia and some rare other alterations. In cases of more severe side effects the therapy should be interrupted. Recently, Saito et al. [13] reported interferon-associated retinopathy occurring in a dose-dependent manner in patients with chronic hepatitis C receiving a uniform dosage of natural interferon-α.

2.1.1. Effect of alcohol on interferon treatment

The progression of liver lesions caused by combined factors of alcohol and HCV infection is much more aggressive than that found in the alterations produced by either alcohol or HCV alone. In alcoholics infected with HCV the ALT activities and HCV-RNA levels in serum are usually higher, and the histologic activity and the fibrosis of the liver are more remarkable than in nonalcoholics. Both alcoholics with HCV infection and HCV-infected patients with excessive alcohol intake are more likely to develop cirrhosis due to the additive effects of alcohol and HCV. Several studies have demonstrated that alcohol consumption accelerates the natural histologic progression of HCV infection [14]. The development of cirrhosis is more common and faster in HCV-infected patients with life long drinking habits or even transient heavy alcohol intake since HCV contamination or during the period of HCV infection [15]. Wiley et al. [16] demonstrated a linear relationship between fibrosis grade (1–4) and years of exposure in a cohort of 176 patients. In 86 patients with HCV infection the fibrosis score was in a mean 0.3/year and in 90 HCV-positive patients declaring alcohol consumption over 40 g/day it was found 0.5/year.

In view of the above-mentioned effect of alcohol on both HCV-RNA levels in serum and the histologic activity and fibrosis, it is not surprising that alcohol intake during antiviral treatment reduced the efficacy of interferon therapy [**?**]. In clinical studies the effect of interferon was impaired by heavy alcohol consumption (>60 g/day) which led to a decreased number of patients with sustained response. That is why the interferon treatment is not recommended in heavy drinkers, or it is necessary to suggest low alcohol intake before and during the treatment [18].

2.1.2. Long-term follow up

Long-term outcome of chronic hepatitis C after interferon treatment is not well known. Gallego et al. [19] recently assessed the outcome of 79 patients with chronic hepatitis C. These patients were treated with lymphoblastoid interferon between 1990 and 1992. They found the 8 year probability of survival in 92.3%. Their most important conclusions are: (1) in sustained response to interferon there was no progression in liver disease, (2) among patients with chronic hepatitis C not responding to interferon the 8 year probability of progression to cirrhosis and hepatocellular carcinoma is about 20% and 3.2%, respectively, (3) the degree of liver fibrosis is the only predictive factor of progression to cirrhosis.

Bruno et al. [10] analysed 47 sustained responders from two interferon trials involving 235 chronic hepatitis C patients. They have found that sustained responders to interferon attain a remarkable and progressive improvement in liver histology, which may become normal in at least half of the subjects who were cleared from the virus. The persistence of HCV RNA involves a risk of late disease reactivation, but as long as ALT levels remain within the normal range, the histology also improves in viremic patients. Disease progression may still be arrested after the development of cirrhosis, but a residual risk of hepatocellular carcinoma remains. Accordingly, regular ultrasound examination should not be discarded in the management of cirrhotic patients, even in those showing persistently normal ALT and undetectable HCV-RNA levels after interferon treatment [20].

2.1.3. Interferon in the prevention of liver cancer

Key and urgent clinical question is whether all patients with HCV-induced liver cirrhosis should receive interferon to prevent liver cancer, or whether antiviral therapy should only be applied to a subgroup of high-risk patients [21].

Camma et al. [22] recently published a paper for answering this question. They analysed the results of three randomized controlled trials and 15 unrandomized controlled studies, including 4614 patients. As a conclusion they summarized: interferon prevents or delays the development of hepatocellular carcinoma in patients with HCV-related liver cirrhosis. The magnitude of the overall effect is low and observed benefit might be due to spurious associations. The preventive effect is stronger among sustained responders to interferon which intrinsically represents a little proportion of all cirrhotics.

2.2. Combined therapy with interferon and ribavirin

In recent years beside interferon monotherapy other treatment modalities are being on trial. Most important of these is ribavirin (1-beta-D-ribofuranosyl-1,2,4,-triazole-3-carboxamide), a guanosine analogue product [23]. There are a growing number of publications suggesting that ribavirin, when administered in combination with interferon-α, can reach healing in chronic hepatitis C in greater proportion, than each medicine separately.

In part (approximately 30–40%) of the patients with chronic hepatitis C, interferon therapy is effective (Fig. 1). However, the other 60–70% of the patients show only a partial or no response to interferon or clinical and laboratory symptoms reappear following cessation of treatment, that is, a relapse occurs. In these cases a combined therapy with interferon-α-2b (or interferon-α-2a) and ribavirin is the treatment of choice.

Ribavirin, a guanosine analogue, exerts significant activity against both RNA and DNA viruses, including the flavovirus family. It is able to inhibit the viral RNA polymerase, as well as to inhibit the synthesis of viral mRNA and viral protein, it has an immunomodulatory effect and it decreases the development of proinflammatory cytochines of macrophage origin, but does not inhibit the TH1 function. Its favourable feature is the possibility of oral administration; the effective dose is 1000–1200 mg daily, divided in two equal parts. Simultaneously given with interferon it has a long-term synergic effect. This drug only rarely has a side effect. There can be a feeling of mild abdominal discomfort of patients in the first week, as well as some mild haemolytic anaemia because its cumulation in the erythrocyte membrane, further low-grade hyperuricemia.

It can be effective in non-responding or relapsing cases in connection with interferon treatment, and it can also be administered, when interferon therapy is contraindicated, for instance in the presence of thyroid antibodies or hypersplenia. In chronic HCV infection, ribavirin therapy was first administered by Reichard et al. [23]. They observed a reduction of ALT values. Later it was confirmed also in placebo-controlled studies, with the demonstration of a diminishing histological activity, in addition. As for HCV-RNA titre, ribavirin monotherapy caused no significant change. The effects of interferon and ribavirin are synergical. During a long-term study with combined treatment, in 40% of the cases a lasting disappearance from the serum of HCV RNA was observed accompanied by a significant improvement in the inflammatory reaction of the liver.

In the first two studies, data of altogether 375 randomized, and independently participating patients were analysed. Interferon-α therapy was administered parenterally, in a dose of 3.0 MU three times a week, combined with either ribavirin or placebo. The dose of ribavirin was 1000–1200 mg/day, administered perorally. The detectable eradication of the hepatitis C virus (determined by HCV-RNA test, when the number of HCV-RNA copies was less than 100/ml) was 48.6% with combined interferon and ribavirin treatment. The most frequent side effects were the occurrence of influenza-like symptoms (headache, weakness, myalgia, and fever), as well as a reversible haemolysis [24,25].

In the last years several studies have been carried out with interferon-α plus ribavirin combined therapy. As a conclusion it can be stated that the responder rate is about

TABLE 4

Recommendation of EASL for chronic hepatitis C

Naive patients, ribavirin not contraindicated
Genotype 1 and high level of viraemia: interferon-α + ribavirin for 12 months
Genotypes 2–3 as well as genotype 1 with low level of viraemia: interferon-α monotherapy (tiw) for 12 months
Relapsers to interferon monotherapy
Ribavirin not contraindicated: interferon-α + ribavirin for 6 months
Ribavirin contraindicated: high-dose interferon for 12 months

doubled in patients treated for one year as compared to that in those treated for half a year (Fig. 2). The sustained response was 18% in genotype 1 and 30% in genotypes 2–3 after half a year treatment, and the response rate was much higher after one year combined therapy, that is 32% in patients with genotype 1 and 80% in patients with genotypes 2–3. Our clinical studies with interferon plus ribavirin combined therapy in Hungary showed similar results. After one year of treatment 56% of the patients became HCV-RNA-negative with normal ALT level. However, two years after cessation of the therapy a third of them relapsed [26,27].

2.2.1. Recommendation of the European Association for the Study of Liver (EASL)

Beside the diagnosis of chronic hepatitis C it is important to know the stage and grade of the disease as well as the baseline viral concentration and genotype before the treatment. Careful analysis of liver biopsy can be recommended in defining the stage of disease, detecting of cirrhosis and ruling out concomitant diseases causing liver damage. It can also provide a useful baseline measure of disease severity and progression. The sero-diagnostic algorithm and the treatment options in case of anti-HCV positive reaction are shown in Fig. 3.

Baseline viral concentration and genotyping should be considered prior to therapy. HCV genotype is a key parameter in detecting response to interferon treatment. Patients with HCV genotypes 2–3 have been shown to have better response rates than patients with genotype 1.

In 1999 the European Association for the Study of Liver (EASL) at the International Consensus Conference determined the current recommendations for chronic hepatitis C [28]. The recommendations for optimal treatment of naive patients are based on genotypes and baseline viral concentration. A summary of these recommendations is presented in Table 4. Patients having genotype 2 or 3 regardless of baseline viral concentration and those having genotype 1 with a baseline viral concentration less than 2 M copies/ml without contraindications for either interferon or ribavirin should be treated for 6 months with combined interferon and ribavirin therapy. The dose of interferon is 3 MU three times a week (tiw) and that of the ribavirin is 1000–1200 mg/day. Genotype 1 patients with a high baseline viral titre (higher than 2 M copies/ml) should be treated for 12 months with the combination of interferon and ribavirin.

Patients having contraindication for ribavirin should be treated with interferon (3 MU tiw) monotherapy for 12 months. For patients relapsed after interferon monotherapy

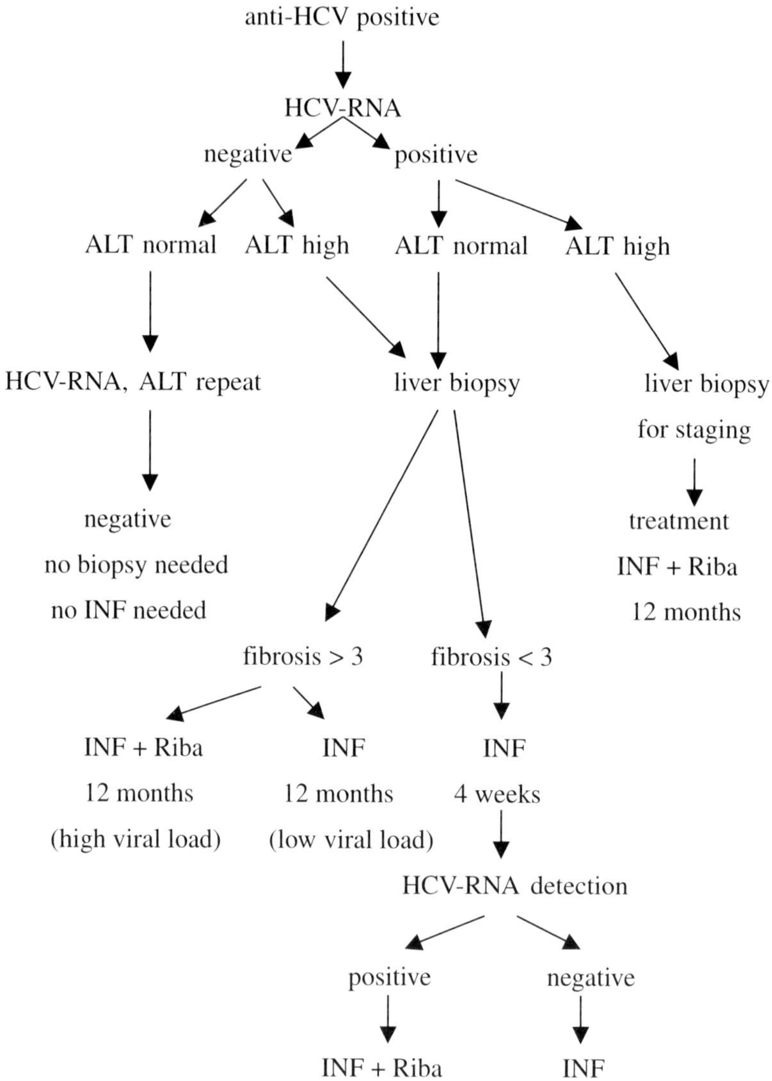

Fig. 3. Sero-diagnostic algorythm and treatment options in case of anti-HCV positive reaction.

there are two options according to the EASL recommendations: a higher dose of interferon for 12 months or a combination therapy of interferon and ribavirin for 6 months. After 3 months of re-treatment HCV RNA should be assessed to determine if combined re-treatment is worthwhile.

2.2.2. Therapy of chronic hepatitis C in children

The most effective method of treatment for chronic hepatitis C in children has yet not been established. Woynarowski et al. [29] treated 24 children with either interferon (3

MU tiw) for 12 months (14 cases) or interferon (3 MU tiw) and ribavirin (15 mg kg^{-1} day^{-1} maximal dose up to 600 mg/day) for 12 months (10 cases). They found that the combined interferon + ribavirin therapy was superior to interferon monotherapy at the end of the 6-months posttreatment follow up. The sustained response was 7/10 (70%) in combination therapy and 2/11 (18%) in interferon monotherapy.

2.2.3. Treatment of patients with HCV recurrency after liver transplantation
In patients with liver transplantation for end-stage liver disease induced by HCV infection, HCV recurrency can develop almost in all the cases. For preventing HCV re-infection after transplantation, interferon therapy is not necessarily effective. Some data suggest it to enhance rejection. Sporadic results so far indicate that in chronic hepatitis C developed after liver transplantation combined interferon-α-2b and ribavirin therapy reduces progression of hepatitis in the transplant, and significantly diminishes clinical symptoms and laboratory abnormalities of the patient [30]. Long-term sustained response can be found only in 20–40% of the cases. Our ongoing clinical trials [31] also show that the treatment with interferon-α plus ribavirin combined therapy is as effective as in patients with chronic hepatitis C without liver transplantation.

3. PEGYLATED INTERFERON

Pegylated (polyethylene glycol, PEG, coated) forms of standard interferon represent the most recent advance in the treatment of hepatitis C. Standard interferon preparations are rapidly cleared from the body, with an elimination half-life about 4 h. Because the short half-life it is necessary to apply the medication at least 3 times a week. Its rapid clearance may potentially limit its efficacy. Pegylation of proteins is a well-established method for delaying their clearance, and as a result, increasing exposure and enhancing efficacy compared with non-pegylated proteins. PEG is used as a protein-modifying agent because it is inert, water-soluble, relatively nontoxic and can be made to almost any size varying the number of repeating oxyethylene units. Two kinds of pegylated interferons have been introduced for the treatment of chronic hepatitis C. Schering Plough has developed a pegylated form of interferon-α-2b (Peginterferon) with a molecular weight of 12,000 Da [32] and the Roche has produced a new pegylated form of interferon-α-2a with a molecular weight of 40,000 Da [33].

Manns et al. [34] analysed the data of 1529 patients with chronic hepatitis C from 62 centres in nine countries in order to determine the optimal dose of Peginterferon and ribavirin. The best sustained virological response was found with the therapy of Peginterferon-α-2b 1.5 μg/kg + ribavirin > 10.6 mg/kg. The overall sustained viral response was 61%, that of genotype 1 was found to be 48% and that of genotypes 2–3 was 88% (Fig. 2). The final conclusions of this clinicopharmacological study are as follows. (1) Peginterferon-α-2b 1.5 μg/kg + ribavirin is significantly more effective than Peginterferon-α-2b 0.5 μg/kg ribavirin or interferon-α-2b 3 MU + ribavirin. (2) Weight-adjusted dosing for both Peginterferon-α-2b + ribavirin will maximize the sustained virologic response rate. (3) Peginterferon-α-2b 1.5 μg/kg + ribavirin > 10.6 mg/kg is the optimal dosing strategy to maximize the sustained virologic response rate in all patients but particularly in those with genotype 1.

4. OTHER TREATMENT MODALITIES, FUTURE POSSIBILITIES

Ursodeoxycholic acid (UDCA) is administered as basic therapy in primary biliary cirrhosis and primary sclerotizing cholangitis. It has been used with good results for dissolution of cholesterol biliary stones, either as monotherapy or in combination with lithotripsy. Its mechanism of action has proven to be complex in the studies. Its direct hepato-protective effect, its advantageous features regarding entero-hepatic circulation of biliary acids, as well as its choleretic effect, and immunomodulatory properties concerning the lymphocytes of the organism have been demonstrated.

This latter effect, as well as action on liver cells has been used in chronic viral hepatitis C. When administered as monotherapy — in a dose of 500 mg three times a day — it reduced ALT, AST, γGT and AP values. In combination with interferon treatment, it increased the rate of lasting response to interferon, and reduced the number of relapses. We could also confirm these latter advantageous features, when we applied the UDCA therapy with interferon-α treatment [35]. It can be supposed that the UDCA treatment enhances the interferon-induced elimination of HCV from the organism.

There are data in the literature also on the combination of interferon with thymostimulin [36], as well as about other therapeutic trials as interferon + ribavirin + amantadine [37]. Final results cannot be judged till now. Furthermore there are a growing number of publications dealing with newer experimental therapy modalities in combination with interferon: helicase inhibitors, protease inhibitors, RNA-dependent RNA polymerase inhibitors, IRES (Internal Ribosome Entry Site) inhibitors, antisense nucleotides, DNA vaccines stimulating cytotoxic T-cell activity, as well as dominantly negative mutants. The results are not definitive and the discussion of these treatment modalities is not part of this chapter.

CONCLUSIONS

Standard, first line therapy of choice in chronic hepatitis C is long-term interferon-α treatment either as a monotherapy or a combined treatment with ribavirin. This is an outpatient therapy, and can be realized well in practice with appropriate experience. Indication of therapy should be established in a hepatological centre following an unequivocally confirmed diagnosis. In the case of non-responders to monotherapy with interferon, another treatment modality should be designed and implemented, in concordance with the hepatological centre. That can be primarily a combination of interferon-α-2b and ribavirin. Other nucleoside analogue (famcyclovir, pencyclovir, lamivudin) therapy, as well as concomitant administration of interferon and ursodeoxycholic acid or thymostimulin can be taken in consideration only more rarely. The treatment requires a great deal of patience both from doctor and patient, while plenty of time and careful monitoring are also needed. Possible harmful side effects should be taken in consideration, and high treatment costs could also not be neglected. A successful treatment, however, can restore the health of the patient, and prevent the development of hepatic cirrhosis and a possible hepatocellular cancer.

REFERENCES

[1] De Francesco R. Molecular virology of the hepatitis C virus. J Hepatol 1999; 31(Suppl. 1): 47–53.
[2] Simmonds P. Viral heterogeneity of the hepatitis C virus. J Hepatol 1999; 31(Suppl. 1): 54–60.
[3] Marcellin P. Hepatitis C: the clinical spectrum of the disease. J Hepatol 1999; 31(Suppl. 1): 9–16.
[4] Zeuzem S. Clinical implications of hepatitis C viral kinetics. J Hepatol 1999; 31(Suppl. 1): 61–64.
[5] Samuel D, Feray C. Recurrency of hepatitis C after liver transplantation. J Hepatol 1999; 31(Suppl. 1): 217–221.
[6] Vogel W. Treatment of acute hepatitis C. Hepatology 1999; 31(Suppl. 1): 189–192.
[7] Hoofnagle JH. Therapy of viral hepatitis. Digestion 1998; 59: 563–578.
[8] Benvegnu L, Chemello L, Noventa F, Fattovich G, Pontisso P, Alberti A. Retrospective analysis of the effect of interferon therapy on the clinical outcome of patients with viral cirrhosis. Cancer 1998; 83: 901–909.
[9] Camma C, Di Marco V, Lo Iacono O, Almasio P, Giunta M, Fuschi P et al. Long term course of interferon-treated chronic hepatitis C. J Hepatol 1998; 28: 531–537.
[10] Bruno S, Battezzati PM, Bellati G, Manzin A, Maggioni M, Crosignani A et al. Long term beneficial effects in sustained responders to interferon-alfa therapy for chronic hepatitis C. J Hepatol 2001; 34: 748–755.
[11] Feher J, Lengyel G, Dalmi L, Dávid K, Gervain J, Gógl A et al. Effect of interferon-alfa2b in chronic hepatitis C. Prospective multicenter study in Hungary. (Hung.). Orvosi Hetilap (Hung Med J) 1996; 137: 1179–1185.
[12] Nakamura H, Ito H, Kimura Y, Takeda A, Ogawa H, Kanazawa S et al. The importance of initial daily administration of interferon-alfa for the eradication of hepatitis C: A multicenter randomized trial. Hepatogastroenterology 1998; 45: 1045–1055.
[13] Saito H, Ebinuma H, Nagata H, Inagaki Y, Saito Y, Wakabayashi K et al. Interferon associated retinopathy in a uniform regime natural interferon-α therapy for chronic hepatitis C. Liver 2001; 21: 1982–1987.
[14] Degos F. Hepatitis C and alcohol. J Hepatol 1999; 31(Suppl. 1): 113–118.
[15] Corrao G, Arico S. Independent and combined action of hepatitis C infection and alcohol consumption on the risk of symptomatic liver cirrhosis. Hepatology 1998; 27: 914–919.
[16] Wiley TE, McCarthy M, Breidi I, McCarthy M, Layden TJ. Impact of alcohol on histological and clinical progression of hepatitis C infection. Hepatology 1998; 28: 805–809.
[17] Mochida S, Ohnishi M, Matsuo K, Kakihara F, Fujiwara K. Effect of alcohol intake on the efficacy of interferon therapy in patients with chronic hepatitis C as evaluated by multivariate logistic regression analysis. Alcohol Clin Exp Res 1996; 20: 371A–377A.
[18] Oshita M, Hayashi N, Kasahara A, Hagiwara H, Mita E, Naito M et al. Increased serum hepatitis C virus RNA levels among alcoholic patients with chronic hepatitis C. Hepatology 1994; 20: 1115–1130.
[19] Gallego A, Torras X, Sancho-Poch FJ, Enriques J. Long term follow up of patients with chronic hepatitis C after interferon therapy. J Hepatol 2001; 34(Suppl. 1): 234 (Abstr.).
[20] Nalpas B, Desenclos JC, Delaroque-Astagneau E, Drucker J. Management of hepatitis C by European hepatologists. J Hepatol 1999; 34(Suppl. 1): 141–145.
[21] Kashara A, Hayashi N, Mochizuki K, Takayamagi M, Yoshioka K, Kakumu S et al. Risk factors for hepatocellular carcinoma and its incidence after interferon treatment in patients with chronic hepatitis C. Hepatology 1998; 27: 1394–1402.

[22] Camma C, Giunta M, Andreone P, Craxi A. Interferon and prevention of hepatocellular carcinoma in viral cirrhosis: an evidence based approach. J Hepatol 2001; 34: 593–602.
[23] Reichard O, Norkrans G, Fryden A, Braconier JH, Sonnerborg A, Weiland A. Randomised, double-blind, placebo controlled trial of interferon-alfa-2b with and without for chronic hepatitis C. Lancet 1998; 351: 83–87.
[24] McHutchinson JG, Gordon SC, Schiff ER, Schiffmann ML, Lee WM, Rustgi VK et al. Interferon alfa-2b or in combination with ribavirin as initial treatment for chronic hepatitis C. New Engl J Med 1998; 339: 1485–1492.
[25] Poynard T, Marcellin P, Lee SL, Niederau C, Minu GS, Ideo G. et al. Randomized trial of interferon alfa-2b plus ribavirin for 48 weeks versus interferon alfa-2b plus ribavirin for 24 weeks for chronic infection with hepatitis C virus. Lancet 1998; 352: 1426–1432.
[26] Fehér J, Lengyel G, Bálint T and the Multicenter Study Group. Interferon-alfa-2b and ribavirin combined treatment in chronic hepatitis C. Results of 100 patients treated for one year. (Hung.) Orvosi Hetilap (Hung Med J), 1999; 140: 1235–1238.
[27] Pár A, Telegdy L, Gógl A and the Multicenter Study Group. Interferon treatment of patients with chronic viral hepatitis in Hungary. 5 year observations. Multicentric Study (Hung.). Orvosi Hetilap (Hung Med J) 1999; 140: 1227–1233.
[28] EASL International Consensus Conference on Hepatitis C. Consensus Statement. J Hepatol 1999; 31(Suppl. 1): 3–8.
[29] Woynarowski M, Socha J, Kuydowicz J, Wisocki J, Shuzewski W, Mizerski J et al. Interferon + ribavirin vs interferon alone treatment of children with chronic HCV infection. J Hepatol 2001; 34(Suppl. 1): 139–140.
[30] Lavezzo B, Rizzetto M. Treatment of recurrent hepatitis C virus infection after liver transplantation. J Hepatol 1999; 31(Suppl. 1): 222–226.
[31] Lengyel G, Nemes B, Kóbori L, Fehérvári J, Görög D, Sárvári E. et al. Combined interferon and ribavirin treatment in HCV recurrence after liver transplantation. 43rd Annual Meeting of the Hungarian Society of Gastroenterology. Balatonaliga, 5–9 June 2001, Newsletter 2001; 8: 120 (Abstr.).
[32] McHutchison J, Manns M, Harvey J, Albrecht JK. Adherence to therapy enhances sustained response in chronic hepatitis C patients receiving PEG-interferon alfa-2b plus ribavirin. J Hepatol 2001; 34(Suppl. 1): 2–3 (Abstr.).
[33] Ferenci P, Tauber R, Hackl F, Jessner W, Hegenbarth K, Munda-Steindl P et al. Viral kinetics on treatment with pegylated (PEG 40 KD) interferon (INF) alfa-2a in patients infected with HCV subtype 1. J Hepatol 2001; 34(Suppl. 1): 131–132 (Abstr.).
[34] Manns M, Hutchison JGMc, Gordom S, Rutsgi V, Lee MV, Ling M et al. Pegylated interferon alfa-2b (PEG INF) plus ribavirin (R) for treatment of chronic hepatitis C. Optimization of ribavirin dose. J Hepatol 2001; 34(Suppl. 12): 236 (Abstr.).
[35] Lengyel G, Fehér J. Clinical observations with combined therapy of ursodeoxycholic acid and interferon-alfa in chronic hepatitis C. Progr Hepato-pharmacol 1997; 2: 71–78.
[36] Sherman KE, Sherman SN. Interferon plus thymosin-α-1 treatment of chronic hepatitis C infection: a meta-analysis. In: Shinazi RF, Sommadossi JP, Thomas HC, editors. Therapies for viral hepatitis. International Medical Press Publisher, 1998; pp. 379–383.
[37] Stauber R, Munda-Steidl F, Hackl F, Schütze K, Datz C et al. Induction treatment of chronic hepatitis C with daily interferon plus ribavirin plus amantadine is effective in non-responders to interferon plus ribavirin. J Hepatol 2001; 34(Suppl. 1): 134–135 (Abstr.).

Molecular Biology and Immunology in Hepatology
Edited by T. Tsuji, T. Higashi, M. Zeniya and K.-H. Meyer zum Büschenfelde

CHAPTER 6

New Therapeutic Strategy for Chronic Hepatitis C

Norio Hayashi and Akinori Kasahara

Department of Molecular Therapeutics, Department of General Medicine, Osaka University Graduate School of Medicine, Osaka, Japan

INTRODUCTION

Infection with hepatitis C virus (HCV) is a major public health problem worldwide. The prevalence of HCV infection based on antibody to HCV ranges from 1 to 2% in developed countries. HCV has been identified as the major causative agent of chronic liver disease. Mortality associated with chronic hepatitis C results mainly from the development of liver fibrosis and the subsequent occurrence of cirrhosis, with complications such as hepatocellular carcinoma (HCC). HCC is one of the most common malignancies, especially in Southeast Asia. In Japan, HCC is the third leading cause of death from cancer, and its incidence has increased more than two-fold over the last 10 years. Moreover, the incidence of HCC is predicted to continue to increase and reach a plateau in 2010 in Japan. Thus, there is a pressing need for efficacious treatment for chronic hepatitis C to delay or prevent the development of HCC.

1. INTERFERON THERAPY

Interferon is widely used for the treatment of both chronic hepatitis B and chronic hepatitis C. The interferons are a family of cytokines that are naturally occurring proteins secreted by many mammalian cells and induce anti-viral, anti-tumor and immunomodulatory activities. The only therapy of proven benefit for patients with chronic hepatitis C is interferon. Three types of interferon-α including recombinant interferon-α2a, -2b and natural interferon and interferon-β have been widely used in Japan. Although some differences have been noted among these interferons, there is little evidence that any form of interferon-α or -β is superior in terms of efficacy or tolerability in the treatment of chronic hepatitis C.

1.1. Recommendations for use of interferon therapy

Interferon therapy is indicated for patients with chronic HCV infection who have the greatest risk for progression to cirrhosis and development of HCC. These patients are characterized by persistent elevation of serum alanine aminotransferase (ALT) levels and detectable serum HCV RNA. Particularly, recommended as candidates for therapy are patients showing portal or bridging fibrosis and at least moderate inflammation and necrosis, because they have a high risk of progressing to liver cirrhosis or developing HCC in a short period. However, a sustained response is common in patients with both elevated ALT levels and histologically mild chronic hepatitis C. Therefore, treatment at this point in the disease is predicted to significantly improve long-term survival. On the other hand, treatment is not indicated for patients with persistently normal ALT, most of whom show histological features of mild to moderate active chronic hepatitis [1], because a virological sustained response is rare and some patients develop persistent elevation of ALT after interferon treatment [2]. Further studies are necessary to determine whether interferon therapy is warranted for such patients.

1.2. Results of interferon therapy with different treatment schedules

Many investigators have reported this therapy to be effective for decreasing serum ALT [3,4], reducing and eliminating HCV RNA levels [4,5], and improving liver histology [6,7] in patients with chronic hepatitis C. An independent meta-analysis [8] of all randomized clinical trials of IFN α-2b in western patients with chronic hepatitis C, who were randomly allocated to receive at least 2 million units (MU) IFN α-2b three times a week for 24 weeks, showed that a biochemical response at the end of therapy was observed in 47% of the treated patients compared 4% of the controls. The biochemical responses were sustained for at least 6 months in 23% of the treated patients compared with 5% of the controls. A virological response at the end of treatment was observed in 29% of the treated patients compared to 5% of the controls, and a virological sustained response at 6 months after therapy was documented in 8% of the treated patients compared to 1% of the controls. Thus, interferon therapy was associated with significant biological and virological improvement when compared with no treatment. When therapy is stopped, however, serum ALT concentrations rise to pretreatment values in at least 50% of the patients who respond to the drug, so that the rate of the biochemical sustained response is only 15–30% [3,4,9,10].

Controlled studies have shown that high doses [9–11] of interferon, a long period of therapy [12–14] and the administration of a large total dose are all associated with a higher cure rate, but these treatments can cause more adverse effects and certainly cost more than the standard schedule. In Japan, the standard schedule of interferon treatment is to give 6–10 MU of interferon-α every day for the first 2–4 weeks and then three times a week for the following 20–22 weeks, because medical expenses can be covered by medical health insurance only if the treatment is shorter than 6 months. The final goal of interferon treatment for chronic hepatitis C is to eradicate HCV, but, despite the fact that a higher rate of complete response with HCV eradication is noted for non-1b HCV genotypes and a low viral load [6,15,16], patients with chronic hepatitis C in Japan are indiscriminately subjected to 6-month courses of interferon therapy. Moreover, at present, although patients in whom serum HCV RNA level does not decrease and/or ALT does not normalize during interferon treatment are considered to be resistant to interferon, they are usually offered the standard schedule of interferon treatment and complete it. On the other hand, for patients with a low viral load, a small dose of interferon as well as a shorter period of therapy are reported to be as effective as a large dose for eradicating HCV [17]. Thus, the optimal schedule of interferon treatment may vary from one patient to another and should be established according to patients' characteristics, such as serum HCV RNA level and HCV genotype.

Even when interferon-α was administered every day for the first 4 weeks and then three times a week for the following 20 weeks (total dose of interferon was 528 MU) for 79 patients with genotype 1b of HCV and a high viral load, the rates of biochemical sustained response and HCV eradication were 8 and 4%, respectively. However, biochemical transient response was observed in 61% of these patients, and the remaining 31% of them were non-responders, who did not respond to interferon.

We examined the efficacy of interferon-α (HLBI) treatment in 605 patients with chronic hepatitis C according to treatment regimens, HCV genotypes and HCV RNA levels. In summary, 6-month courses of interferon-alone therapy for patients with genotype 1b of HCV and a high viral load are not useful for HCV eradication, but are useful for ALT normalization during interferon therapy, indicating that the aim of interferon-alone therapy for these patients is the normalization of ALT. On the other hand, HCV eradication is expected in 30–40% of patients with genotype 1b and a low viral load, and in 55% of patients with genotype 2a and a low viral load, demonstrating that interferon therapy for these patients should aim at HCV eradication.

1.3. Prolonged interferon treatment

Recently, there have been reports of the therapeutic efficacy increasing with a higher total dose of interferon and prolonged interferon therapy [6,10,12–14]. Interferon treatment for 12–24 months is documented to result in an approximately two-fold increase in biochemical and virological responses. This therapy is effective, especially in HCV genotype 1b patients with a high viral load [18]. Thus, longer courses of interferon treatment have been approved as standard therapy in the USA and most of Europe. Therefore, treatment with a 12-month course of interferon should be introduced for HCV genotype 1b patients with a high viral load and its medical expenses should be covered by health insurance in Japan.

2. CLINICAL OUTCOME AFTER INTERFERON TREATMENT

2.1. Long-term biochemical and virological outcome

Several studies of interferon-treated chronic hepatitis C patients demonstrate that relapse is extremely rare when ALT levels are within the normal range and serum HCV RNA is undetectable at the end of therapy and for 6–12 months thereafter. Therefore, the combination of persistently normal ALT and negative HCV RNA at 6–12 months after stopping interferon therapy can be safely assumed to identify patients in whom HCV infection has been eradicated [6,19–21].

HCV is not eradicated in all the biochemical sustained responders. Serum HCV RNA remained undetectable in approximately 76% of them at 6 months after cessation of therapy [21]. The remaining 24% had HCV but sustained normal ALT. The risk of HCV RNA persistence was greater in biochemical sustained responders with a high viral load and those treated with a smaller amount of interferon. A large cohort study showed that ALT normalization continued for more than 2 years (26–80 months) after cessation of therapy in about 60% of biochemical sustained responders, even when HCV RNA remained detectable. Thus, some patients can display year-long persistence of normal ALT despite the continuation of HCV viremia after interferon therapy, while the HCV immune complex continues to be dominant in the circulation [22]. However, the loss of immune complex predominance in HCV populations was shown to be associated with biochemical relapse [22].

2.2. *Histological outcome after interferon*

Many studies have revealed histological changes in patients receiving interferon-α. These studies showed improvement in histologic necro-inflammatory lesions in patients who had normalized ALT levels after interferon therapy [6,7]. However, liver fibrosis has been reported to be unchanged, even in patients who responded to therapy, when histologic activity and fibrosis were assessed according to the scoring system of Knodell et al. [23]. The Knodell scoring system is not sensitive enough to detect small changes in fibrosis. When a new 'hepatic fibrosis score' was used, treatment with interferon was shown to be able to alleviate fibrosis in addition to necrosis and inflammation in patients with negative HCV RNA at the end of therapy [7,24]. Patients with HCV eradication were demonstrated to show further improvements in both inflammation and fibrosis. Moreover, during the long-term follow-up, interferon treatment for chronic hepatitis C was reported to reduce the natural fibrosis progression rate independently of the genotype and an early response to interferon [25]. In a 10-year follow-up study after interferon-α therapy [26], patients with HCV eradication were diagnosed as having normal livers or mild, non-specific inflammatory changes of the liver. By using colorimetrical quantitation of liver collagen, a significant decrease in the Disse space collagen was also reported at the end of therapy and 6–18 months later [27]. Thus, most of studies have found a significant decrease in the fibrosis score as well as the Disse space collagen and necro-inflammatory scores in patients with sustained virological response, except for the study of Marcellin and colleagues [28].

Transforming growth factor-β1 (TGF-β1) is a polypeptide which promotes fibrogenesis and extracellular matrix accumulation. Hepatic expression of mature TGF-β1 in transgenic mice has been shown to result in hepatic fibrosis [29]. Interferon is demonstrated to be an anti-fibrotic agent. With respect to the relationship between TGF-β1 and interferon-α therapy, patients who responded to interferon treatment show normalization of indicators of fibrogenesis (serum levels of procollagen type III peptide and type IV collagen 7s and expression of type I procollagen messenger RNA in the liver) and normal amounts of liver TGF-β1 mRNA at the end of therapy [30,31]. Moreover, α-smooth muscle actin-expressing cells responsible for liver fibrosis have also been shown to decrease in responders to interferon [32]. Thus, interferon-α-induced suppression of hepatic TGF-β1 production as well as reduced necroinflammatory activity may inhibit proliferation and collagen synthesis in hepatic stellate cells, leading to a decrease in fibrogenesis.

2.3. Development of HCC

To evaluate the effect of interferon treatment on the incidence of HCC among patients with chronic hepatitis C, a randomized controlled trial should be conducted. However, since interferon therapy has already been established as a standard modality of radical therapy for chronic hepatitis C patients, a prospective randomized trial, including untreated control patients, cannot be done. There have been three retrospective studies using control patients who did not receive interferon [33–35]. Two of the studies [33,34] demonstrated that interferon significantly decreased the risk for developing HCC among patients with chronic hepatitis C who showed a persistent normal ALT level after the completion of therapy. However, interferon did not significantly reduce the risk for HCC among those who did not respond to the therapy compared with the control patients [33,34]. The effect of interferon-α on the incidence of HCC in patients with compensated type C cirrhosis has been assessed in randomized controlled trials [36,37] and in observational studies using a control group [38–42]. Two of these studies [37,38] concluded that interferon therapy did not have a significant beneficial effect for preventing the development of HCC in these patients.

When the cumulative incidence of HCC was compared according to the ALT response to interferon therapy in chronic hepatitis C patients, its incidence in biochemical transient responders was almost equal to that in biochemical sustained responders and was significantly higher in biochemical non-responders than in biochemical sustained and transient responders (Fig. 1) [21,43]. Cox regression analysis showed that age, ALT response to interferon and gender were independent significant risk factors in the development of HCC. The risk of HCC was 8-fold higher for biochemical non-responders than for biochemical sustained responders, but it was not elevated

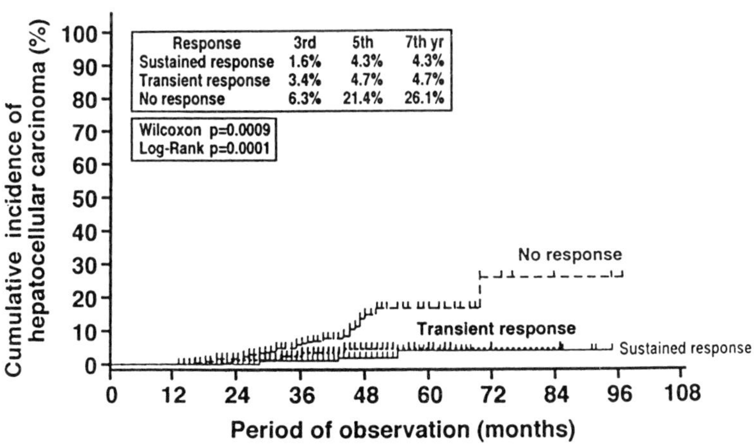

Fig. 1. Cumulative incidence of HCC after interferon treatment in the patients with type C chronic hepatitis.

in biochemical transient responders compared with biochemical sustained responders [21], Thus, the risk of HCC development is significantly low in chronic hepatitis C patients in whom interferon is effective for normalizing ALT, even when HCC is not eradicated.

The cumulative survival of patients given interferon treatment is higher compared to those without it. When the cumulative survival is compared according to ALT responses to interferon, it is higher in biochemical sustained responders and transient responders than in non-responders and those without interferon treatment. None of the biochemical sustained or transient responders died of liver-related disease after interferon therapy. The risk of death is one-fifth in biochemical sustained responders and transient responders compared with biochemical non-responders and patients not given interferon treatment.

These results suggest that the aim of interferon therapy for chronic hepatitis C should not only be HCV eradication but also ALT normalization during interferon therapy, even if HCV is not eradicated, in order to reduce the incidence of HCC and improve survival. However, the seventh-year cumulative appearance rates of clinically and ultrasonographically evident liver cirrhosis in biochemical sustained responders, transient responders and non-responders were estimated to be 16, 35 and 65%, respectively, suggesting that the evolution of the disease was observed more often in biochemical transient responders than in biochemical sustained responders [21]. Consequently, the cumulative incidence of HCC may increase, displaying a hyperbolic curve, in biochemical transient responders in the near future. From these results, retreatment with interferon of chronic hepatitis C patients showing ALT relapse after the initial interferon therapy is necessary to delay or prevent the progression to liver cirrhosis and development of HCC.

When the cumulative HCC appearance rates were compared according to the averaged ALT levels during long-term follow-up after interferon treatment in patients without HCV eradication, its incidence significantly increased in the order of the averaged ALT after the interferon therapy. The lower the averaged ALT after interferon therapy was, the lower the cumulative incidence of HCC was, as described previously. Thus, under the present circumstance that medical expenses of retreatment with interferon cannot be covered by health insurance, alternative treatments for maintaining ALT values within the normal range are needed to reduce the incidence of HCC development, when there is persistent elevation of ALT.

CONCLUSIONS

At present, the only therapy of proven benefit in the treatment of chronic hepatitis C is interferon. It can induce clearance of HCV, normalization of serum ALT concentrations and improvement of liver histology, leading to delay or prevention of the development of HCC. Also, even if HCV is not eradicated with interferon therapy, the clinical goal of delaying or preventing the development of HCC may be achieved by reducing serum ALT levels. Therefore, chronic hepatitis C patients with elevated serum ALT, for whom interferon therapy is not contraindicated, should be started on interferon therapy, because the pre-treatment prognostic factors thus far identified cannot be used to distinguish non-responders from others.

REFERENCES

[1] Naito M, Hayashi N, Hagiwara H, Hiramatsu N, Kasahara A, Fusamoto H et al. Serum hepatitis C virus RNA quantity and histological features of hepatitis C virus carriers with persistently normal ALT levels. Hepatology 1994; 19: 871–875.

[2] Sangiovanni A, Morales R, Spinzi G, Rumi M, Casiraghi A, Ceriani R et al. Interferon alfa treatment of HCV RNA carriers with persistently normal transaminase levels: a pilot randomized controlled study. Hepatology 1998; 27: 853–856.

[3] Davis GL, Balart LA, Schiff ER, Lindsay K, Bodenheimer HC, Rerrilo RP et al. Treatment of chronic hepatitis C with recombinant interferon alpha. A multicenter randomized controlled trial. New Engl J Med 1989; 321: 1501–1506.

[4] Di Bisceglie AM, Martin P, Kassianides C, Lisker-Melman M, Murray L, Waggoner J et al. Recombinant interferon alpha therapy for chronic hepatitis C. A randomized, double blind placebo-controlled trial. New Engl J Med 1989; 321: 1506–1510.

[5] Hagiwara H, Hayashi N, Mita E, Takehara T, Kasahara A, Fusamoto H et al. Quantitative analysis of hepatitis C virus RNA in serum during interferon alfa therapy. Gastroenterology 1993; 104: 877–883.

[6] Kasahara A, Hayashi N, Hiramatsu N, Oshita M, Hagiwara H, Katayama K et al. Ability of prolonged interferon treatment to suppress relapse after cessation of therapy in patients with chronic hepatitis C: A multicenter randomized controlled trial. Hepatology 1995; 21: 291–297.

[7] Hiramatsu N, Hayashi N, Kasahara A, Hagiwara H, Takehara T, Haruna Y et al. Improvement of liver fibrosis in chronic hepatitis C patients treated with natural interferon alpha. J Hepatol 1995; 22: 135–142.

[8] Carithers RL Jr, Emerson SS. Therapy of hepatitis C. Meta-analysis of interferon alfa-2b trials. Hepatology 1997; 26: S83–S88.

[9] Causse X, Godinot H, Chevallier M, Chossegros P, Zoulim Fouzan D et al. Comparison of 1 or 3 MU of interferon alfa-2b and placebo in patients with chronic non-A, non-B hepatitis. Gastroenterology 1991; 101: 497–502.

[10] Poynard T, Leroy V, Cohard M, Thevenot T, Mathurin P, Opolon P et al. Meta-analysis of interferon randomized trials in the treatment of viral hepatitis: effects of dose and duration. Hepatology 1996; 24: 778–789.

[11] Chemello L, Cavaletto L, Casarin C, Bonetti P, Bernardinello E, Pontisso P et al. Persistent hepatitis C viremia predicts late relapse after sustained response to interferon-α in chronic hepatitis C. Ann Intern Med 1996; 124: 1058–1060.

[12] Poynard T, Bedossa P, Chevallier M, Mathurin P, Lemonnier C, Trepo C et al. A comparison of three interferon alfa-2b regimens for the long-term treatment of chronic non-A, non-B hepatitis. Multicenter Study Group. New Engl J Med 1995; 332: 1457–1462.

[13] Lin R, Roach E, Zimmerman M, Strasser S, Farrell GC. Interferon alfa-2b for chronic hepatitis C: effects of dose increment and duration of treatment on response rates. Results of the first multicenter Australian trial. Australia Hepatitis C Study Group. J Hepatol 1995; 23: 487–496.

[14] Saracco G, Borghesio E, Mesina P, Solinas A, Spezia C, Macor F et al. Prolonged treatment (2 years) with different doses (3 versus 6 MU) of interferon alpha-2b for chronic hepatitis C. Results of a multicenter randomized trial. J Hepatol 1997; 27: 56–62.

[15] Mita E, Hayashi N, Hagiwara H, Ueda K, Kanazawa Y, Kasahara A et al. Predicting interferon therapy efficacy from hepatitis C virus genotype and RNA titer. Dig Dis Sci 1994; 39: 977–982.

[16] Yoshioka K, Kakumu S, Wakita T, Ishikawa T, Itoh Y, Takayanagi M et al. Detection

of hepatitis C virus by polymerase chain reaction and response to interferon therapy: relationship to genotypes of hepatitis c virus. Hepatology 1992; 16: 293–299.

[17] Fukuda M, Chayama K, Tsubota A, Kobayashi M, Hashimoto M, Miyano Y et al. Predictive factors in eradicating hepatitis C virus using a relatively small dose of interferon. J Gastroenterol Hepatol 1998; 13: 412–418.

[18] Yuki N, Hayashi N, Kasahara A, Hagiwara H, Takehara T, Oshita M et al. Pretreatment viral load and response to prolonged interferon-α course for chronic hepatitis C. J Hepatol 1995; 22: 457–463.

[19] Shindo M, Di-Bisceglie AM, Hoofnagle JH. Long-term follow-up of patients with chronic hepatitis C treated with alpha-interferon. Hepatology 1992; 15: 1013–1016.

[20] Lau JYN, Mizokami M, Ohno T, Diamond DA, Kniffen J, Davis GL. Discrepancy between biochemical and virological responses to interferon-α in chronic hepatitis C. Lancet 1993; 342: 1208–1209.

[21] Kasahara A, Hayashi N, Mochizuki K, Takayanagi M, Yoshioka K, Kakumu S et al. Risk factors for hepatocellular carcinoma and its incidence after interferon treatment in patients with chronic hepatitis C. Hepatology 1998; 27: 1394–1402.

[22] Kanto T, Hayashi N, Takehara T, Hagiwara H, Mita E, Oshita M et al. Serial density analysis of hepatitis C virus particle populations in chronic hepatitis C patients treated with interferon-alpha. J Med Virol 1995; 46: 230–237.

[23] Saracco G, Rosina F, Abate ML, Chiandussi L, Gallo V, Ceruti E et al. Long-term follow-up of patients with chronic hepatitis C treated with different doses of interferon-α2b. Hepatology 1993; 18: 1300–1305.

[24] Knodell RG, Ishak KG, Black WC, Chen TS, Craig R, Kaplowitz N et al. Formulation and application of a numerical scoring system for assessing histological activity in asymptomatic chronic active hepatitis. Hepatology 1981; 1: 431–435.

[25] Manabe N, Chevallier M, Chossegros P, Causse X, Guerret S, Trepo C et al. Interferon α-2b therapy reduces liver fibrosis in chronic non-A, non-B hepatitis: a quantitative histological evaluation. Hepatology 1993; 18: 1344–1349.

[26] Sobesky R, Mathurin P, Charlotte F, Moussalli J, Olivi M, Vidaud M et al. Modeling the impact of interferon alfa treatment on liver fibrosis progression in chronic hepatitis C: a dynamic view. Gastroenterology 1999; 116: 378–386.

[27] Lau DTL, Kleiner DE, Ghany MG, Park Y, Schmid P, Hoofnagle JH. 10-year follow-up after interferon-α therapy for chronic hepatitis C. Hepatology 1998; 28: 1121–1127.

[28] Duchatelle V, Marcellin P, Giostra E, Bregeaud L, Pouteau M, Boyer N et al. Changes in liver fibrosis at the end of alpha interferon therapy and 6 to 18 months later in patients with chronic hepatitis C: quantitative assessment by a morphometric method. J Hepatol 1998; 29: 20–28.

[29] Edwards DR, Murphy G, Reynolds JJ, Whitham SE, Docherty AJ, Angel P et al. Transforming growth factor β modulates the expression of collagenase and metalloproteinase inhibitor. EMBO J 1987; 6: 1899–1904.

[30] Sanderson N, Factor V, Nagy P, Kopp J, Kondaiah P, Wakefield L et al. Hepatic expression of transforming growth factor-β1 in transgenic mice results in multiple tissue lesions. Proc Natl Acad Sci USA 1995; 92: 2572–2576.

[31] Castilla A, Prieto J, Fausto N. Transforming growth factor β1 and α in chronic liver disease: effects of interferon alfa therapy. New Engl J Med 1991; 324: 933–940.

[32] Tsushima H, Kawata S, Tamura S, Ito N, Shirai Y, Kiso S et al. Reduced plasma transforming growth-factor-β1 levels in patients with chronic hepatitis C after interferon-α therapy: association with regression of hepatic fibrosis. J Hepatol 1999; 30: 1–7.

[33] Sakaida I, Nagatomi A, Hironaka K, Uchida K, Okita K. Quantitative analysis of liver

fibrosis and stellate cell changes in patients with chronic hepatitis C after interferon therapy. Am J Gastroenterol 1999; 94: 489–496.

[34] Imai Y, Kawata S, Tamura S, Yabuuchi I, Noda S, Inada M et al. Relation of interferon therapy and hepatocellular carcinoma in patients with chronic hepatitis C. Ann Intern Med 1998; 129: 94–99.

[35] Ikeda K, Saitoh S, Arase Y, Chayama K, Suzuki Y, Kobayashi M et al. Effect of interferon therapy on hepatocellular carcinogenesis in patients with chronic hepatitis C: A long-term observation study of 1,643 patients using statistical bias correction with proportional hazard analysis. Hepatology 1999; 29: 1124–1130.

[36] Yoshida H, Shiratori Y, Moriyama M, Arakawa Y, Ide T, Sata M et al. Interferon therapy reduces the risk for hepatocellular carcinoma: National surveillance program of cirrhotic and noncirrhotic patients with chronic hepatitis C in Japan. Ann Intern Med 1999; 131: 174–181.

[37] Nishiguchi S, Kuroki T, Nakatani S, Moriomoto H, Takeda T, Nakajima S et al. Randomized trial of effects of interferon-alpha on incidence of hepatocellular carcinoma in chronic active hepatitis C with cirrhosis. Lancet 1995; 346: 1051–1055.

[38] Valla DC, Chevallier M, Marcellin P, Payen JL, Trepo C, Fonck M et al. Treatment of hepatitis C virus-related cirrhosis: a randomized, controlled trial of interferon alfa-2b versus no treatment. Hepatology 1999; 29: 1870–1875.

[39] Mazzella G, Accogli E, Sottili S, Festi D, Orsini M, Salzetta A et al. Alpha interferon treatment may prevent hepatocellular carcinoma in HCV-related liver cirrhosis. J Hepatol 1996; 24: 141–147.

[40] Fattovich G, Giustina G, Degos F, Diodati G, Tremolada F, Nevens F et al. Effectiveness of interferon alfa on incidence hepatocellular carcinoma and decompensation in cirrhosis type C. European Concerted Action on Viral Hepatitis. J Hepatol 1997; 27: 201–205.

[41] Brunetto MR, Oliveri F, Koehler M, Zahm F, Bonino F (International Interferon-α Hepatocellular Carcinoma Study Group). Effect of interferon-alpha on progression of cirrhosis to hepatocellular carcinoma: a retrospective cohort study. Lancet 1998; 351: 1535–1539.

[42] Serfaty L, Aumaitre H, Chazouilleres O, Bonnand AM, Rosmorduc O, Poupon RE et al. Determinants of outcome of compensated hepatitis C virus-related cirrhosis. Hepatology 1998; 27: 1435–1440.

[43] Okanoue T, Itoh Y, Minami M, Sakamoto S, Yasui K, Sakamoto M et al. Interferon therapy lowers the rate of progression to hepatocellular carcinoma in chronic hepatitis C but not significantly in advanced stage: a retrospective study in 1148 patients. J Hepatol 1999; 30: 653–659.

Molecular Biology and Immunology in Hepatology
Edited by T. Tsuji, T. Higashi, M. Zeniya and K.-H. Meyer zum Büschenfelde

CHAPTER 7

Transgenic Mouse Models for Viral Hepatitis: The Role of Hepatitis Viruses in Hepatocarcinogenesis

Kazuhiko Koike

Department of Infectious Diseases, Internal Medicine, Graduate School of Medicine, University of Tokyo, Tokyo, Japan

INTRODUCTION

Viral hepatitis is defined as a pathologic state triggered by infection with hepatitis viruses that can replicate in the liver of hosts. The pathology may be modified by many factors, such as the expression of viral proteins and their exposure on the surface of hepatocytes, as well as cellular immune responses of the host against them. At present, five hepatitis viruses are known and named by capital letters from A to E. Among them, hepatitis A virus and hepatitis E virus induce acute hepatitis that rarely, if ever, becomes chronic. The outcome of these two hepatitis viruses is uneventful, except in rare cases of fulminant hepatitis. Hepatitis D virus can replicate only when it co-infects hosts with hepatitis B virus (HBV) and has a restriction of epidemiological distribution. Although it aggravates the pathology and the clinical course of chronic hepatitis B, it has limited local implication.

Worldwide, HBV and hepatitis C virus (HCV) persistently infect hundreds of millions of people and induce a spectrum of chronic liver diseases. Hence they impact society in a number of domains including medical, sociologic and economic. Hepatocellular carcinoma (HCC) has become the most frequent cause of death in individuals persistently infected with HBV or HCV; in particular, HCV has gained increasing attention because of its wide and deep penetration into the community, coupled with a very high incidence of HCC in the persistent infection. Once liver cirrhosis is established in hosts infected with HCV, HCC develops at a yearly rate of 5–7% [1]. Knowledge of the mechanism involved in the development of HCC in chronic HCV infection, therefore, is urgently required for the prevention of HCC.

1. PATHOGENESIS OF HCC IN PERSISTENT HEPATITIS VIRUS INFECTIONS

How hepatitis viruses induce HCC is not yet clear, despite the fact that more than 95% of patients with HCC in Japan are infected with HBV or HCV, or both [2,3]. Infections with these two hepatitis viruses are also common in patients with HCC in other countries, albeit to lesser extents. Evidence of concurrent or past HBV infection is demonstrated even in the remaining 5% of patients with HCC in Japan [3,4], which has been categorized in non-B, non-C HCC. Furthermore, co-infection with HBV and HCV is frequent in patients with HCC [4,5]. These lines of evidence obligate hepatologists to a burning task of looking for a role of hepatitis viruses in hepatocarcinogenesis. Inflammation induced by hepatitis viruses, manifesting itself in various forms of hepatitis, needs to be taken into consideration in the study for carcinogenic capacity of hepatitis viruses. It has been repeatedly proposed that necrosis of hepatocytes due to chronic inflammation and ensuing regeneration that follows would enhance mutagenesis in host cells, the accumulation of which might culminate in HCC. The theory presupposes an indirect involvement of hepatitis viruses in HCC via hepatic inflammation. It leaves us specialists in hepatology with a serious question, however: can inflammation per se result in HCC in such a high incidence? The proposal for a secondary role of hepatitis viruses would have to be weighed against an extremely rare occurrence of HCC in patients with autoimmune hepatitis in whom severe inflammation of the liver goes on indefinitely.

These backgrounds and reasonings lead one to the possibility that activity of viral proteins may play a role in the induction of HCC. The possibility has been evaluated by introducing genes of HBV or HCV into hepatocytes in culture with little success. One of the difficulties with cultured cells is that a carcinogenic capacity of hepatitis viruses, if any, would be weak and take a long time to manifest itself. Actually, it takes 30–40 years for HCC to develop in individuals infected with HCV. Another constraint common to studies for carcinogenesis is the development of HCC by transformed cells that might have gone out of growth control and escaped surveillance of the host. Should it be the case, the analysis of transformed cells would not been sufficient for bringing the mystery of carcinogenesis into the light. Based on these viewpoints, we started tackling the carcinogenesis in chronic viral hepatitis by the technology of transgenic mouse.

2. APPLICATION OF TRANSGENIC MICE TO MOLECULAR MEDICAL ANALYSIS OF VIRAL HEPATITIS

Transgenic mice are produced by introducing exogenous genes into fertilized eggs. The technology of transgenic mice crystallized, for the first time in 1985, by the production of a phenotype in mice genetically engineered with the human growth hormone gene [6]. Since then, the technology has ignited an enormous explosion of studies; it has become a standard technique. As of April 2001, a survey of the PubMed database by keywording ‘transgenic mouse’ hits more than 17,000 publications; this will increase at an accelerated rate in the future.

The technology of transgenic mice involves the introduction of exogenous genes with a dominant trait into animals. A number of transgenic mice have been produced for studies of many diseases by introducing various genes of viral origins, in particular [7,8]. The virus represents a simple organism composed only of viral proteins and nucleic acids. In infected cells, viral genes are released from viral particles and they are then transcribed for replication and translation of viral proteins. Because these series of processes, including introduction of genes followed by transcription and translation, are faithfully mimicked in transgenic mice, they are suitable as a model of diseases induced by viral infections. The establishment of the technology for transgenic mouse has offered incomparable opportunities for answering in vivo many questions raised in a variety of biological fields, which had been accomplished exclusively in vitro until the transgenic mouse entered the scene.

We have produced transgenic mice in which the core gene, envelope gene and non-structural gene of HCV, as well as the X gene of HBV, were introduced primarily for studying the mechanism of hepatocarcinogenesis. It is of particular note that every viral gene is under the control of expression with the same enhancer and promoter. This has made it feasible to compare in vivo functions among various viral proteins. As salient results of our studies, both HCV core protein and HBx protein have been found capable of inducing HCC due to carcinogenic potentials of these two products of viral genes.

3. HCV TRANSGENIC MOUSE

3.1. Establishment of transgenic mice introduced with the HCV core gene

As illustrated in Fig. 1A, the transgenic mouse with the HCV core gene was engineered by introducing the core gene excised from cDNA of the HCV genome of genotype 1b [9] that was placed under transcriptional control of the HBV X gene [10,11]. Because HCV is an RNA virus, exogenous control of its transcription is required. We used the one for the HBV X gene to this effect; we have confirmed an excellent performance of it in transgenic mice (vide infra). We introduced viral genes into the C57BL/6 strain (commonly known as B6), which is renowned for its rare spontaneous occurrence of HCC [12]. Five transgenic mice were obtained by introduction of the HCV core gene. Two mice randomly selected from them were crossed with B6 mice to produce a colony of transgenic mice engineered to possess the HCV core gene in their own chromosome.

The two strains of transgenic mice thus obtained were named C21 and C49, respectively. The expression of HCV core protein in the liver started right after birth and continued for at least 23 months thereafter. By Western blot analysis, the degrees of expression of HCV core protein in their livers were comparable with those in the liver of patients with HCV-associated HCC (Fig. 1B) [11,13]. Similar degrees of expression were also confirmed by determination of HCV core protein in the liver by fluorescence enzyme immunoassay. Levels of HCV core protein in transgenic mice ranged from 13 to 804 pg/mg protein which were included in the range of patients with HCV-associated HCC spanning 6–1,000 pg/mg protein [13]. The lack of overexpression of HCV core protein in transgenic mice validates an extrapolation of the results with an experimental system in mice into HCV-associated HCC in humans.

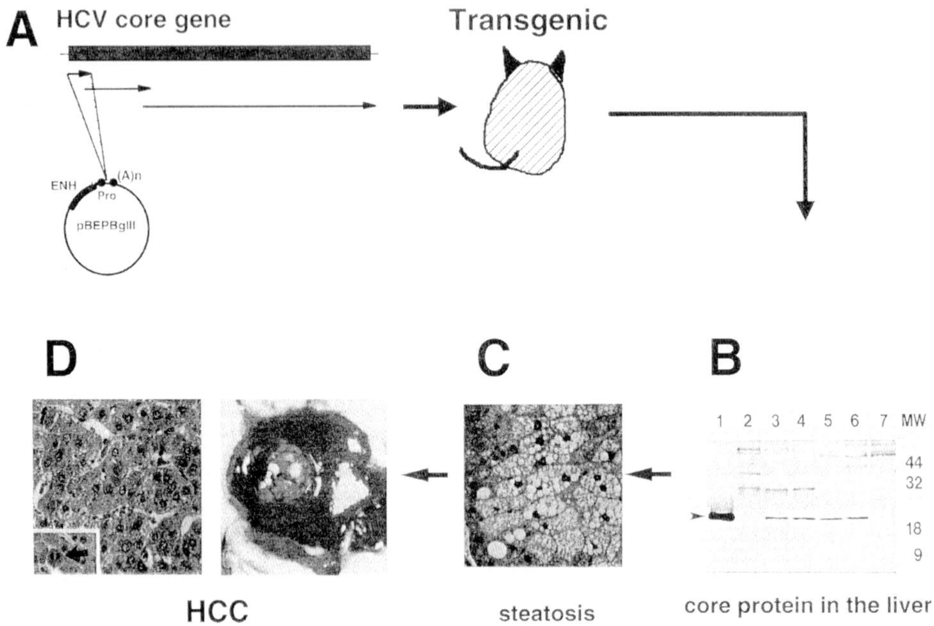

Fig. 1. Development of HCC in HCV core gene transgenic mice. (A) The core gene of HCV was introduced into mouse eggs under a transcriptional regulatory element from HBV. (B) The core protein was expressed at levels similar to those in the liver of chronic hepatitis C patients. These mice developed hepatic steatosis early in life (C) and HCC later in life (D), indicating a direct role of HCV in hepatocarcinogenesis. HCC, hepatocellular carcinoma; HCV, hepatitis C virus.

3.2. Early development of steatosis characteristic of chronic hepatitis C in transgenic mice having the HCV core gene

As shown in Fig. 1C, transgenic mice with the HCV core gene developed steatosis in the liver starting as early as 3 months of age [10]. Steatosis in the liver has been reported as a characteristic of chronic hepatitis C along with the formation of lymphoid follicles and damage to the bile ducts [14]. The steatosis in transgenic mice is slowly progressive with no significant elevation in alanine aminotransferase (ALT) in the serum. Of note, no significant inflammation was observed in the liver.

There are conflicting views with regard to an involvement of HCV in the development of steatosis. There are Western pathologists who are for this claim, but it is refuted by some researchers represented by Japanese pathologists. We have evaluated the association of steatosis with the expression of HCV core protein in 43 patients with chronic hepatitis C. Amounts of core protein were determined by Western blotting, and they were compared with scores of steatosis estimated in the liver. Factors influencing steatosis were body mass index (BMI), levels of ALT and triglycerides in serum, as well as the amount of HCV core protein in the liver. By multivariate analysis, BMI, ALT levels and HCV core protein were independent factors contributing to steatosis. Hence, the HCV core protein is confirmed as a factor influencing the development of steatosis in chronic hepatitis C [15].

3.3. Development of HCC in transgenic mice harboring the HCV core gene

For the evaluation of the long-term effects of HCV core protein expressed in transgenic mice, livers were removed from two strains of mice (C21 and C49) at 3, 6, 9, 12 and 16 months of age for histological examination. Evident steatosis unaccompanied by inflammatory or tumorigenic changes was observed in the liver of transgenic mice until the age of 9 months; it was also found in mice examined at the age of 12 months. Large HCCs, such as the one shown in Fig. 1D, developed, however, in mice by 16 months of age [11].

Encouraged by these results, we followed transgenic mice with the HCV core gene for liver pathology until 16–23 months of age. Hepatic nodules were displayed by approximately one-third of male transgenic mice. There were nodules arising as highly differentiated HCCs in trabecular structures. Most hepatic nodules disclosed a pathology characterized by 'nodule in nodule', and HCC with low degrees of differentiation developed within adenoma as well as in HCC of higher stages of differentiation. Typically, a cluster of cancer cells (area 3 in Fig. 2) arose in adenoma (area 2); together, they pressed aside adjacent non-tumorous hepatocytes (area 1).

Although plenty of lipid droplets were found in cells forming adenoma, just as in non-tumorous cells, they were rarely observed in HCC cells. These histological features closely resembled those seen in HCC developing in chronic hepatitis C, in which prominent lipid droplets are found in small differentiated HCC and its precursors, while poorly differentiated HCC without lipid droplets elicits in differentiated HCC [16].

We went on to evaluate incidence of HCC in the two independent strains of transgenic mice. The incidence rates of HCC in male transgenic mice in C21 and C49 strains were 26% (11 of 43) and 32% (6 of 19), respectively, and significantly higher than those in non-transgenic male mice serving as controls ($P < 0.01$ and $P < 0.005$, respectively). No HCC developed in any of 56 male littermates at the same ages that were not transgenic, standing in agreement with an extremely low incidence of HCC in B6 mice in previous reports. Female transgenic mice, in contrast to males, developed HCC infrequently (4% or 1 in 27 in C21 strain and 15% or 3 in 20 in C49 strain). In humans with chronic hepatitis C, likewise, females are at much less risk than males for developing HCC.

It must be stressed that we did not observe development of adenoma or HCC in any of more than 100 transgenic mice to which the HCV envelope gene was introduced throughout the follow-up of 24 months [17,18]. These transgenic mice possessed the complete envelope gene covering both E1 and E2 regions, and expressed the envelope protein coded for by it over the lifetime. Several strains of transgenic mice have been reported into which HCV genes were engineered. They fail to demonstrate a direct role of HCV in the induction of HCC. The strains with the HCV core gene reported by others had very low expression of viral core protein that was hardly detectable by anti-HCV core antibodies in wide clinical use [19–21]. With such a poor expression of HCV core protein, the development of HCC in them is hardly expected. The HCC eliciting in both

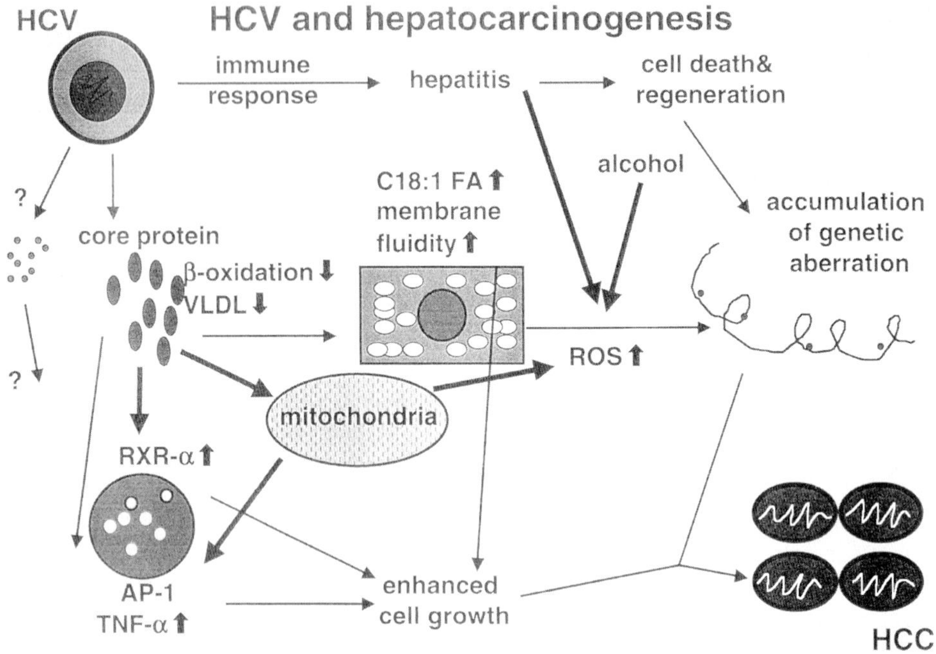

Fig. 2. Mechanism of hepatocarcinogenesis in HCV infection. The core protein is localized in the nuclei and mitochondria of hepatocytes in addition to the cytoplasm. The core protein may interact with nuclear factors, thereby deregulating the cell growth and death. The core protein may also affect cell growth by inducing accumulation of reactive oxygen species (ROS) and lipid in the hepatocytes. Lipids such as free fatty acids are now known to be ligands for some nuclear receptors. ROS is known to cause genetic aberrations and modify the expression of cytokines such as TNF-α.

strains of transgenic mice we engineered (C21 and C49) is summed up as follows. It is composed of acidophilic cells in trabeculae and with evidence of chromosomal division. By immunological analysis, the expression of HCV core protein is higher in tumor cells than in the surrounding normal hepatocytes, in the absence of lymphocyte infiltration, suggestive of hepatitis. In support of this, transgenic mice of 16–19 months of age had ALT levels of 136±116 IU/l, no different from 122±92 IU/L in control, non-transgenic B6 mice. Taken altogether, 'chronic hepatitis' accompanied by continuing death and regeneration of hepatocytes would not be an absolute prerequisite for the development of HCC. Rather, HCV by itself should have a potential for inducing HCC.

3.4. Mechanism for hepatocarcinogenesis in transgenic mice harboring the HCV core gene

It is hard to sort out the mechanism for carcinogenesis even for our simple model in transgenic mice with the expression of the HCV core gene alone. One activity of the core protein would be to modify the expression of cellular genes and to interact with intracellular proteins. For an example, tumor necrosis factor (TNF)-α is known to have such multipotent activities; an intranuclear receptor, for TNF-α has been demonstrated as evidence for its interaction with biologically active substances. Another possible pathway would be an increased production of reactive oxygen species (ROS) in the liver. We would like to draw particular attention to the fact that the production of ROS is increased in our model of transgenic mice in the absence of inflammation in the liver (hepatitis) [22,23]. This reflects a state of hyperproduction of free radicals in the liver, or predisposition thereof, staged by HCV core protein without any inflammation intervening. If hepatic inflammation occurs in HCV infection in the liver, the production of free radicals would be enhanced to an extent that it cannot be scavenged any longer by the physiological antagonistic system. This indicates that inflammation given rise to by HCV would be different in its quality from other hepatitis represented by autoimmune hepatitis. Such a mechanism may be able to explain an extremely high incidence of HCC developing in the background of chronic hepatitis C [24].

4. HBV TRANSGENIC MOUSE

4.1. Transgenic mice harboring the HBV X gene

Previous sections have focused on a role of HCV core protein in the induction of HCC in persistently infected individuals. How, then, is HBV involved in the development of HCC in the chronic hepatitis it induces? We and others have already shown, even prior to hepatocarcinogenesis of the HCV core protein, that the product of the HBV X gene (HBx protein) is capable of inducing HCC in chronic hepatitis B [25–29].

Transgenic mice with the expression of the HBV X gene have been engineered by the introduction of the X gene, and its promoter as well as enhancers and the poly(A) signal excised from HBV DNA of subtype *adr*. The HBx protein was expressed in hepatocytes in the vicinity of central veins soon after the birth in a level that remained unchanged until 24 months of age. After 3 months of age, hepatocytes in a precancerous stage emerged in mice that contained abundant glycogen particles in the cytoplasm. More than 80% of transgenic mice with the HBV X gene in two independent strains developed adenoma and HCC at the age of 13 months and thereafter. Hence, the HBx protein has the capacity to induce HCC in the liver of mice [24,25].

4.2. Sequential changes in the liver of transgenic mice with the HBV X gene

In transgenic mice incorporated with the HBV X gene, HBx protein is expressed soon after birth and HCC develops at the age of 13 months and older. These two events are intervened by a latency when pathologic hepatocytes enriched with respect to cytoplasmic glycogen accumulate around the central vein. These pathologic cells invariably appear in areas of the liver with a high expression of HBx protein. The pathology characterized by glycogen-rich hepatocytes is considered to represent a precancerous state, because: (1) a heightened synthesis of DNA is observed in hepatocytes with the expression of HBx protein; and (2) nuclei of hepatocytes rich in cytoplasmic glycogen particles exhibit numerous states of aneuploidy in addition to diploid and quadriploid nuclei.

The capacity of HBx protein for enhancing the synthesis of DNA has also been observed in cultured cell systems [30]. Together, these lines of evidence point to accelerated proliferation of hepatocytes and rapid cell cycle given rise to by the HBx protein. Such activities of the HBx protein in transgenic mice are taken even more seriously, in view of low reproductive capacity of hepatocytes surrounding the central vein, if it were not for promoting factors.

With the knowledge of the HBx protein capable of activating cell proliferation, taken along with an accelerated DNA synthesis after an age of 2 months and older, one wonders why HCC never develops until 13 months of age in the face of such stimuli in favor of increased cell proliferation.

4.3. Mechanism for hepatocarcinogenesis stimulated by the HBx protein

The answer to the aforementioned query is apoptosis occurring pari passeau with cell proliferation. Sequential analysis of the liver histology of transgenic mice incorporated with the HBV X gene, with special reference to the morphology of nuclei, has unfolded highly specific characteristics. They include numerous pathologic hepatocytes having peculiar nuclei with chromatin aggregates attracted around the nucleus. Such unusual hepatocytes were very frequently seen over the entire liver in mice at a precancerous state. By analysis with the TUNEL method, the liver of transgenic mice with the expression of HBx protein revealed hepatocytes staining positive far TUNEL approximately 20-fold more than normal mice serving as controls. Furthermore, pathologic cells with chromatin aggregates around the nucleus were positive for TUNEL. Very intriguingly, TUNEL-positive cells decreased remarkably in number after 10 months of age, well before the development of HCC [27].

The obtained results indicate that, in the precancerous state of transgenic mice harboring the HBV X gene, the cell proliferation induced by HBx protein would be compensated by apoptosis of hepatocytes. In other words, the equilibrium maintained between proliferation and apoptosis of hepatocytes may prevent inappropriate excessive proliferation of hepatocytes, and by inference, hepatocarcinogenesis. Unlimited proliferation of hepatocytes may start, if and once such equilibrium is disrupted. The induction of apoptosis by HBx protein is demonstrated, also, in hepatocytes in culture [31]. Taken altogether, the HBx protein would have dual activities, one for proliferating cells and the other for inducing apoptosis, thereby providing hepatocytes with conditions in favor of the replication of HBV. By doing so, the HBx protein may circumvent very cunningly crisis in the fate of HBV as ramifications of hepatocarcinogenesis, which inevitably results in death of the host as well as the virus itself.

5. HEPATOCARCINOGENESIS INDUCED BY HEPATITIS VIRUSES: A MECHANISM DISTINCT FROM THE PROPOSAL BY VOGELSTEIN

The results of our studies on transgenic mice have indicated a carcinogenic potential of HCV core protein as well as HBV X protein expressed in vivo. HCV and HBV, therefore, are directly involved in the development of HCC.

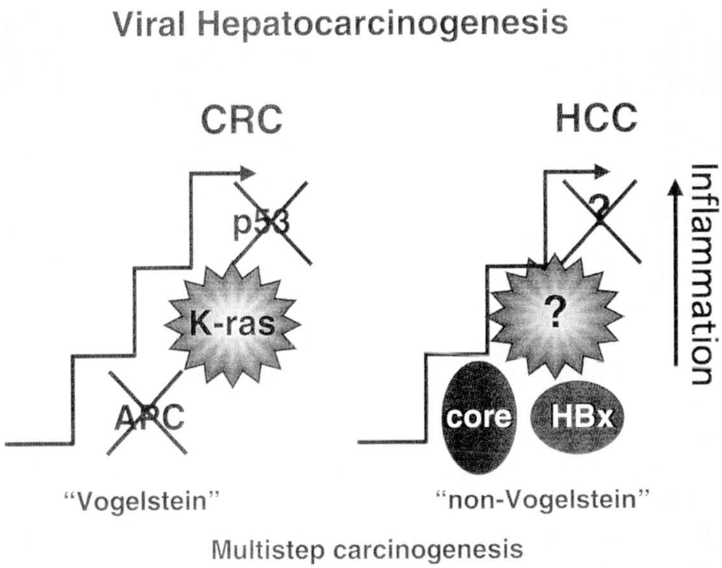

Fig. 3. The role of hepatitis viruses in multistep hepatocarcinogenesis. Similar to pathogenesis of cancers like colorectal cancer ('Vogelstein-type' carcinogenesis), the accumulation of genetic aberrations may be necessary in the multistage carcinogenesis of HCC. However, the presence of the HCV core or HBx protein, which has an oncogenic potential, may allow some of the multiple steps in hepatocarcinogenesis to be skipped. Unlike colorectal cancer, HCC may develop in the absence of a complete set of genetic aberrations in association with HCV or HBV infection ('non-Vogelstein-type' carcinogenesis). HCC, hepatocellular carcinoma; CRC, colorectal cancer.

In researches of carcinogenesis, the theory of Vogelstein et al. has gained a wide popularity. They propose a development of colorectal cancer by accumulation of mutations occurring in cellular genes [32]. They have deduced that mutations in the APC gene for inactivation, those in K-Ras for activation and those in the p53 gene for inactivation accumulate, which cooperate toward the development of colorectal cancer [33]. Their theory has been extended to carcinogenesis of the other cancers, as well.

On the basis of results we obtained for the induction of HCC by HCV core gene and HBV X gene, we would like to introduce a mechanism different from that of Vogelstein et al. for the hepatocarcinogenesis occurring in infections with hepatitis viruses. We do admit multi-stages in the induction of all cancers; it would be mandatory for hepatocarcinogenesis that many mutations accumulate in hepatocytes. Some of these stages might be skipped in the development of HCC in infections with HCV and HBV, however, to which HCV core protein and HBx protein, respectively, would contribute (Fig. 3). The overall effects achieved by the expression of these viral proteins would be the induction of HCC, even in the absence of a complete set of genetic aberrations, required for carcinogenesis.

Such a non-Vogelstein process for induction of HCC taken into consideration, a plausible explanation may be offered for many unusual events happening in carriers of hepatitis viruses. Now it does not seem so difficult to understand why HCC develops in persistent HCV infection with an outstandingly high incidence and in multicentric nature, and how it occurs in young individuals with chronic HBV infection unaccompanied by liver injuries, and elicits itself in the liver rated F0 or F1 by staging of fibrosis.

SUMMARY

Overwhelming lines of epidemiological evidence have indicated that chronic infection with HCV or HBV poses a major risk toward development of HCC. In the pathogenesis of HCC associated with HBV or HCV, it remains controversial whether these hepatitis viruses play a direct role or merely serve for an indirect role. By virtue of the transgenic mouse established by us, it has become evident that the product of the HBx protein and the core protein of HCV have an oncogenic potential, although the pathways through which these two viral proteins operate may differ. The findings in our studies indicate that HBV and HCV are directly involved in hepatocarcinogenesis, albeit that other factors, such as continued cell death and regeneration associated with chronic hepatitis may play a role, as well. Combined, our results suggest that there would be a mechanism for the development of HCC in persistent infection with hepatitis viruses that is distinct from those for the other cancers. Similar to the pathogenesis of other malignancies represented by colorectal cancer, the accumulation of a set of genetic aberrations may also be necessary for a multi-stage development of HCC. However, HBx protein and HCV core protein, to which an oncogenic potential is ascribed, may allow some of the multiple stages skipped in hepatocarcinogenesis. Unlike other cancers, therefore, infection with HBV or HCV may be capable of eliciting HCC in the absence of a complete set of genetic aberrations. Such a scenario would explain the unusually high incidence and multicentric nature of HCC developing in chronic hepatitis B or C.

REFERENCES

[1] Ikeda K, Saitoh S, Suzuki Y, Kobayashi M, Tsubota A, Koida I et al. Disease progression and hepatocellular carcinogenesis in patients with chronic viral hepatitis: a prospective observation of 2215 patients. J Hepatol 1988; 28: 930–938.

[2] Kiyosawa K, Sodeyama T, Tanaka E, Gibo Y, Yoshizawa K, Nakano Y et al. Interrelationship of blood transfusion, non-A, non-B hepatitis and hepatocellular carcinoma: analysis by detection of antibody to hepatitis C virus. Hepatology 1990; 12: 671–675.

[3] Yotsuyanagi H, Shintani Y, Moriya K, Fujie H, Tsutsumi T, Kato T et al. Virological analysis of non-B, non-C hepatocellular carcinoma in Japan: frequent involvement of hepatitis B virus. J Infect Dis 2000; 181: 1920–1928.

[4] Koike K, Yasuda K, Yotsuyanagi H, Moriya K, Hino K, Iino S et al. Dominant replication of either virus in dual infection with hepatitis viruses B and C. J Med Virol 1955; 45: 236–239.

[5] Shintani Y, Yotsuyanagi H, Moriya K, Fujie H, Tsutsumi T, Takayama T et al. Significance of hepatitis B virus DNA detected in hepatocellular carcinoma in patients with hepatitis C. Cancer 2000; 88: 2478–2486.

[6] Hammer RE, Brinster RL, Rosenfeld MG, Evans RM, Mayo KE. Expression of human growth hormone-releasing factor in transgenic mice results in increased somatic growth. Nature 1985; 315: 413–416.

[7] Hanahan D. Dissecting multistep tumorigenesis in transgenic mice. Annu Rev Genet 1988; 22: 479–519.

[8] Chisari FV. Hepatitis B virus transgenic mice: insights into the virus and the disease. Hepatology 1995; 22: 1316–1325.

[9] Takeuchi K, Kubo Y, Boonmer S, Watanabe Y, Katayama T, Choo QL et al. The putative nucleocapsid and envelope protein genes of hepatitis C virus determined by comparison of the nucleotide sequences of two isolates derived from an experimentally infected chimpanzee and healthy human carriers. J Gen Virol 1990; 71: 3027–3033.

[10] Moriya K, Yotsuyanagi H, Shintani Y, Fujie H, Ishibashi K, Matsuura Y et al. Hepatitis C virus core protein induces hepatic steatosis in transgenic mice. J Gen Virol 1997; 78: 1527–1531.

[11] Moriya K, Fujie H, Shintani Y, Yotsuyanagi H, Tsutsumi T, Matsuura Y et al. Hepatitis C virus core protein induces hepatocellular carcinoma in transgenic mice. Nature Med 1988; 4: 1065–1068.

[12] Smith GS, Walford RL, Mickey MR. Lifespan and incidence of cancer and other diseases in selected long-lived inbred mice and their F1 hybrids. J Natl Cancer Inst 1973; 50: 1195–1213.

[13] Koike K, Tustsumi T, Fujie H, Shintani Y, Moriya K. Role of hepatitis viruses in hepatocarcinogenesis. Oncology 2002; in press.

[14] Lefkowitch JH, Schiff ER, Davis GL, Perrillo RP, Lindsay K, Bodenheimer HC Jr. et al. Pathological diagnosis of chronic hepatitis C: a multicenter comparative study with chronic hepatitis B. Gastroenterology 1993; 104: 595–603.

[15] Fujie H, Yotsuyanagi H, Moriya K, Shintani Y, Tsutsumi T, Takayama T et al. Steatosis and intrahepatic hepatitis C virus in chronic hepatitis. J Med Virol 1999; 59: 141–145.

[16] Nakashima O, Sugihara S, Kage M, Kojiro M. Pathomorphologic characteristics of small hepatocellular carcinoma: a special reference to small hepatocellular carcinoma with distinct margins. Hepatology 1995; 22: 101–105.

[17] Koike K, Moriya K, Ishibashi K, Matsuura Y, Suzuki T, Saito I et al. Expression of hepatitis C virus envelope proteins in transgenic mice. J Gen Virol 1995; 76: 3031–3038.

[18] Koike K, Moriya K, Yotsuyanagi H, Shintani Y, Fujie H, Ishibashi K et al. Sialadenitis resembling Sjogren's syndrome in mice transgenic for hepatitis C virus envelope genes. Proc Natl Acad Sci USA 1997; 94: 233–236.

[19] Matsuda J, Suzuki M, Nozaki C, Shinya N, Tashiro K, Mizuno K et al. Transgenic mouse expressing a full-length hepatitis C virus cDNA. Jpn J Cancer Res 1998; 89: 150–158.

[20] Pasquinelli C, Shoenberger JM, Chung J, Chang KM, Guidotti LG, Selby M et al. Hepatitis C virus core and E2 protein expression in transgenic mice. Hepatology 1997; 25: 719–727.

[21] Kawamura T, Furusaka A, Koziel MJ, Chung RT, Wang TC, Schmidt EV et al. Transgenic expression of hepatitis C virus structural proteins in the mouse. Hepatology 1997; 25: 1014–1021.

[22] Moriya K, Todoroki T, Tsutsumi T, Fujie H, Shintani Y, Miyoshi H et al. Increase of carbon 18 mono-unsaturated fatty acids in the liver of hepatitis C: Analysis in transgenic mice and humans. Biophys Biochem Res Commun 2001; 281: 1207–1212.

[23] Moriya K, Nakagawa K, Santa T, Shintani Y, Fujie H, Miyoshi H et al. Oxidative stress in the absence of inflammation in the liver of a mouse model for hepatitis C virus-associated hepatocellular carcinoma. Cancer Res 2001; in press.

[24] Koike K. Transgenic mouse models of viral hepatitis: Insight into viral hepatocarcinogenesis. Viral Hepatitis Rev 1999; 5: 177–203.
[25] Kim CM, Koike K, Saito I, Miyamura T, Jay G. HBx gene of hepatitis B virus induces liver cancer in transgenic mice. Nature 1991; 351: 317–320.
[26] Koike K, Moriya K, Iino S, Yotsuyanagi H, Endo Y, Miyamura T et al. High-level expression of hepatitis B virus HBx gene and hepatocarcinogenesis in transgenic mice. Hepatology 1994; 19: 810–819.
[27] Koike K, Moriya K, Yotsuyanagi H, Shintani Y, Fujie H, Tsutsumi T, Kimura S. Compensatory apoptosis in preneoplastic liver of transgenic mouse model for hepatocarcinogenesis. Cancer Lett 1998; 134: 181–186.
[28] Koike K. Hepatitis B virus HBx gene and hepatocarcinogenesis. Intervirology 1995; 38: 134–142.
[29] Yu DY, Moon HB, Son JK, Jeong S et al. Incidence of hepatocellular carcinoma in transgenic mice expressing the hepatitis B virus X-protein. J Hepatol 1999; 31: 123–132.
[30] Koike K, Moriya K, Yotsuyanagi H, Iino S, Kurokawa K. Induction of cell cycle progression by hepatitis B virus HBx gene expression in quiescent mouse fibroblasts. J Clin Invest 1994; 94: 44–49.
[31] Shintani Y, Yotsuyanagi H, Moriya K, Fujie H, Tsutsumi T, Kanegae Y et al. Induction of apoptosis upon the switch-on of the hepatitis B virus X gene mediated by Cre/loxP recombinase system. J Gen Virol 1999; 80: 3257–3266.
[32] Vogelstein B, Kinzler KW. The multistep nature of cancer. Trends Genet 1993; 9: 138–141.
[33] Kinzler KW, Vogelstein B. Lessons from hereditary colorectal cancer. Cell 1996; 87: 159–170.

Molecular Biology and Immunology in Hepatology
Edited by T. Tsuji, T. Higashi, M. Zeniya and K.-H. Meyer zum Büschenfelde

CHAPTER 8

Gene Therapy of Viral Hepatitis

Hubert E. Blum

*Department of Medicine II, University of Freiburg,
Freiburg, Germany*

INTRODUCTION

More than 300 million people worldwide are chronically infected with hepatitis B virus (HBV) [1] and more than 100 million people with hepatitis C virus (HCV) [2–5]. Chronic viral hepatitis is associated with a broad spectrum of clinical presentations that can range from an asymptomatic natural course with a normal life expectancy to progressive liver disease and substantial morbidity and mortality from the complications of liver cirrhosis and hepatocellular carcinoma (HCC) [1–4,6]. Current therapeutic options for chronic hepatitis B include interferon-alpha and nucleoside analogues [7–9], for chronic hepatitis C interferon-alpha in combination with ribavirin [2,5,10]. Despite recent progress in the treatment and management of patients with chronic hepatitis B or C, apart from special subgroups of patients, the biochemical, virological and histological response rate is not more than 50%. Therefore, alternative novel antiviral strategies need to be developed and explored. Among these, gene therapy of viral hepatitis is an attractive concept, based on the fact that viral hepatitis can be viewed as an acquired monogenetic disease.

Gene therapy is defined as the introduction of new genetic material into a target cell with a therapeutic benefit to the individual. Based on this definition cell or organ transplantation is not considered as gene therapy. For the molecular therapy of HBV and HCV infection several genetic antiviral strategies aimed at blocking viral gene expression or function as well as therapeutic DNA vaccination are being explored. Ribozymes, antisense oligonucleotides and interfering peptides or proteins, including aptamers strongly inhibit viral replication and gene expression in experimental systems in vitro and in some models in vivo. Further, molecular strategies to treat or prevent the long-term sequelae of chronic viral hepatitis, i.e., liver cirrhosis and HCC, are being developed and experimentally tested. Despite exciting recent developments, a number of issues, such as gene transfer, stability, toxicity, resistance and safety, need to be resolved before gene therapy of viral hepatitis B or C and its sequelae will complement existing therapeutic and preventive strategies. In the following the basic concepts as well as the current state of gene therapy of chronic viral hepatitis will be briefly discussed.

1. BASIC CONCEPTS OF GENE THERAPY

Based on the genetic classification of diseases as hereditary monogenetic, acquired monogenetic or acquired complex genetic (Table 1), gene therapy involves four concepts: gene repair or substitution for the therapy of hereditary monogenetic diseases, gene repair or substitution, block of gene expression or function and DNA vaccination for acquired monogenetic diseases, gene augmentation and DNA vaccination for acquired complex genetic diseases (Table 2). In the context of this review, gene therapy is defined as the introduction of nucleic acids into cells or tissues with a therapeutic benefit [11].

1.1. Gene repair or substitution

An increasing number of inherited genetic diseases as well as some acquired genetic diseases have been molecularly defined as a defect of a single gene. In principle, the aim of gene therapy for these monogenetic diseases is the targeted substitution of the defective cellular gene by the corresponding normal homologue with production of the physiological gene product. Given the complexity of gene regulation in normal cells, the conceptually simple approach of gene substitution is difficult to effectively translate into experimental or clinical applications. Alternatively, strategies are aimed at the repair of mutations at the DNA or RNA level. In this context, it has been recently shown that

TABLE 1

Genetic basis of liver diseases (selection)

Genetic classification	Liver diseases
Hereditary monogenetic	Alpha-1-antitrypsin deficiency Arginase deficiency Arias syndrome Crigler–Najjar syndrome type I Cystic fibrosis Familial hypercholesterolemia Gaucher's disease Hemophilia A and B Hunter's disease Ornithine transcarbamylase deficiency Phenylketonuria Sly's disease Tyrosinemia Wilson's disease
Acquired monogenetic	Hepatitis A–E HCC
Acquired complex genetic	Liver fibrosis/cirrhosis HCC

TABLE 2

Concepts of gene therapy

Diseases	Gene therapy
Inherited monogenetic	Gene repair Gene replacement
Acquired monogenetic	Gene repair Gene replacement Block of gene expression or function DNA vaccination
Acquired complex genetic	Gene augmentation DNA vaccination

oligodeoxynucleotides may allow site-directed repair of point mutations [12–16]. At the RNA level, *trans*-splicing group I ribozymes have been shown to specifically modify cellular RNA species [17,18].

1.2. Block of gene expression or function

For diseases caused by the expression of acquired genes, such as viral DNA or RNA genomes, blocking gene expression or function can be an effective therapeutic approach. Several strategies can be employed: interfering with the transcription of genes by sequestration of transcription factors via binding to nucleic acids introduced into or synthesized in the cells (decoy strategy) [19,20], binding of single-stranded nucleic acids to double-stranded DNA, forming a triple helix structure [19,20], hybridization of RNA molecules possessing endonuclease activity (ribozymes) to target RNA molecules, resulting in sequence-specific RNA cleavage [21,22], blocking translation through binding of antisense oligonucleotides to RNA [19,20,23,24], and intracellular synthesis of peptides or proteins which interfere with their normal counterpart (dominant negative mutant strategy) [25], including the synthesis of intracellular antibodies ('intracellular immunization'). The peptide aptamer system is another novel genetic approach for the identification of peptides that inhibit target proteins at the intracellular level [26–31].

1.3. Gene augmentation

Complex genetic diseases are among the most prevalent clinical problems. In this situation, gene augmentation is aimed at the local expression of a therapeutic gene product that is physiologically not expressed or expressed at therapeutically insufficient levels. This strategy is being explored, among others, for the treatment of malignant diseases. The therapeutic principle is frequently a cytotoxin that ultimately leads to the elimination of the target cells. In this context, the introduction of a 'suicide gene' holds great promise. For example, as a genetic prodrug therapy, the intracellular expression of a gene encoding varizella zoster virus or herpes simplex virus thymidine kinase (VZVtk or HSVtk), followed by the administration of ganciclovir that is converted in the transduced cell to ganciclovir triphosphate, results in inhibition of alpha-DNA polymerase, DNA chain termination and death of the target cell [32,33].

1.4. DNA vaccination

The direct gene transfer into muscle [34] represents an exciting new development and elegant application of gene therapy [35,36]. The therapeutic DNA vaccine acts via the intracellular plasmid-derived synthesis of a protein which enters the MHC class I and MHC class II pathways [35]. Only proteins that originate within the cell can be processed by MHC class I molecules that carry fragments of the protein to the cell surface. There they stimulate $CD8^+$ cytotoxic T cells, resulting in cell-mediated immunity. In principle, this strategy is applicable to the treatment of diseases which are associated with the (over-)expression of disease-specific antigens, including tumor-specific antigens, that may serve as targets for $CD8^+$ cytotoxic T cells.

2. GENE THERAPY OF VIRAL HEPATITIS

Antiviral strategies are aimed at one or several steps of the viral life cycle: attachment of the virus to the cell membrane, internalization and uncoating, viral replication and gene expression, virus assembly and finally virion export. In view of the limited efficacy of currently available therapies of chronic viral hepatitis B or C [2,37], several genetic antiviral strategies are being explored. Apart from DNA vaccination [35,36,38–41], an attractive genetic antiviral concept is blocking viral gene expression or function at different levels of the viral life cycle.

2.1. Block of gene expression or function

In the following, we will briefly describe the current concepts, experimental results and potential applications of gene therapy for chronic viral hepatitis B or C, using ribozymes, antisense oligonucleotides and interfering peptides or proteins, including dominant negative (DN) mutants and aptamers.

2.1.1. Ribozymes

Ribozymes (‘ribonucleic acid enzymes’) were originally discovered as naturally occurring RNA molecules that catalyze the sequence-specific cleavage of RNA and RNA splicing reactions [21,22]. This catalytic activity is the major attraction of the ribozyme concept since one ribozyme can cleave many target RNAs. The hammerhead ribozyme consists of antisense flanking sequences mediating its binding to the target RNA as well as a conserved catalytic domain. Ribozymes that cleave RNA are being developed as inhibitors of gene expression and viral replication. Several studies have clearly demonstrated that hammerhead ribozymes can specifically cleave HBV RNA [42–49] or HCV RNA in vitro [50–57]. In vivo, an efficient ribozyme-mediated cleavage of HBV RNA could not be demonstrated to date. For HCV infection, the elimination of HCV RNA in infected hepatocytes by ribozymes has recently been reported. Phase I/II studies of an anti-HCV ribozyme (HepatzymeTM) have shown that the drug is safe and can be given as a daily at-home self-injection. Phase II studies are scheduled to investigate the efficacy of HepatzymeTM as monotherapy and in combination with interferon-alpha.

2.1.2. Antisense oligonucleotides

Antisense nucleic acids are designed to specifically bind to RNA, resulting in the formation of RNA–DNA (antisense DNA) or RNA–RNA hybrids (antisense RNA) with an arrest of RNA replication, reverse transcription or mRNA translation [19,20,23,24, 58]. Antisense effects can be potentiated by degradation of RNA in RNA–DNA hybrids by cellular RNases H. The antisense strategy has been successfully applied in vitro to HBV [59–67] and HCV infection [68–78], respectively.

In addition, studies in nude mice [79], in the duck hepatitis B virus (DHBV) [80] and the woodchuck hepatitis virus (WHV) model of HBV infection [81] demonstrated the in vivo applicability of this approach. While no toxic effects have been observed in these experiments, the contribution of non-antisense effects to the inhibition of viral replication or gene expression has not been systematically assessed in most studies. Independent of the antisense or non-antisense mechanism of the biological effects, an in vitro screening procedure for the identification of functionally active oligonucleotides [82,83] should greatly facilitate the design of oligonucleotide-based antiviral therapies.

2.1.3. Interfering peptides or proteins

The intracellular synthesis of interfering peptides or proteins, including single-chain or whole non-secreted antibodies, is aimed at the specific interference with the assembly or function of viral structural or non-structural proteins. The potential advantage of DN mutants and intracellular immunization over ribozymes or antisense oligonucleotides is their relative independence from viral sequence variations, minimizing the risk of selecting or accumulating 'therapy escape' mutants. This approach has proven effective for both mammalian and avian hepadnaviruses in cell culture experiments. Thus, the fusion of different polypeptides of various lengths to the carboxy-terminus of the viral core protein yields DN mutants [84–88]. These DN mutants are species-specific and suppress viral replication by at least 90% at an effector to target ratio of 1 : 10. Moreover, the non-secretory form of the hepatitis B e antigen (HBeAg) was shown to effectively inhibit viral replication and may indeed act as a natural regulator of HBV propagation [89–91], including the synthesis of intracellular antibodies. Intracellular immunization by intracellular expression of a single-chain antibody against HBV core protein has been experimentally explored [92]. Different from HBV, in HCV infection the DN mutant strategy has not been explored to a greater extent.

Recently, peptide aptamers targeting the HBV core protein have been identified as a new class of molecules with antiviral activity [31]. Also for the treatment of HCV infection aptamers are being evaluated [93,94].

2.1.4. DNA vaccination

Therapeutic DNA vaccination has been experimentally explored as an antiviral strategy in HBV [95–104] as well as HCV infection [105–107].

3. CURRENT ISSUES AND PERSPECTIVES

Genetically, human diseases can be classified into three major categories: (1) hereditary monogenetic diseases that are caused by a single gene defect and erited by the Mendelian rules; (2) acquired monogenetic diseases that include infections as well as some malignancies; (3) acquired complex genetic diseases which are associated with the acquisition and sequential accumulation of several genetic alterations during life-time, only some of which have been identified to date. Based on this genetic classification of diseases gene therapy involves four concepts: gene repair or substitution for the therapy of hereditary monogenetic diseases, block of gene expression or function as well as DNA vaccination for acquired monogenetic diseases and gene repair or substitution, gene augmentation and DNA vaccination for acquired complex genetic diseases.

From a genetic point of view, viral hepatitis B and C are acquired monogenetic diseases that are potentially treatable by gene therapy. Genetic antiviral strategies presently being explored are among others ribozymes, antisense oligonucleotides, interfering peptides or proteins, including DN mutants and intracellular immunization, as well as DNA vaccination. While their therapeutic potential has been clearly demonstrated in vitro, experimental studies in established or novel animal models, e.g., DHBV, WHV, nude and transgenic mouse models, will be central for the evaluation of the major current issues of gene therapy in vivo.

With the completion of the sequence of the human genome [108,109] molecular medicine and gene therapy will increasingly become part of our patient management, complementing existing diagnostic, therapeutic and preventive strategies. Despite exciting developments in molecular therapy of liver diseases, the systematic implementation of strategies to prevent or treat chronic liver diseases, including vaccination against HBV infection, reduction of alcohol consumption, elimination of aflatoxin B_1 contamination, treatment of chronic hepatitis B or C, hemochromatosis and others are of highest priority in clinical practice and have been shown to effectively reduce liver-related morbidity and mortality. Along these lines, the worldwide immunization against HBV as well as the development of a vaccine against HCV infection are of paramount clinical and epidemiological importance. Recent advances in vaccine development, including oral immunization against HBV using HBsAg transgenic plants [110] and DNA vaccination against HBV infection, including topical application of HBV DNA to the skin [111–113], and against HCV infection [114–125] will eventually allow the universal vaccination against HBV and HCV infection.

REFERENCES

[1] Lee WM. Hepatitis B virus infection. N Engl J Med 1997; 337: 1733–1745.

[2] Liang TJ, Rehermann B, Seeff LB, Hoofnagle JH. Pathogenesis, natural history, treatment, and prevention of hepatitis C. Ann Intern Med 2000; 132(4): 296–305.

[3] Seeff LB, Miller RN, Rabkin CS, Buskell-Bales Z, Straley-Eason KD, Smoak BL et al. 45-year follow-up of hepatitis C virus infection in healthy young adults. Ann Intern Med 2000; 132(2): 105–111.

[4] Seeff LB, Hollinger FB, Alter HJ, Wright EC, Cain CM, Buskell ZJ et al. Long-term

mortality and morbidity of transfusion-associated non-A, non-B, and type C hepatitis: A National Heart, Lung, and Blood Institute collaborative study. Hepatology 2001; 33(2): 455–463.
[5] Lauer GM, Walker BD. Hepatitis C virus infection. N Engl J Med 2001; 345(1): 41–52.
[6] Di Bisceglie AM. Natural history of hepatitis C: its impact on clinical management. Hepatology 2000; 31(4): 1014–1018.
[7] Malik AH, Lee WM. Chronic hepatitis B virus infection: treatment strategies for the next millennium. Ann Intern Med 2001; 132: 723–731.
[8] Torresi J, Locarnini S. Antiviral chemotherapy for the treatment of hepatitis B virus infections. Gastroenterology 2000; 118(2 Suppl. 1): S83–103.
[9] Lok AS, Heathcote EJ, Hoofnagle JH. Management of hepatitis B: 2000 — summary of a workshop. Gastroenterology 2001; 120(7): 1828–1853.
[10] Davis GL. Current therapy for chronic hepatitis C. Gastroenterology 2000; 118(2 Suppl. 1): S104–114.
[11] Morgan RA, Anderson WF. Human gene therapy. Annu Rev Biochem 1993; 62: 191–217.
[12] Kren BT, Cole-Strauss A, Kmiec EB, Steer CJ. Targeted nucleotide exchange in the alkaline phosphatase gene of HuH-7 cells mediated by a chimeric RNA/DNA oligonucleotide. Hepatology 1997; 25: 1462–1468.
[13] Kren BT, Bandyopadhyay P, Steer CJ. In vivo site-directed mutagenesis of the factor IX gene by chimeric RNA/DNA oligonucleotides [see comments]. Nat Med 1998; 4(3): 285–290.
[14] Bandyopadhyay P, Ma X, Linehan-Stieers C, Kren BT, Steer CJ. Nucleotide exchange in genomic DNA of rat hepatocytes using RNA/DNA oligonucleotides. Targeted delivery of liposomes and polyethyleneimine to the asialoglycoprotein receptor. J Biol Chem 1999; 274(15): 10163–1072.
[15] Kren BT, Metz R, Kumar R, Steer CJ. Gene repair using chimeric RNA/DNA oligonucleotides. Semin Liver Dis 1999; 19(1): 93–104.
[16] Kren BT, Parashar B, Bandyopadhyay P, Chowdhury R, Chowdhury JR, Steer CJ. Correction of the UDP-glucuronosyltransferase gene defect in the Gunn rat model of Crigler–Najjar syndrome type I with a chimeric oligonucleotide. Proc Natl Acad Sci USA 1999; 96: 10349–10354.
[17] Sarver N, Cairns S. Ribozyme trans-splicing and RNA tagging: following the messenger. Nat Med 1996; 2: 641–642.
[18] Jones JT, Lee SW, Sullenger BA. Tagging ribozyme reaction sites to follow trans-splicing in mammalian cells. Nat Med 1996; 2: 643–648.
[19] Helene C. Rational design of sequence-specific oncogene ibitors based on antisense and antigene oligonucleotides. Eur J Cancer 1991; 27(11): 1466–1471.
[20] Helene C, Toulme JJ. Specific regulation of gene expression by antisense, sense and antigene nucleic acids. Biochim Biophys Acta 1990; 1049(2): 99–125.
[21] Haseloff J, Gerlach WL. Simple RNA enzymes with new and highly specific endoribonuclease activities. Nature 1988; 334(6183): 585–591.
[22] Thompson JD, Macejak D, Couture L, Stinchcomb DT. Ribozymes in gene therapy. Nat Med 1995; 1(3): 277–278.
[23] Calabretta B. Inhibition of protooncogene expression by antisense oligodeoxynucleotides: biological and therapeutic implications. Cancer Res 1991; 51(17): 4505–4510.
[24] Tseng BY, Brown, K.D. Antisense oligonucleotide technology in the development of cancer therapeutics. Cancer Gene Ther 1994; 1: 65–71.
[25] Herschkowitz I. Functional inactivation of genes by dominant negative mutations. Nature 1987; 329: 219–222.

[26] Colas P, Cohen B, Jessen T, Grishina I, McCoy J, Brent R. Genetic selection of peptide aptamers that recognize and ibit cyclin-dependent kinase 2. Nature 1996; 380(6574): 548–550.
[27] Cohen BA, Colas P, Brent R. An artificial cell-cycle ibitor isolated from a combinatorial library. Proc Natl Acad Sci USA 1998; 95(24): 14272–14277.
[28] Kolonin MG, Finley RL Jr. Targeting cyclin-dependent kinases in Drosophila with peptide aptamers. Proc Natl Acad Sci USA 1998; 95(24): 14266–14271.
[29] Butz K, Denk C, Ullmann A, Scheffner M, Hoppe-Seyler F. Induction of apoptosis in human papilloma viruspositive cancer cells by peptide aptamers targeting the viral E6 oncoprotein. Proc Natl Acad Sci USA 2000; 97(12): 6693–6697.
[30] Hoppe-Seyler F, Butz K. Peptide aptamers: powerful new tools for molecular medicine. J Mol Med 2000; 78(8): 426–430.
[31] Butz K, Denk C, Fitscher B, Crnkovic-Mertens I, Ullmann A, Schröder CH et al. Peptide aptamers targeting the hepatitis B virus core protein: a new class of molecules with antiviral activity. Oncogene 2001; 20(45): 6579–6586.
[32] Caruso M, Panis Y, Gagandeep S, Houssin D, Salzmann J-L, Klatzmann D. Regression of established macroscopic liver metastases after in situ transduction of a suicide gene. Proc Natl Acad Sci USA 1993; 90: 7024–7028.
[33] Martin LA, Vile R, Lemoine NR, Sikora K, Pandha HS. Genetic prodrug activation therapy. Lancet 1997; 350: 1793–1794.
[34] Wolff JA, Malone RW, Williams P, Chong W, Acsadi G, Jani A et al. Direct gene transfer into mouse muscle in vivo. Science 1990; 247: 1465–1468.
[35] McDonnell WM, Askari FK. DNA vaccines. N Engl J Med 1996; 334(1): 42–45.
[36] Pardoll DM, Beckerleg AM. Exposing the immunology of naked DNA vaccines. Immunity 1995; 3: 165–169.
[37] Hoofnagle JH, Di Bisceglie AM. The treatment of chronic viral hepatitis. N Engl J Med 1997; 336: 347–356.
[38] Blau HM, Springer ML. Muscle mediated gene therapy. N Engl J Med 1995; 333(23): 1554–1556.
[39] Kumar V, Sercarz E. Genetic vaccination: the advantages of going naked. Nat Med 1996; 2: 857–859.
[40] Condon C, Watkins SC, Celluzzi CM, Thompson K, Falo LD Jr. DNA-based immunization by in vivo transfection of dendritic cells. Nat Med 1996; 2: 1122–1128.
[41] Conry RM, Widera G, Lobuglio AF, Fuller JT, Moore SE, Barlow DL et al. Selected strategies to augment polynucleotide immunization. Gene Ther 1996; 3: 67–74.
[42] Von Weizsäcker F, Blum HE, Wands JR. Cleavage of hepatitis B virus RNA by three ribozymes transcribed from a single DNA template. Biochem Biophys Res Commun 1992; 189(2): 743–748.
[43] Beck J, Nassal M. Efficient hammerhead ribozyme-mediated cleavage of the structured hepatitis B virus encapsidation signal in vitro and in cell extracts, but not in intact cells. Nucl Acids Res 1995; 23: 4954–4962.
[44] Kim YK, Junn E, Park I, Lee Y, Kang C, Ahn JK. Repression of hepatitis B virus X gene expression by hammerhead ribozymes [published erratum appears in Biochem Biophys Res Commun 1999; 259(1): 231]. Biochem Biophys Res Commun 1999; 257(3): 759–765.
[45] Zu Putlitz J, Yu Q, Burke JM, Wands JR. Combinatorial screening and intracellular antiviral activity of hairpin ribozymes directed against hepatitis B virus. J Virol 1999; 73(7): 5381–5387.
[46] Welch PJ, Tritz R, Yei S, Barber J, Yu M. Intracellular application of hairpin ribozyme genes against hepatitis B virus. Gene Ther 1997; 4(7): 736–743.

[47] Ruiz J, Wu CH, Ito Y, Wu GY. Design and preparation of a multimeric self-cleaving hammerhead ribozyme. Biotechniques 1997; 22(2): 338–345.
[48] Feng Y, Kong YY, Wang Y, Qi GR. Inhibition of hepatitis B virus by hammerhead ribozyme targeted to the poly(A) signal sequence in cultured cells. Biol Chem 2001; 382(4): 655–660.
[49] Weinberg M, Passman M, Kew M, Arbuthnot P. Hammerhead ribozyme-mediated inhibition of hepatitis B virus X gene expression in cultured cells. J Hepatol 2000; 33(1): 142–151.
[50] Welch PJ, Tritz R, Yei S, Leavitt M, Yu M, Barber J. A potential therapeutic application of hairpin ribozymes — in vitro and in vivo studies of gene therapy for hepatitis C virus infection. Gene Ther 1996; 3: 994–1001.
[51] Lieber A, He C-Y, Polyak SJ, Gretch DR, Barr D, Kay MA. Elimination of hepatitis C virus RNA in infected human hepatocytes by adenovirus-mediated expression of ribozymes. J Virol 1996; 70: 8782–8791.
[52] Sakamoto N, Wu CH, Wu GY. Intracellular cleavage of hepatitis C virus RNA and inhibition of viral protein translation by hammerhead ribozymes. J Clin Invest 1996; 98: 2720–2728.
[53] Welch PJ, Yei S, Barber JR. Ribozyme gene therapy for hepatitis C virus infection. Clin Diagn Virol 1998; 10(2–3): 163–171.
[54] Ohkawa K, Yuki N, Kanazawa Y, Ueda K, Mita E, Sasaki Y et al. Cleavage of viral RNA and inhibition of viral translation by hepatitis C virus RNA-specific hammerhead ribozyme in vitro. J Hepatol 1997; 27(1): 78–84.
[55] Macejak DG, Jensen KL, Jamison SF, Domenico K, Roberts EC, Chaudhary N et al. Inhibition of hepatitis C virus (HCV)-RNA-dependent translation and replication of a chimeric HCV poliovirus using synthetic stabilized ribozymes. Hepatology 2000; 31(3): 769–776.
[56] Lee PA, Blatt LM, Blanchard KS, Bouhana KS, Pavco PA, Bellon L et al. Pharmacokinetics and tissue distribution of a ribozyme directed against hepatitis C virus RNA following subcutaneous or intravenous administration in mice. Hepatology 2000; 32(3): 640–646.
[57] Oketani M, Asahina Y, Wu CH, Wu GY. Inhibition of hepatitis C virus-directed gene expression by a DNA ribonuclease. J Hepatol 1999; 31(4): 628–634.
[58] Wagner RW. Gene inhibition using antisense oligodeoxynucleotides. Nature 1994; 372(6504): 333–335.
[59] Goodarzi G, Gross SC, Tewari A, Watabe K. Antisense oligodeoxyribonucleotides ibit the expression of the gene for hepatitis B virus surface antigen. J Gen Virol 1990; 71: 3021–3025.
[60] Blum HE, Galun E, Weizsäcker F, Wands JR. Inhibition of hepatitis B virus by antisense oligodeoxynucleotides. Lancet 1991; 337(8751): 1230.
[61] Wu GY, Wu CH. Specific inhibition of hepatitis B viral gene expression in vitro by targeted antisense oligonucleotides. J Biol Chem 1992; 267(18): 12436–12439.
[62] Nakazono K, Ito Y, Wu CH, Wu GY. Inhibition of hepatitis B virus replication by targeted pretreatment of complexed antisense DNA in vitro. Hepatology 1996; 23: 1297–1303.
[63] Offensperger WB, Offensperger S, Blum HE. Antisense therapy of hepatitis B virus infection. Mol Biotechnol 1998; 9(2): 161–170.
[64] Soni PN, Brown D, Saffie R, Savage K, Moore D, Gregoriadis G et al. Biodistribution, stability, and antiviral efficacy of liposome-entrapped phosphorothioate antisense oligodeoxynucleotides in ducks for the treatment of chronic duck hepatitis B virus infection. Hepatology 1998; 28(5): 1402–1410.
[65] Zoulim F, Trepo C. New antiviral agents for the therapy of chronic hepatitis B virus infection. Intervirology 1999; 42(2–3): 125–144.

[66] Offensperger WB, Thoma C, Moradpour D, von Weizsäcker F, Offensperger S, Blum HE. Antisense oligonucleotide therapy of hepadnavirus infection. Methods Enzymol 2000; 314: 524–536.
[67] Robaczewska M, Guerret S, Remy JS, Chemin I, Offensperger WB, Chevallier M et al. Inhibition of hepadnaviral replication by polyethylenimine-based intravenous delivery of antisense phosphodiester oligodeoxynucleotides to the liver. Gene Ther 2001; 8(11): 874–881.
[68] Wakita T, Wands JR. Specific inhibition of hepatitis C virus expression by antisense oligodeoxynucleotides. In vitro model for selection of target sequence. J Biol Chem 1994; 269(19): 14205–14210.
[69] Mizutani T, Kato N, Saito S, Ikeda M, Sugiyama K, Shimotohno K. Characterization of hepatitis C virus replication in cloned cells obtained from a human T-cell leukemia virus type 1-infected cell line, MT-2. J Virol 1996; 70(10): 7219–7223.
[70] Alt M, Renz R, Hofschneider PH, Paumgartner G, Caselmann WH. Specific inhibition of hepatitis C viral gene expression by antisense phosphorothioate oligodeoxynucleotides. Hepatology 1995; 22(3): 707–717.
[71] Seki M, Honda Y. Phosphorothioate antisense oligodeoxynucleotides capable of inhibiting hepatitis C virus gene expression: in vitro translation assay. J Biochem 1995; 118: 1199–1204.
[72] Hanecak R, Brown-Driver V, Fox MC, Azad RF, Furusako S, Nozaki C et al. Antisense oligonucleotide inhibition of hepatitis C virus gene expression in transformed hepatocytes. J Virol 1996; 70: 5203–5212.
[73] Vidalin O, Major ME, Rayner B, Imbach JL, Trepo C, Inchauspe G. In vitro inhibition of hepatitis C virus gene expression by chemically modified antisense oligodeoxynucleotides. Antimicrob Agents Chemother 1996; 40: 2337–2344.
[74] Alt M, Eisenhardt S, Serwe M, Renz R, Engels JW, Caselmann WH. Comparative ibitory potential of differently modified antisense oligodeoxynucleotides on hepatitis C virus translation. Eur J Clin Invest 1999; 29(10): 868–876.
[75] Lehmann TJ, Eisenhardt S, Engels JW. Thermodynamic studies on hairpin forming antisense-oligodeoxynucleotides directed against hepatitis C virus RNA. Nucleosides Nucleotides 1999; 18(6–7): 1689–1691.
[76] Brown-Driver V, Eto T, Lesnik E, Anderson KP, Hanecak RC. Inhibition of translation of hepatitis C virus RNA by 2-modified antisense oligonucleotides. Antisense Nucleic Acid Drug Dev 1999; 9(2): 145–154.
[77] Zhang H, Hanecak R, Brown-Driver V, Azad R, Conklin B, Fox MC et al. Antisense oligonucleotide inhibition of hepatitis C virus (HCV) gene expression in livers of mice infected with an HCV-vaccinia virus recombinant. Antimicrobiol Agents Chemother 1999; 43(2): 347–353.
[78] Wu CH, Wu GY. Targeted inhibition of hepatitis C virus-directed gene expression in human hepatoma cell lines. Gastroenterology 1998; 114(6): 1304–1312.
[79] Yao Z, Zhou Y, Feng X, Chen C, Guo J. In vivo inhibition of hepatitis B viral gene expression by antisense phosphorothioate oligodeoxynucleotides in athymic nude mice. J Viral Hepat 1996; 3: 19–22.
[80] Offensperger WB, Offensperger S, Walter E, Teubner K, Igloi G, Blum HE et al. In vivo inhibition of duck hepatitis B virus replication and gene expression by phosphorothioate modified antisense oligodeoxynucleotides. EMBO J 1993; 12(3): 1257–1262.
[81] Bartholomew RM, Carmichael EP, Findeis MA, Wu CH, Wu GY. Targeted delivery of antisense DNA in woodchuck hepatitis virus-infected woodchucks. J Viral Hepat 1995; 2: 273–278.

[82] Branch AD. A hitchhiker's guide to antisense and nonantisense biochemical pathways. Hepatology 1996; 24: 1517–1529.
[83] Tuerk C, Gold L. Systematic evolution of ligands by exponential enrichment: RNA ligands to bacteriophage T4 DNA polymerase. Science 1990; 249: 505–510.
[84] Delaney MA, Goyal S, Seeger C. Design of modified core genes that ibit replication of woodchuck hepatitis virus. In: Hollinger FB, Lemon SM, Margolis H, editors. Viral hepatitis and liver disease. Baltimore, MD: Williams and Wilkins, 1991; pp. 667–668.
[85] Scaglioni PP, Melegari M, Wands JR. Characterization of hepatitis B virus core mutants that ibit viral replication. Virology 1994; 205(1): 112–120.
[86] Scaglioni P, Melegari M, Takahashi M, Chowdhury JR, Wands J. Use of dominant negative mutants of the hepadnaviral core protein as antiviral agents. Hepatology 1996; 24: 1010–1017.
[87] Von Weizsäcker F, Wieland S, Blum HE. Inhibition of viral replication by genetically engineered mutants of the duck hepatitis B virus core protein. Hepatology 1996; 24: 294–299.
[88] Von Weizsäcker F, Köck J, Wieland S, Offensperger WB, Blum HE. Dominant negative mutants of the duck hepatitis B virus core protein interfere with RNA pregenome packaging and viral DNA synthesis. Hepatology 1999; 30(1): 308–315.
[89] Scaglioni PP, Melegari M, Wands JR. Posttranscriptional regulation of hepatitis B virus replication by the precore protein. J Virol 1997; 71: 345–353.
[90] Buckwold VE, Xu Z, Chen M, Yen TSB, Ou J-H. Effects of a naturally occurring mutation in the hepatitis B virus basal core promoter on precore gene expression and viral replication. J Virol 1996; 70: 5845–5851.
[91] Guidotti LG, Ishikawa T, Hobbs MV, Matzke B, Schreiber R, Chisari FV. Intracellular inactivation of the hepatitis B virus by cytotoxic T lymphocytes. Immunity 1996; 4: 25–36.
[92] Yamamoto M, Hayashi N, Takehara T, Ueda K, Mita E, Tatsumi T et al. Intracellular single-chain antibody against hepatitis B virus core protein ibits the replication of hepatitis B virus in cultured cells. Hepatology 1999; 30(1): 300–307.
[93] Hwang J, Fauzi H, Fukuda K, Sekiya S, Kakiuchi N, Shimotohno K et al. The RNA aptamer-binding site of hepatitis C virus NS3 protease. Biochem Biophys Res Commun 2000; 279(2): 557–562.
[94] Fukuda K, Vishnuvardhan D, Sekiya S, Hwang J, Kakiuchi N, Taira K et al. Isolation and characterization of RNA aptamers specific for the hepatitis C virus nonstructural protein 3 protease. Eur J Biochem 2000; 267(12): 3685–3694.
[95] Schirmbeck R, Bohm W, Ando K, Chisari FV, Reimann J. Nucleic acid vaccination primes hepatitis B virus surface antigen specific cytotoxic T lymphocytes in nonresponder mice. J Virol 1995; 69(10): 5929–5934.
[96] Vitiello A, Ishioka G, Grey HM, Rose R, Farness P, LaFond R et al. Development of a lipopeptide based therapeutic vaccine to treat chronic HBV infection, I. Induction of a primary cytotoxic T lymphocyte response in humans. J Clin Invest 1995; 95(1): 341–349.
[97] Kuhöber A, Pudollek HP, Reifenberg K, Chisari FV, Schlicht HJ, Reimann J et al. DNA immunization induces antibody and cytotoxic T cell responses to hepatitis B core antigen in H-2b mice. J Immunol 1996; 156: 3687–3695.
[98] Davis HL, Schirmbeck R, Reimann J, Whalen RG. DNA-mediated immunization in mice induces a potent MHC class I-restricted cytotoxic T lymphocyte response to the hepatitis B envelope protein. Hum Gene Ther 1995; 6: 1447–1456.
[99] Mancini M, Hadchouel M, Davis HL, Whalen RG, Tiollais P, Michel M-L. DNA-mediated immunization in a transgenic mouse model of the hepatitis B surface antigen chronic carrier state. Proc Natl Acad Sci USA 1996; 93: 12496–12501.

[100] Sallberg M, Hughes J, Javadian A, Ronlov G, Hultgren C, Townsend K et al. Genetic immunization of chimpanzees chronically infected with the hepatitis B virus, using a recombinant retroviral vector encoding the hepatitis B virus core antigen. Hum Gene Ther 1998; 9(12): 1719–1729.
[101] Pancholi P, Lee DH, Liu Q, Tackney C, Taylor P, Perkus M et al. DNA prime/canarypox boost-based immunotherapy of chronic hepatitis B virus infection in a chimpanzee. Hepatology 2001; 33(2): 448–454.
[102] Bocher WO, Dekel B, Schwerin W, Geissler M, Hoffmann S, Rohwer A et al. Induction of strong hepatitis B virus (HBV) specific T helper cell and cytotoxic T lymphocyte responses by therapeutic vaccination in the trimera mouse model of chronic HBV infection. Eur J Immunol 2001; 31(7): 2071–2079.
[103] Heathcote J, McHutchison J, Lee S, Tong M, Benner K, Minuk G et al. A pilot study of the CY-1899 T-cell vaccine in subjects chronically infected with hepatitis B virus. The CY1899 T Cell Vaccine Study Group. Hepatology 1999; 30(2): 531–536.
[104] Lu M, Hilken G, Kruppenbacher J, Kemper T, Schirmbeck R, Reimann J et al. Immunization of woodchucks with plasmids expressing woodchuck hepatitis virus (WHV) core antigen and surface antigen suppresses WHV infection. J Virol 1999; 73(1): 281–289.
[105] Lagging LM, Meyer K, Hoft D, Houghton M, Belshe RB, Ray R. Immune responses to plasmid DNA encoding the hepatitis C virus core protein. J Virol 1995; 69(9): 5859–5863.
[106] Major ME, Vitvitski L, Mink MA, Schleef M, Whalen RG, Trepo C et al. DNA based immunization with chimeric vectors for the induction of immune responses against the hepatitis C virus nucleocapsid. J Virol 1995; 69(9): 5798–5805.
[107] Tokushige K, Wakita T, Pachuk C, Moradpour D, Weiner DB, Zurawski Jr. VR et al. Expression and immune response to hepatitis C virus core DNA-based vaccine constructs. Hepatology 1996; 24: 14–20.
[108] Consortium IHGS. Initial sequencing and analysis of the human genome. Nature 2001; 409: 860–921.
[109] Venter JC, Adams MD, Myers EW, Li PW, Mural RJ, Sutton GG et al. The sequence of the human genome. Science 2001; 291: 1304–1351.
[110] Richter LJ, Thanavala Y, Arntzen CJ, Mason HS. Production of hepatitis B surface antigen in transgenic plants for oral immunization. Nat Biotechnol 2000; 18(11): 1167–1171.
[111] Fan H, Lin Q, Morrissey GR, Khavari PA. Immunization via hair follicles by topical application of naked DNA to normal skin. Nat Biotechnol 1999; 17(9): 870–872.
[112] Siegel F, Lu M, Roggendorf M. Coadministration of gamma interferon with DNA vaccine expressing woodchuck hepatitis virus (WHV) core antigen enhances the specific immune response and protects against WHV infection. J Virol 2001; 75(11): 5036–5042.
[113] Roh S, Lee YK, Ahn BY, Kim K, Moon A. Induction of CTL responses and identification of a novel epitope of hepatitis B virus surface antigens in C57BL/6 mice immunized with recombinant vaccinia viruses. Virus Res 2001; 73(1): 17–26.
[114] Forns X, Payette PJ, Ma X, Satterfield W, Eder G, Mushahwar IK et al. Vaccination of chimpanzees with plasmid DNA encoding the hepatitis C virus (HCV) envelope E2 protein modified the infection after challenge with homologous monoclonal HCV. Hepatology 2000; 32(3): 618–625.
[115] Lazdina U, Hultgren C, Frelin L, Chen M, Lodin K, Weiland O et al. Humoral and CD4(+) T helper (Th) cell responses to the hepatitis C virus non-structural 3 (NS3) protein: NS3 primes Th1-like responses more effectively as a DNA-based immunogen than as a recombinant protein. J Gen Virol 2001; 82(Pt 6): 1299–1308.
[116] Nemchinov LG, Liang TJ, Rifaat MM, Mazyad HM, Hadidi A, Keith JM. Development of a plant-derived subunit vaccine candidate against hepatitis C virus. Arch Virol 2000;

145(12): 2557–2573.

[117] Duenas-Carrera S, Alvarez-Lajonchere L, Alvarez-Obregon JC, Herrera A, Lorenzo LJ, Pichardo D et al. A truncated variant of the hepatitis C virus core induces a slow but potent immune response in mice following DNA immunization. Vaccine 2000; 19(7–8): 992–997.

[118] Pancholi P, Liu Q, Tricoche N, Zhang P, Perkus ME, Prince AM. DNA prime-canarypox boost with polycistronic hepatitis C virus (HCV) genes generates potent immune responses to HCV structural and nonstructural proteins. J Infect Dis 2000; 182(1): 18–27.

[119] Gordon EJ, Bhat R, Liu Q, Wang YF, Tackney C, Prince AM. Immune responses to hepatitis C virus structural and nonstructural proteins induced by plasmid DNA immunizations. J Infect Dis 2000; 181(1): 42–50.

[120] Houghton M, Gordon EJ, Bhat R, Liu Q, Wang YF, Tackney C et al. Strategies and prospects for vaccination against the hepatitis C viruses. Curr Top Microbiol Immunol 2000; 242(1): 327–339.

[121] Nishimura Y, Kamei A, Uno-Furuta S, Tamaki S, Kim G, Adachi Y et al. A single immunization with a plasmid encoding hepatitis C virus (HCV) structural proteins under the elongation factor 1-alpha promoter elicits HCV-specific cytotoxic T-lymphocytes (CTL). Vaccine 1999; 18(7–8): 675–680.

[122] Hu GJ, Wang RY, Han DS, Alter HJ, Shih JW. Characterization of the humoral and cellular immune responses against hepatitis C virus core induced by DNA-based immunization. Vaccine 1999; 17(23–24): 3160–3170.

[123] Fournillier A, Depla E, Karayiannis P, Vidalin O, Maertens G, Trepo C et al. Expression of noncovalent hepatitis C virus envelope E1–E2 complexes is not required for the induction of antibodies with neutralizing properties following DNA immunization. J Virol 1999; 73(9): 7497–7504.

[124] Cho JH, Lee SW, Sung YC. Enhanced cellular immunity to hepatitis C virus nonstructural proteins by codelivery of granulocyte macrophage-colony stimulating factor gene in intramuscular DNA immunization. Vaccine 1999; 17(9–10): 1136–1144.

[125] Weiner AJ, Paliard X, Selby MJ, Medina-Selby A, Coit D, Nguyen S et al. Intrahepatic genetic inoculation of hepatitis C virus RNA confers cross-protective immunity. J Virol 2001; 75(15): 7142–7148.

Liver Cirrhosis

Molecular Biology and Immunology in Hepatology
Edited by T. Tsuji, T. Higashi, M. Zeniya and K.-H. Meyer zum Büschenfelde

CHAPTER 9

Reversibility of Liver Cirrhosis: Evidence from Clinical and Basic Research

Akiharu Watanabe

Third Department of Internal Medicine, Faculty of Medicine, Toyama Medical and Pharmaceutical University, Toyama, Japan

INTRODUCTION

In chronic liver diseases, irrespective of its cause, the development of liver fibrosis is the greatest problem because of progression to liver cirrhosis. With progression of liver fibrosis, extracellular matrix such as types I, III, and IV collagens, laminin, fibronectin and others deposits in Disse's space, and sinusoidal endothelial cells form a basement membrane similar to that in general vascular endothelial cells, resulting in a phenomenon called sinusoidal capillarization [1].

Clarification of the types and roles of cells producing extracellular matrix, and the molecular mechanism and its control system of matrix synthesis and degradation has led to the development of drugs for liver fibrosis [2]. This was initiated by clinical improvement and disappearance of liver fibrosis observed after treatment of chronic hepatitis C with interferon (IFN) [3]. Though the reversibility of liver cirrhosis cannot be discussed based on improvement of liver fibrosis alone, liver cirrhosis cannot be reversed without improvement in liver fibrosis. Liver cirrhosis is regarded as reversible only when the following findings are obtained: (1) normalization of all parameters of liver function tests; (2) disappearance of clinical symptoms; (3) disappearance of histological findings of liver cirrhosis, i.e., restoration of the normal hepatic lobular architecture and disappearance of regenerating nodules; and (4) normalization of the portal pressure and disappearance of collateral vessels (portosystemic shunting) even if it is functional disappearance.

1. DIAGNOSTIC CRITERIA OF LIVER CIRRHOSIS

In the diagnosis of liver cirrhosis, morphological criteria, i.e., diffuse liver fibrosis and resulting remodeling of the hepatic lobular architecture and formation of regenerating nodules (pseudolobules), have been considered to be important. In addition, with progression of liver cirrhosis, the diameter and number of pores in sinusoidal endothelial cells decrease, and a basement membrane forms (formation of continuous endothelial cell with type IV collagen and laminin) immediately below sinusoidal endothelial cells (sinusoidal capillarization). These changes are clinically very important. When various molecules, such as glucose and bilirubin in the blood, pass through sinusoids, these changes obstruct their diffusion through numerous pores in sinusoidal endothelial cells to hepatic cells via Disse's space. In addition, these molecules exchange between intrahepatic circulating blood and hepatic cells are inhibited, inducing further hepatocyte damage, which may be involved in the progression of liver fibrosis (vicious circle). In the cirrhotic liver, sinusoidal stricture occurs because of contraction of perisinusoidal stellate cells [4] and enlargement of Disse's space due to fiber deposition, and then the portal pressure increases (portal hypertension). As a result, collateral vessels (portosystemic shunts) such as esophageal varices form.

Liver morphology and function in liver cirrhosis vary depending upon its clinical state and pathophysiologic conditions. Even in the same liver, morphological findings differ among areas. Therefore, the morphological diagnosis of liver cirrhosis has limitations. Despite recent advances in diagnostic imaging (noninvasive) methods, such as high performance ultrasonography, CT and MRI of the liver, there is no clinically applicable international diagnostic criteria for liver cirrhosis independent of morphological findings of the liver.

In advanced liver cirrhosis with atrophy accompanied by typical nodule formation and highly developed collateral circulation, its diagnosis is easy based on clinical findings, examination results and laboratory data. However, in recent years, opportunities to follow-up patients with chronic hepatitis for a long period have been increasing, and during this follow-up, the transition period from chronic hepatitis to liver cirrhosis has been evaluated [5]. Therefore, differentiation between chronic hepatitis and early liver cirrhosis or pre-cirrhosis is difficult. The answer to the question "Is liver cirrhosis a reversible disease?" may change whether only advanced liver cirrhosis alone is defined as liver cirrhosis in the narrow sense (terminal stage of liver disease and irreversible pathophysiologic condition of the liver).

From these aspects, it is necessary to establish the diagnostic criteria for liver cirrhosis that are also useful for evaluating liver reserve function and prognosis from clinical findings. As such attempts, some equations for discriminating chronic hepatitis from liver cirrhosis have been proposed [6]. Ikeda et al. [7] proposed the following discriminant and showed its usefulness: $Z = 0.12 \times (\gamma\text{-globulin, \%}) + 0.001 \times (\text{hyaluronic acid, } \mu g/l) - 0.075 \times (\text{platelet count, } \times 10^4/\mu l) - 0.413 \times \text{sex (male, 1; female 2)} - 2.005$. The Japanese Society of Gastroenterology is also evaluating the clinical diagnostic criteria for liver cirrhosis, making efforts to establish new diagnostic principles mainly for a classification according to long-term prognosis [8].

2. DIFFICULTY IN DIAGNOSING LIVER CIRRHOSIS — EVALUATION OF THE TRANSITION PERIOD FROM CHRONIC HEPATITIS TO LIVER CIRRHOSIS

With marked advances in hepatology, the causes of liver diseases have been clarified, and findings of liver biopsy under ultrasonography, which can be readily and safely performed, have become important in evaluating the effectiveness of radical treatment. Detailed long-term observation of the course of chronic hepatitis by this method has allowed evaluation of the transition period from chronic hepatitis to liver cirrhosis. Therefore, we have increased the opportunity of encountering patients with lesions that can be interpreted as both progressed hepatitis and early cirrhosis.

The progression process from chronic hepatitis to liver cirrhosis is morphologically continuous, and a line differentiating between them cannot be drawn. First, findings resembling liver cirrhosis appear in parts of hepatitis lesions. These cirrhotic parts gradually increase, and eventually, the entire liver becomes cirrhotic. Therefore, the differentiation between chronic hepatitis showing remodeling of the hepatic lobular architecture and early liver cirrhosis is difficult. In their differentiation, attention should be paid to the fact that fibrous connection between portal areas (P–P) or between portal areas and central venous areas (P–C) is not equal to remodeling of the hepatic lobular architecture. For correct evaluation of this state, an adequate amount of liver biopsy tissue should be obtained so that the distribution of P–C fibrosis and the mutual relationship among P–C fibrotic lesions can be evaluated at a low magnification of microscope. In liver biopsy under ultrasonograpy using a thin Majima needle (17 gauge) [9], pseudolobule formation in macronodular liver cirrhosis sometimes cannot be confirmed, and diffuse liver fibrosis and the presence of regenerating nodules in the entire liver cannot be accurately evaluated in biopsied liver (about 1/50,000 of the whole liver weight). Therefore, a thick biopsy needle is necessary to obtain adequate tissue for accurate pathological diagnosis. A previous study [10] evaluated the consistency between the degree of fibrosis examined by biopsy under laparoscopy using a Silverman needle (14 gauge) and that examined by biopsy of the same site using a Majima needle. The inconsistency rate was 61.1% at 300–400 code number of the liver surface, and the degree of fibrosis was underestimated by liver biopsy using a 17-gauge needle. Attention should be also paid that fibrosis is generally less advanced in deep areas of the liver than in their shallow areas closer to the liver surface that can be laparoscopically observed.

3. PARAMETERS FOR EVALUATION OF 'IMPROVEMENT IN LIVER FIBROSIS'

For follow-up of the pathology of liver fibrosis and evaluation of treatment effects by comparing pre- and post-treatment states, an objective evaluation method that can be commonly performed at institutions is necessary. This is because the degree of improvement in liver fibrosis may differ according to the evaluation methods.

3.1. Fiber-stained specimens of liver tissue

In general, the degree of liver fibrosis has qualitatively been evaluated in fiber-stained specimens of liver tissue (azan staining for collagen fibers; elastica staining for elastic fibers, silver impregnation method for reticular fibers). In Japan, the degree of fibrosis has been expressed as the stage according to a new histological diagnostic criterion of chronic hepatitis (new Inuyama's Classification) [11]. The progression of fibrosis from early fibrosis in portal areas, through lobular remodeling, to liver cirrhosis consists of the following five stages: F0, no fibrosis; F1, fibrous extension of portal areas: F2, bridging fibrosis; F3, bridging fibrosis accompanied by lobular strain and F4, nodule formation tendency in the entire liver (completion of nodular hypertrophy) defined as liver cirrhosis.

However, since histological evaluation always produces differences according to the diagnostic standards and ability of individual pathologists, objectivity and high reproducibility are required. Previous studies have shown that staging of fibrosis is universal and produces no marked differences in interpretation among pathologists compared with the vague histological criteria of the activity of necrosis and inflammatory reactions [12]. Of course, fibrosis in liver biopsy specimens should be comprehensively evaluated based on findings in the entire liver, not in areas with the most advanced fibrosis.

Internationally, the histological activity index (HAI) score proposed by Knodell et al. [13] is frequently used. For example, the following scoring is done for 'IV. fibrosis in portal areas': no fibrosis (0), mild fibrosis (1), moderate fibrosis (3), and severe fibrosis (4). However, many authors consider this method to be inappropriate for evaluating liver pathology (fibrosis) before and after IFN therapy for chronic hepatitis [12], suggesting that addition of the score for the three activity categories and that for one fibrosis category is a problem.

Quantitative morphometry by fiber staining has higher quality and is used as a sensitive histological evaluation method before and after treatment [14]. In the conventional method, the area of fibrotic parts is quantitatively measured in azan staining specimens using an image cytometer [15]. In another method, the change per year in the amount of intrahepatic fibers is calculated based on fiber-stained specimens of liver tissue obtained by repeated liver biopsy, and the period (year) until recovery to a normal liver is estimated by extrapolation of this value [16].

There is also a method in which the area showing collagen fiber deposition within a certain area in Sirius (Fast) red staining specimens is obtained as a fibrosis rate using a computer automatic image (analysis) processor [14]. In another method, many areas around the central vein or Zone 2 are randomly selected (magnified 400 times), and the ratio of collagen deposition in Disse's space to that in all areas with collagen deposition is calculated [14].

3.2. Blood biochemistry

Since measurement of type I collagen propeptide as a serum marker of liver fibrosis by radioimmunoassay in 1974, measurement has become possible for extracellular matrix components that appear in the blood (various types of collagen, laminin, fibronectin, hyaluronic acid), soluble receptors (fibronectin receptors = Integrin β1), components in the extracellular matrix synthesis and degradation system (matrix metalloproteinase, MMP; and tissue inhibitor of metalloproteinase, TIMP) and cytokine in their regulation system (TGF-β). Using these markers, the degree of improvement in liver fibrosis after treatment can be evaluated. For example, in patients with chronic hepatitis who markedly responded to IFN therapy, the concentrations of blood type III procollagen N peptide (PIIIP), type IV collagen and laminin, and serum hyaluronic acid have been reported to decrease to the normal state [17].

3.3. Biochemistry using liver tissue

Measurement of total collagen in biopsied liver tissue by quantifying hydroxyproline has long been performed. There is also a liver collagen quantification method by dye binding in which liver biopsy sections (15 μm in thickness) are stained with Fast green–Sirius red, and dye is extracted from a certain amount of stained tissue, and its optical intensity is measured by spectrophotometry [18].

3.4. Urinary pyridinoline

Pyridinoline resulting from specific crosslinking of mature collagen increases due to liver fibrosis, and its level in liver tissue is associated with the degree of fibrosis and the degree of the reversibility of the fibrosis process. Pyridinoline is excreted as a degradation product of mature collagen into urine, and therefore, the degree of liver fibrosis can be monitored by measurement of the urinary pyridinoline concentration by high performance liquid chromatography (HPLC) or an immunological method [19].

4. IS ADVANCED CHRONIC HEPATITIS (PRE-CIRRHOSIS) OR EARLY LIVER CIRRHOSIS REVERSIBLE?

Studies have evaluated changes in liver fibrosis after IFN therapy for chronic hepatitis C by follow-up liver biopsy performed for some years after treatment mainly in patients showing persistent HCV-RNA negative conversion (marked responses). In patients with marked responses, fibers became smaller and the margins of portal areas became smooth first after treatment, and then collagen fibers and reticular fibers decrease after 3–5 years, and bridging fibrosis accompanied by lobular strain became thin (improvement rate, 67% after 4–6 years) [20,21]. It has been reported that improvement from F3 to F2 according to the new Inuyama's Classification required 3 years or more, but intrahepatic fibers markedly decreased in even F4 cases (liver cirrhosis) [22,23]. In addition, long-term observation in the US [3] showed that similar findings were obtained by examination of liver fibrosis performed after 6–13 years (mean, 10 years) in patients who markedly responded to IFN therapy, and marked fibrosis disappeared in one patient (score 3 → 0).

Significant improvement in liver fibrosis after IFN therapy has also been shown by biochemical quantification of liver collagen and morphological measurement. Reichard et al. [24] reported significant improvement in both necrosis and inflammation scores for liver fibrosis and decreases in the serum types PIIIP and IV collagen (7S) concentrations in patients with marked responses to IFN. In another study, 90 patients with compensatory liver cirrhosis (Child A) were randomly divided into two groups undergoing and not undergoing IFN therapy, and the course was observed until 5–6 years after administration (HCV complete elimination rate, 16%) [25]. In the IFN therapy group, the serum type IV collagen (7S) concentration significantly decreased though no significant improvement was observed in Knodell's HAI score.

In patients with alcoholic liver cirrhosis, long-term abstinence from drinking results in morphological improvement in the liver, a reduction in portal pressure, and definite

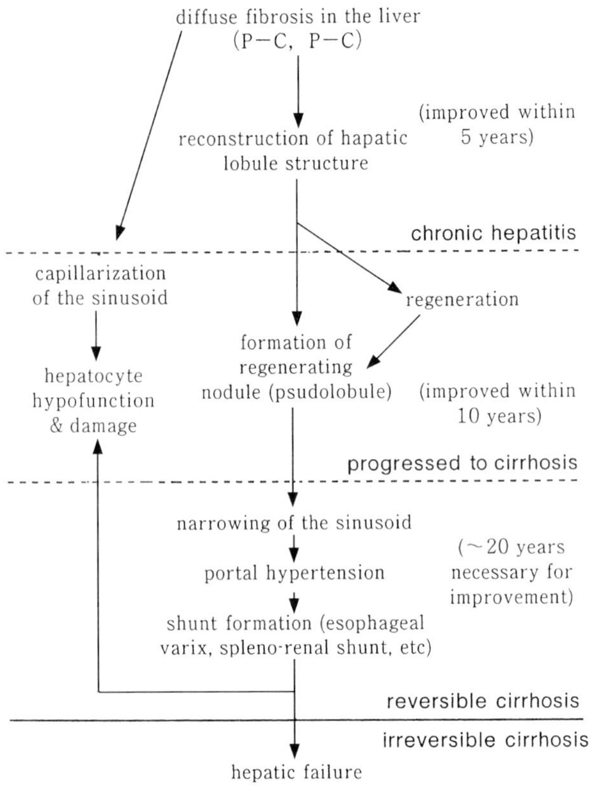

Fig. 1. Reversibility of liver cirrhosis by the anti-fibrotic therapy and the periods (years) necessary for disappearance of the findings.

endoscopic improvement in esophageal varices [26]. This morphological and hemodynamic improvement in the liver increases protein synthesis ability and nearly normalizes the indocyanine green (ICG) retention rate in routine liver function tests.

Thus, there has been increasing evidence to suggest that early liver cirrhosis histologically improves, when causes of liver injury are eliminated after long-term treatment, to a state that does not allow a diagnosis of liver cirrhosis (Fig. 1). Sinusoidal capillarization and remodeling of the hepatic lobular architecture are repaired, and regenerating nodules are laparoscopically flattened, and esophageal varices endoscopically disappear [26].

5. MECHANISM OF IMPROVEMENT IN LIVER FIBROSIS AND ANTI-FIBROSIS DRUGS

The mechanism of the reversibility of liver fibrosis has been evaluated in terms of molecular biology and cytology. The order and time course of clinical improvement in sinusoidal capillarization, remodeling of the hepatic lobular architecture, portal hypertension, and collateral circulation should be also clarified. In addition, studies are necessary to determine whether the results of treatment with anti-fibrosis drugs obtained in vitro and experimental systems can be also obtained in vivo (there is complicated crosstalk in both the synthesis and degradation systems) and to develop methods of increasing the anti-fibrosis drug concentration around stellate cells as the site of the production and degradation of extracellular matrix. In treatment methods controlling cytokines, such as TGF-β that promote fibrosis, the physiological action of cytokine is markedly affected, and therefore, side effects should be carefully evaluated.

It may also be necessary to study and develop anti-fibrosis drugs inhibiting the progression (aggravation) of liver fibrosis while continuously administering a compound experimentally inducing liver fibrosis. This is corresponding to clinical failure of radical treatment of causes. Furthermore, anti-fibrosis drugs accelerating improvement in liver cirrhosis after elimination of causes (virus elimination or abstinence from drinking) are also necessary in the management of hepatitis patients.

5.1. Mechanism of improvement in liver fibrosis

In alcoholic liver disease, the cause of the disease can be eliminated by withdrawal of alcohol. Therefore, this disease is a good model in studies in time series on the mechanism of improvement in liver fibrosis in humans. In alcoholic liver cirrhosis, with a decrease in the stainability of α-smooth muscle actin, a marker of activation of stellate cells, 4–10 weeks after stopping drinking, decreases are observed in the stainability of type IV collagen that had deposited in sinusoidal walls as well as the stainability of laminin and hyaluronic acid [27]. Sinusoidal capillarization also improves in a short period after stopping drinking. In alcoholic liver cirrhosis, a short period after stopping drinking, the interstitium bordering pseudolobules has been replaced by elastic fibers strongly stained with Victoria blue, which appear to be old residual fibrotic lesions difficult to disappear [26]. Blood biochemical examination shows rapid normalization of the concentrations of type IV collagen, laminin, and hyaluronic acid after stopping drinking [27]. The serum MMP-2 level further increases, while the serum TIMP-2 level decreases after stopping drinking. Thus, after stopping drinking, activation of stellate cells subsides, and the synthesis system and the system inhibiting degradation are rapidly inactivated while the degradation system is strongly activated. This may promote the degradation of the basement membrane components.

When liver fibrosis is induced in rats by continuous administration of carbon tetrachloride (CCl_4), and its administration is discontinued, liver fibrosis rapidly improves and disappears. The mechanism of this phenomenon may be an increase in MMP gene expression and a decrease in TIMP expression, resulting in relative predominance of the degradation system [28]. After in situ hybridization, MMP-13 mRNA is markedly positive (stellate cells) in fibrous septal areas that are in contact with liver cells.

It is an interesting problem to what degree the pathologic condition of liver cirrhosis improves after correction of liver hemodynamics, i.e., portal blood flow factors. This is a theme that essentially differs from the theme "Is liver cirrhosis a reversible disease?". However, it is also important to answer the question, "Does the pathophysiology of liver cirrhosis reversibly improve?". In patients with non-compensatory liver cirrhosis, reversible improvement to compensatory liver cirrhosis is possible by reducing portal pressure and extrahepatic shunt blood flow (disappearance of esophageal varices) by partial splenic arterial embolization, and this effect can be maintained for a long period [29]. However, there are few studies on changes in liver fibrosis observed with this improvement.

5.2. Development of drugs for liver fibrosis

Liver fibrosis results from the imbalance between synthesis and degradation. Therefore, the amount of fibers in the liver decreases if degradation exceeds synthesis (Fig. 2).

IFN-γ directly acts on activated stellate cells, making them a state near the static phase, which inhibits extracellular matrix production (reduces the production of type I procollagen mRNA) [30]. Compared with IFN-γ, IFN-α has a mild action but also reduces types I, III, IV procollagen mRNA in vivo by reducing TGF-β1 mRNA in the liver [31]. HGF reduces the mRNA levels of procollagen, TGF-β1, and desmins, and increases MMP activity, exerting anti-fibrosis action [32].

On the other hand, there have been extensive studies on drugs that inhibit the extracellular matrix synthesis system and promote its degradation system, or inhibit and inactivate the synthesis of cytokines promoting liver fibrosis. Inhibitors of prolyl 4-hydroxylase (rate-limiting enzyme in the collagen synthesis system) are prodrugs activated in the liver and have anti-fibrosis effects on experimental liver fibrosis models [33]. Glycyrrhizin and glycine contained in Strong Neo-Minophagen C act on human stellate cells, inhibiting collagen production [34]. Proteoglycans (decholin) that binds to TGF-β, neutralizing antibody for TGF-β1, and soluble TGF-β2 receptors inhibit collagen production [35]. Inhibitors of angiotensin II receptors localized in stellate cells, which reduce portal pressure, inhibit the autocrine system of TGF-β, improving liver fibrosis in human chronic hepatitis [36].

6. IS LIVER CIRRHOSIS ACCOMPANIED BY THICK COLLATERAL VESSELS REVERSIBLE?

A study on detailed changes on the liver surface and in liver histological findings in alcoholic liver cirrhosis after stopping drinking showed improvement in some patients, but not in others [26]. These findings led to a conclusion that the reversibility of liver cirrhosis is markedly affected by the degree of development of collateral circulation. After stopping drinking, the interstitial width decreases with regeneration, which makes pseudolobules roundish, and endoscopy can confirm improvement in not only vasodilation in the round ligament and falciform ligament of the liver, but also esophageal varices [26]. However, in many patients with liver cirrhosis showing thick collateral vessels resulting from portal hypertension, even long-term follow up (3–9 years; mean 6 years) after stopping drinking shows inadequate improvement in liver function and still abnormal ICG retention rates. Irreversible circulatory impairment may cause gradual progression of liver cirrhosis, eventually leading to liver failure. Therefore, the dividing point in the degree of collateral vessel formation between

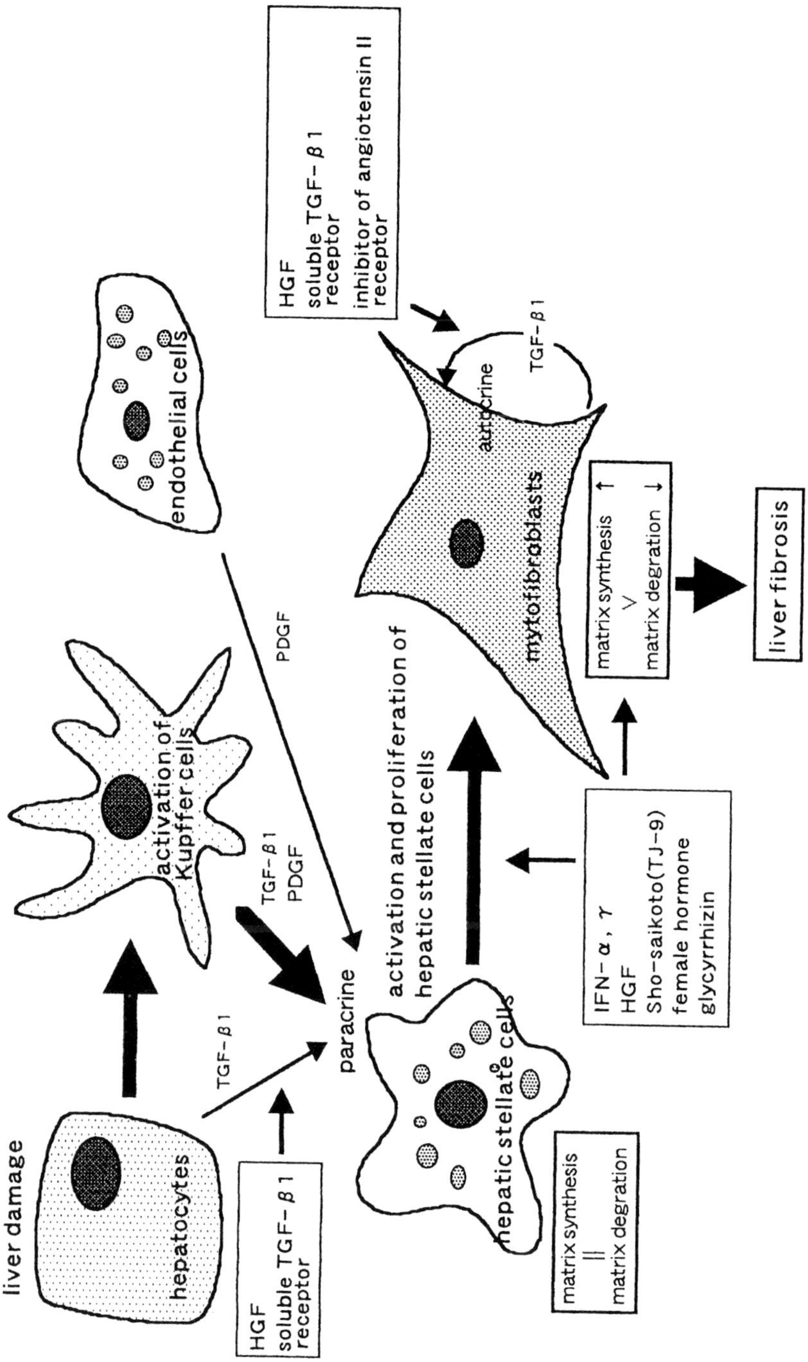

Fig. 2. Mechanisms of liver fibrogenesis and therapeutic agents for blocking these fibrogenesis processes.

reversible and irreversible cirrhosis should be quantitatively evaluated in terms of the thickness and blood flow of collateral vessels. At present, there appears to be a divide for the reversibility of alcoholic liver cirrhosis.

7. ASSOCIATION WITH LIVER CARCINOGENESIS

There is a high correlation between the progression of liver fibrosis and the incidence of hepatocellular carcinoma [37]. The degree of prevention of hepatocellular carcinoma that can be achieved by improving liver fibrosis is a problem. Before evaluating this problem, it is necessary to determine whether the virus disappears or remains after cure of viral liver cirrhosis. In a long-term follow-up study, three patients with type B liver cirrhosis who showed negative conversion of HBs antigen after a maximum period of 13 years underwent liver biopsy 1–15 years (mean 5 years) after negative conversion, and liver fibrosis resolved in all of them, and findings of liver cirrhosis disappeared in 1 of them after 5 years [38]. However, all patients were persistently positive for HBV-DNA in liver tissue and showed remaining slight inflammatory findings in portal areas. The second liver biopsy was performed 11–19 years after diagnosis in two patients with type C liver cirrhosis who were positive for HCV antibody and negative for blood HCV-RNA, but showed a decrease in the HCV antibody titer during subsequent long-term follow-up. Disappearance of histological findings of liver cirrhosis, normalization of results of liver function tests, and disappearance of esophageal varices were observed in both patients, but intrahepatic HCV-RNA was persistently positive in one patient. Even if liver cirrhosis improves after such spontaneous virological remission (virus elimination after a spontaneous course), the possibility of persistence of intrahepatic HBV and HCV infection is high.

In another study, liver function was normalized 7.3 years (mean) after diagnosis in 15 of 19 patients with liver cirrhosis in whom improvement in histological findings of the liver was observed by the second or more biopsy [39]. In all three of the 15 patients who showed seroconversion of HBs antigen, two of three with type C who responded to IFN therapy, one of two with type C after stopping drinking, two of two with autoimmune hepatitis (liver cirrhosis) who responded to steroids, hepatocellular carcinoma developed 6 years (mean) after normalization of transaminase (total 8 patients; 42.1%).

Thus, patients who once developed liver cirrhosis are at the risk of developing hepatocellular carcinoma even if improvement is observed in liver function and liver histological findings (liver fibrosis).

CONCLUSION

'Treating liver fibrosis' differs from 'treating liver cirrhosis'. However, the above observations suggest that treatment of liver fibrosis, even if it requires a long period, results in improvement in liver cell function, repair of the hepatic lobular architecture (including sinusoidal capillarization), disappearance of regenerating nodules (pseudolobules), and functional disappearance, even if not anatomical disappearance, of collateral vessels. In advanced liver cirrhosis showing atrophied liver and thick collateral vessels, which represent classical liver cirrhosis, the function and morphology of the liver temporarily improves after elimination of the cause of the disease, but subsequent re-progression is expected, leading to liver failure. Thus, thick collateral vessel formation is a division of the reversibility of liver cirrhosis. Thick collateral vessel formation may indicate the limitations of anti-fibrosis therapy.

At present, liver cirrhosis is a terminal stage of liver disease and is considered to be an advanced irreversible disease that cannot be treated. However, we expect that the opinion that most cases of liver cirrhosis are reversible and can be cured will be commonly accepted in the near future.

REFERENCES

[1] Shaffner F, Popper H. Capillarization of hepatic sinusoids in man. Gastroenterology 1963; 44: 239–242.

[2] Friedman SL. The cellular basis of hepatic fibrosis: mechanisms and treatment strategies. New Engl J Med 1993; 328: 1828–1835.

[3] Lau DT-Y, Kleiner DE, Ghany MG et al. 10-year follow-up after interferon-α therapy for chronic hepatitis C. Hepatology 1998; 28: 1121–1127.

[4] Rockey DC. Vasoactive agents in intrahepatic portal hypertension and fibrosis: Implications for therapy. Gastroenterology 2000; 118: 1262–1265.

[5] Shiratori Y, Imazeki F, Moriyama M et al. Histological improvement of fibrosis in patients with hepatitis C who have sustained response to interferon therapy. Ann Int Med 2000; 132: 517–524.

[6] Cozzolino G, Lonardo A, Francica G et al. Differential diagnosis between hepatic cirrhosis and chronic active hepatitis: specificity and sensitivity of physical and laboratory findings in a series from Mediterranean area. Am J Gastroenterol 1983; 78: 442–445.

[7] Ikeda K, Saitoh S, Kobayashi M et al. Distinction between chronic hepatitis and liver cirrhosis in patients with hepatitis C virus infection. Practical discriminant function using common laboratory data. Hepatol Res 2000; 18: 252–266.

[8] Yang M, Ishibashi T. Clinical diagnostic criteria of liver cirrhosis: its classification from the aspect of the long-term follow-up. Jpn J Gastroenterol 2000; 97(Suppl): A118–A120.

[9] Majima Y, Fujimoto T, Iwai I, Tanaka M, Abe M, Abe H et al. Histological diagnosis of hepatocellular carcinoma by a new technique of ultrasound-guided fine needle biopsy. Acta Hepatol Jpn 1988; 29: 628–636 (in Japanese).

[10] Ito T, Niiyama G, Ifukube S, Kawanaka MK, Takekawa S, Imai N et al. Diagnostic disagreement of liver cirrhosis between laparoscopy and liver histology. Gastroenterology 2000; 31: 184–189 (in Japanese).

[11] Ichida F, Omata M, Tsuji T, Ichida T, Inoue K, Kamimura A et al. Histological classification of chronic hepatitis — New Inuyama Classification. The Proceedings of the 19th Inuyama Symposium, Chugai-Igakusya, Tokyo, 1996; 183–188 (in Japanese).

[12] Maeyama S, Koike A, Sohda F, Ohbe M et al. Evaluation of liver morphology in management and etiology in chronic hepatitis. Minophagen Med Rev 1998; 43: 27–35 (in Japanese).

[13] Knodell RG, Kshak KG, Black WC, Chen TS, Craig R, Kaplowitz N et al. Formulation and application of a numerical scoring system for assessing histologic activity in asymptomatic chronic hepatitis. Hepatology 1981; 1: 431–435.

[14] Manabe N, Chevallier M, Chossegros P, Causse X, Guerret S, Trépo C et al. Interferon-α 2b therapy reduce liver fibrosis in chronic Non-A, Non-B hepatitis; A quantitative histological evaluation. Hepatology 1993; 18: 1334–1349.

[15] Kobayashi T, Sakamoto T, Katayama K, Amano H, Enomoto K, Ohishi K et al. Estimation of liver fibrogenesis in type C chronic hepatitis patients with hepatocellular carcinoma. Acta Hepatol Jpn 2000; 41(Suppl. 2): A453 (in Japanese).

[16] Moriyama M, Shimizu T, Arakawa Y. Is liver cirrhosis reversible? — From the scoring of liver fibrosis. Acta Hepatol Jpn 2000; 41(Suppl. 2): A347 (in Japanese).

[17] Murakami Y, Ikuta Y, Koda M, Kawasaki H. Serum type III procollagen peptide, type IV collagen 7S domain, central triple-helix of type IV collagen and tissue inhibitor of metalloproteinase in patients with chronic viral liver disease: relationship to liver histology. Hepatology 1994; 20: 780–787.

[18] Jiménez W, Parés A, Caballeria J, Torres M et al. Measurement of fibrosis in needle liver biopsies: evaluation of a colorimetric method. Hepatology 1985; 5: 815–818.

[19] Grenard P, Blanquier B, Richard-Blum SR. Urinary excretion of the collagen cross-link pyridinoline increases during liver fibrogenesis. J Hepatol 1997; 26: 1356–1362.

[20] Yokosuka O, Fujiwara K. Improvement of liver fibrosis 3–5 years after effective treatment of chronic hepatitis by interferon. In: Toda G, Omata M, Okazaki I et al., editors. Is interferon therapy effective for liver fibrosis in type C chronic hepatitis? Tokyo: Chugai-Igakusha, 1996; pp. 88–91 (in Japanese).

[21] Kobayashi M, Kumada H. Effect in the course of type C chronic hepatitis. Acta Hepatol Jpn 1998; 39(Suppl. 1): 96 (in Japanese).

[22] Moriyama M, Arakawa Y. Prognosis of patients with type C chronic hepatitis treated by interferon. Acta Hepatol Jpn 1998; 39(Suppl. 2): 43 (in Japanese).

[23] Sato A, Suzuki H. Long-term prognosis of patients with type C chronic hepatitis treated by interferon. Acta Hepatol Jpn 1998; 39: 789–791 (in Japanese).

[24] Reichard O, Glaumann H, Norkrans G, Wejstál R, Fryden A, Schvarcz R et al. Histological outcome in patients with chronic hepatitis C given a 60-week interferon alfa-2b treatment course. Liver 1994; 14: 169–174.

[25] Nishiguchi S, Nakatani S, Kuroki T. Preventive effect of hepatocellular carcinoma by treatment of IFN in type C liver cirrhosis. In: Yamanaka M, Takikawa H, editors. Frontier of Hepatology. Tokyo: Chugai-Igakusha, 1997; pp. 116–120 (in Japanese).

[26] Otake H. Diagnostic problems of clinical criteria for liver cirrhosis — from a view point of laparoscopy. Gastroenterology 2000; 31: 165–174 (in Japanese).

[27] Tutsumi M, Takase S. Reversibility of liver fibrosis in alcoholic liver injury. Acta Hepatol Jpn 2000; 41: 621–622 (in Japanese).

[28] Okazaki I, Hozawa S, Ishikawa A, Watanabe T. Final purpose of liver fibrosis research: Development of treatment for liver cirrhosis. Saishin Igaku 2000; 55: 1725–1734 (in Japanese).

[29] Hirata K, Abe H, Miyoshi K. Reversible improvement of liver cirrhosis by partial splenic artery embolization. Acta Hepatol Jpn 2000; 41(Suppl. 2): A348 (in Japanese).

[30] Baroni GS, D'Ambrosio L, Curto P, Casini A, Mancini R, Jezequel AM et al. Interferon gamma decreases hepatic stellate cell activation and extracellular matrix deposition in rat liver fibrosis. Hepatology 1996; 23: 1189–1199.

[31] Granstein RD, Flotte TJ, Amento EP. Interferon and collagen production. J Invest Dermatol 1990; 95: 75S–80S.

[32] Matsuda Y, Mtsumoto K, Ichida T, Nakamura T. Hepatocyte growth factor suppresses the onset of liver cirrhosis and abrogates lethal hepatic dysfunction in rats. J Biochem 1995; 118: 643–649.

[33] Bickel M, Baringhaus K-H, Gerl M, Gunzler V, Kanta J, Schmidts L et al. Selective inhibition of hepatic collagen accumulation in experimental liver fibrosis in rats by a new prolyl 4-hydroxylase inhibitor. Hepatology 1998; 28: 404–411.

[34] Yamauchi M, Takahashi A, Toda G. Effect of glycirrhitin and glycine on collagen production in human Ito's cells. Acta Hepatol Jpn 2000; 41(Suppl. 2): A348 (in Japanese).
[35] Strobel D, Wittekind C, Ruoslahti E et al. In vivo application of a neutralising TGF-beta antibody in experimental liver fibrosis. J Hepatol 1993; 18(Suppl. 1): S63.
[36] Kawada S, Sakuda S. Development of new anti fibrotic therapy for blocking angiotensin II (AT) receptor. Acta Hepatol Jpn 2000; 41(Suppl. 2): A347 (in Japanese).
[37] Sakaida I, Hironaka K, Uchida K, Suzuki C, Kayano K, Okita K. Fibrosis accelerates the development of enzyme-altered lesions in the rat liver. Hepatology 1998; 28: 1247–1252.
[38] Yuki Y, Kato M. Long-term follow-up of spontaneous virological remission in type B and C liver cirrhosis. Acta Hepatol Jpn 2001; 41(Suppl. 2): A347 (in Japanese).
[39] Yakura M, Harada E. Study of cirrhotic patients who showed improvement of liver histology. Acta Hepatol Jpn; 41(Suppl. 2): A347 (in Japanese).

Hepatocellular Carcinoma

Molecular Biology and Immunology in Hepatology
Edited by T. Tsuji, T. Higashi, M. Zeniya and K.-H. Meyer zum Büschenfelde

CHAPTER 10

Treatment of Hepatocellular Carcinoma: Diverse Strategies Based on Underlying Liver Diseases

Masao Omata

Department of Gastroenterology, University of Tokyo, Tokyo, Japan

1. INCREASE IN HEPATOCELLULAR CARCINOMA

The annual mortality rate in Japan is currently about 900,000 per annum, with hepatocellular carcinoma (HCC) accounting for more than 30,000 of these deaths. Studies conducted 10 years previously indicated that hepatitis Type B and Type C accounted for 18 and 59% of the total number of cases of HCC, respectively. A further study at this university conducted 8 years ago indicated that hepatitis Type B and Type C accounted for 11 and 83% of the total number of cases, respectively, indicating an increase in the ratio of Type C to Type B. These data underscore the importance of the hepatitis virus as an etiological factor in the pathogenesis of HCC with 94% of tumors involving viral infection.

Looking at the 94% of patients with HCC due to viral infection, one can obtain an overall perspective of hepatitis by distinguishing the virus types. In Japan, the populations of patients with Type B and Type C viral infections are each estimated to number 1,500,000 persons, though there is an 8 : 1 ratio for Type C to Type B with regard to the incidence of HCC. It is obvious, at the present time, that the incidence of HCC is caused mostly by Type C hepatitis virus.

2. COURSE OF HEPATIC FIBROSIS AND CARCINOGENESIS

After returning from the US in 1979, the author undertook clinical work in the hepatic outpatient department. Typically, patients were healthy Japanese with an average age of 40 years who felt subjectively well. However, they exhibited slightly abnormal liver function tests, such as an elevated transaminase (GPT) levels of about 100 U/l. These patients underwent a liver biopsy and pathological examination of the tissue revealed chronic hepatitis (not cirrhosis). They were subsequently followed up (Fig. 1). One hundred and twenty-seven patients had hepatitis Type B and 124 had hepatitis Type C. About 6 years into follow-up, HCC was noted in five Type B patients and

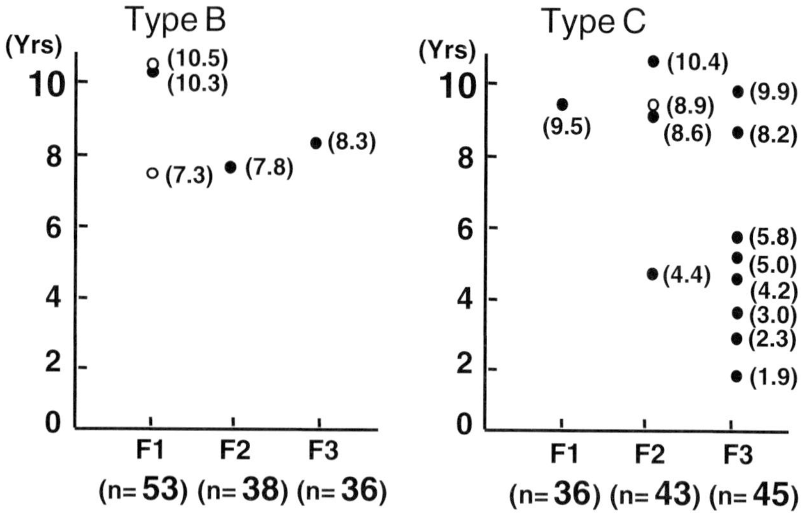

Fig. 1. Hepatocellular carcinoma onset for Types B and C chronic hepatitis patients. •, Liver cirrhosis was present when hepatocellular carcinoma developed; ○, no cirrhosis was present when hepatocellular carcinoma developed.

13 Type C patients (Fig. 1). The calculated annual rates of carcinogenesis for 100,000 people were 647 patients with Type B and 1723 with Type C. Furthermore, it is true that 96–97% of Japanese citizens are thought to be not infected with the hepatitis virus. In those persons without hepatitis, the incidence rate is 1000-fold lower at about 1.7 cases per 100,000 people. It is, therefore, apparent that HCC will be drastically reduced if the hepatitis virus could be effectively eliminated. Interestingly, a recent report of a vaccination program performed in Taiwan indicated that the rate of onset of HCC between the ages of 6 and 17 years had fallen dramatically and was comparable to that of rare cerebral neoplasms [1]. As a single parameter, this figure thus represents the highest rate of carcinogenesis. For example, the relative degree of risk of pulmonary carcinoma for smokers is only 10 times that for non-smokers. The liver is therefore a somewhat unfortunate organ in that it is exposed and vulnerable to two markedly carcinogenic environmental agents viz. the hepatitis B and C viruses. The degree of fibrosis of the liver biopsy was classified as slight (F1), medium (F2), and severe (F3). Thirty-six patients with Type C were classified as F1 (slight) and only one patient developed carcinoma after 9.5 years (Fig. 1). The 45 patients in the F3 subgroup had a much higher rate of HCC with seven individuals developing the disease after short periods of follow-up. Predictably, patients in the F2 (medium fibrosis) subgroup exhibited a moderate incidence of HCC. This trend results from the proposed pathway of development of HCC from chronic hepatitis. This can be envisioned as a stepwise model with progression from mild fibrosis (F1) to hepatic cirrhosis (F4) and eventual HCC (F5) being potentially steady but very slow. This model is applicable to Type C, but not Type B. Indeed, only three of the 53 Type B patients in the chronic hepatitis (F1) subgroup developed HCC. Only one of 36 Type B patients with severe chronic

hepatitis (F3) developed carcinoma. There are two potential mechanisms underlying the development of HCC with Type B hepatitis. Tumors may develop following repeated bouts of necrosis, inflammation and fibrosis culminating in cirrhosis or tumors may occur independently. In Type C, the onset of carcinoma is thought to occur after the development of fibrosis (cirrhosis) lasting over a year. Indeed, cirrhosis or hepatic fibrosis is typically present in liver specimens containing carcinomatous tissue. For example, of the 124 patients with Type C, 13 developed carcinoma, 12 of whom exhibited cirrhosis (F4) (Fig. 1). Accordingly, patients did not develop carcinoma at the F1 stage, but rather developed progressive fibrosis that preceded tumor development, a process that can occur over 10 years.

Of the five patients with Type B hepatitis, two patients (40%) did not exhibit cirrhosis when they developed tumors (Fig. 1). Therefore, the course of carcinogenesis for Types B and C differs substantially.

The annual rates of carcinogenesis per 100,000 patients are about 1700 and 600 for all Type C and Type B patients, respectively. The corresponding figures for the F1, F2, and F3 subgroups of Type C are 457, 1450, and 3005. Expressing the annual rate of carcinogenesis per 100,000 patients as a percentage yields respective numbers of 0.45, 1.5, and 3%. Since the average age of these patients is 40 years, one can calculate the estimated lifetime risk of developing heptocarcinoma. The annual rate of 3% in the 'severe' chronic hepatitis subgroup (F3) gives an estimated lifetime rate of carcinogenesis of 90%. Conversely, the 'slight' chronic hepatitis subgroup (F1) has a carcinogenesis rate of 13–14% such that 86–87% of patients will not develop a tumor. Liver function tests, such as GOT and GPT, cannot be used to identify individuals that are predisposed to the development of cancer in their lifetime. However, if the degree of hepatic fibrosis can be ascertained by analysis of a liver biopsy, then it may be possible to estimate the risk of developing carcinoma over a prolonged period of 30 years in patients with Type C hepatitis.

In contrast, in Type B patients, it remains difficult to predict who will develop carcinoma even following analysis and assessment of a liver biopsy, but Type C patients predominate in clinical practice.

The F classification (for fibrosis classification: F1, slight; F2, medium; F3, severe; and F4, cirrhosis) (new Inuyama classification, histological classification of liver biopsy) allows an appropriate classification for the multistep model proposed earlier. Data derived from the use of this classification are in accordance with the clinical data that indicate the increase in Type C HCC.

3. SUPPRESSION OF THE INDICENCE OF TYPE C HCC USING INTERFERON

One might predict that the elimination of the HCV virus would result in diminished hepatic inflammation and ameliorate the development of Type C-associated HCC. Indeed, if eradication of the virus was associated with either a reduction in fibrosis or prevention of further fibrosis, one might expect a dramatic suppression in tumor development in hepatitis C. Interferon was approved as a therapeutic anti-viral agent in 1992, and has been administered to over 200,000 people in Japan. The therapeutic results of interferon treatment of Type C patients indicate that the reduction in hepatic necrosis and inflammation consequent upon elimination of the virus ameliorates both fibrosis and the rate of carcinogenesis. A prospective–retrospective study of the suppression of carcinogenesis by interferon treatment has been conducted as part of a 10-year plan supported by the Japanese government [2,3]. With the cooperation of multiple centers throughout Japan, 2890 cases were entered to consist of a control group of 490 patients who were not treated with interferon and a treatment group of 2400 patients. Thirty-three percent (789 cases) of treated patients were complete responders (CRs) i.e. the virus was completely eliminated. Comparison of the incidence of carcinogenesis for the treated group and the untreated group (Figs. 2 and 3) indicates that the rate of carcinogenesis for the interferon-treated group significantly decreased to half that of the untreated control group [2]. The treated group may be further divided into subgroups consisting of: (1) patients in whom the virus was eliminated; (2) patients in whom the virus was not eliminated but whose transaminase levels normalized; and (3) patients in whom the virus was not eliminated and whose transaminase levels remained either mildly or markedly elevated. Subgroup analysis indicates that the rate of carcinogenesis for the complete responder subgroup (33% treated patients) where the virus completely disappeared decreased to 20% that in the untreated control group (Table 1). In addition, a comparable fall in the rate of carcinogenesis to 20%

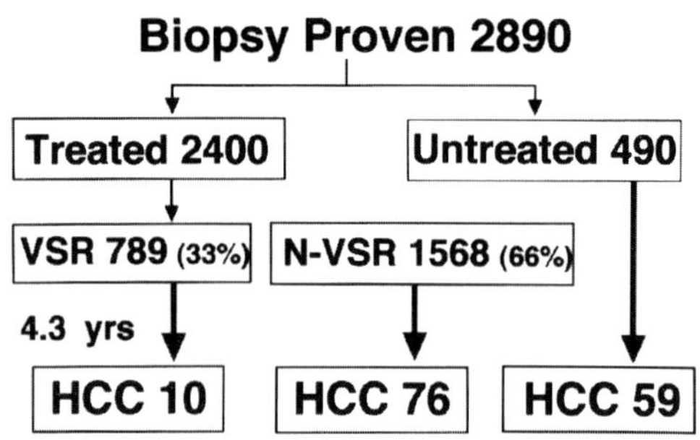

Fig. 2. VSR, virological sustained response — equivalent to complete response; N-VSR, non-VSR; HCC, hepatocellular carcinoma; From [2,3].

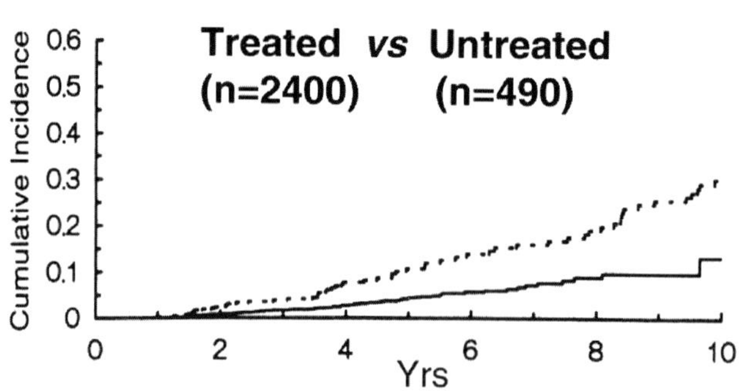

Fig. 3. Incidence of hepatocellular carcinoma over time in control and interferon-treated groups. From [2].

TABLE 1

Change in transaminase and reduced risk of carcinogenesis after treatment and viral elimination

	Response and risk for HCC	
Untreated		1.000
Treated as a whole	(100%)	0.516
VSR/Normal ALT	(33%)	0.197
non-VSR/Normal ALT	(11%)	0.214
non-VSR/Abnormal ALT	(56%)	
Mild elevated	(25%)	0.358
High elevated	(31%)	0.910

Untreated: non-interferon administration group. Treated as a whole: interferon administration group. VSR: virological sustained response (viral elimination group). non-VSR: viral non-elimination group. From ref. [2].

also occurred in the subgroup with persistent viral infection but normal transaminase levels (11% of treated patients) (Table 1). This indicates that the incidence rate of carcinogenesis was drastically decreased in the normalized transaminase group after the treatment (4.3 years). Analysis of the subgroups of patients with persistent viral infection and elevated transaminase levels indicates that those patients with a mild elevation exhibited a rate of carcinogenesis of 36% while patients with a marked elevation of up to twice the normal upper limit exhibited a rate of carcinogenesis of 91%, which is comparable to the untreated control group (Table 1). It is therefore apparent that the return of transaminase values to normal levels during the treatment of Type C patients plays an important role in the suppression of carcinogenesis, which presumably reflects a diminution of ongoing hepatic injury, inflammation, and fibrosis.

4. MITIGATION OF HEPATIC NECROSIS/INFLAMMATION WITH VIRAL ELIMINATION AND ABATEMENT OF FIBROSIS

In order to investigate whether the suppression of carcinogenesis occurred in parallel with inhibition of progressive hepatic injury and subsequent fibrosis, a second liver biopsy was performed in 593 patients in the treatment group and untreated group (mean interval of 3.7 years) and the status of fibrosis was scored [3]. The degree of progression of fibrosis was expressed as the fibrosis progression per year, i.e., an F1 baseline biopsy that progressed to F3 after 4 years would yield a fibrosis progression per year score of +0.5 (i.e. 2 ÷ 4) while a F3 biopsy that improved to an F1 would be −0.5, with the negative sign indicating resolution of fibrosis. This simple index provides useful data on the rate of fibrosis progression in untreated and treated patient populations. The fibrosis progression per year was +0.1 for the 106 cases in the untreated group (Table 2), which would result in a single-stage worsening over a 10-year period. In contrast, 183 treated patients in whom treatment induced elimination of the virus had a value of −0.28, which would result in a single-stage improvement in the hepatic fibrosis score in approximately 4 years. 304 treated patients who exhibited persistence

TABLE 2

Treated cases and the rate of the natural course of hepatic fibrosis progression

	Fibrosis progression rate per year
106 Untreated	$+0.10 \pm 0.22$
183 Eradicated	-0.28 ± 0.33
304 Non-eradicated	$+0.02 \pm 0.36$

Untreated: untreated group. Eradicated: viral elimination group. Non-eradicated: viral non-elimination group. +, worsened; −, improved. From ref. [3].

TABLE 3

Speed of the abatement of fibrosis in cases of viral elimination classified by extent of fibrosis (F4–F1)

Improvement in VSR		
From F4	($n = 24$)	−0.283
From F3	($n = 45$)	−0.374
From F2	($n = 69$)	−0.284
From F1	($n = 42$)	−0.152

VSR, virological sustained response. From ref. [3].

of the virus had a value of +0.02. Thus, the elimination of the virus by interferon treatment results in an impressive resolution of hepatic fibrosis that is not evident if the virus persists (Fig. 4). Furthermore, patients in the complete responder group exhibited comparable fibrosis progression per year scores, irrespective of the score on their initial baseline biopsy (Table 3). This means that virus elimination may even lead to a cure for

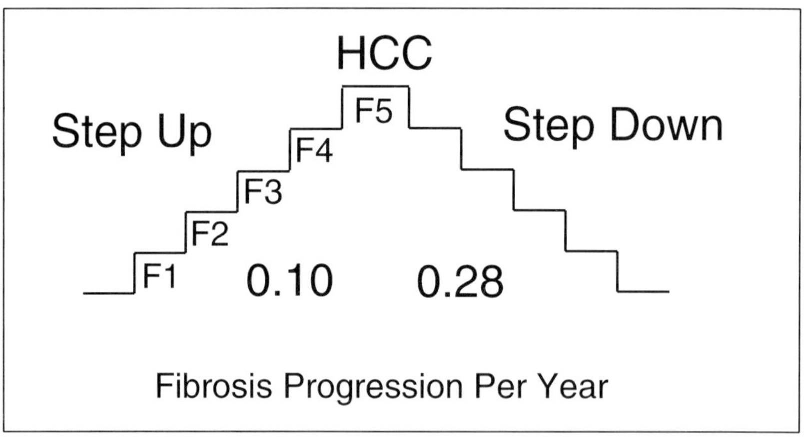

Fig. 4. From Type C hepatitis to hepatocellular carcinoma. Step Up, natural course of Type C chronic hepatitis as seen with a liver biopsy; Step Down, speed of fibrosis amelioration following virus elimination with interferon treatment. From [3].

cirrhosis (F4) (Table 3) [3]. This study was the first to demonstrate the natural history of Type C hepatitis and amelioration of cirrhosis [3]. The fibrosis progression per year score for the treated group where the virus could not be eliminated was +0.02, which essentially indicates a halt to progression of disease (Table 2). It is clear that stopping or ameliorating the progression of fibrosis is important in order to suppress the rate of carcinogenesis in Type C patients.

5. REGULAR MEDICAL CARE FOR HCC

The progression from chronic hepatitis to HCC, its natural course, and treatment results have been presented, but many patients at our institute exhibit more advanced disease, that is, HCC. Patients with HCC number over 400 per annum (8 per week). To date, the University of Tokyo Gastroenterology Department has treated about 1000 cases by percutaneous tumor ablation (PTA). The first 700 cases involved ethanol injection therapy [4], followed by microwave coagulation therapy, and then by radiation frequency ablation (RFA). At our institute, about 89% of all admitted patients receive PTA, while the figure at many other facilities is 10–20% of total patients. However, the increased usage of PTA at this center reflects the increased proportion of patients who are either not treatable by surgery or who wish to undergo non-surgical treatment (PTA) for their disease. The 3- and 5-year survival rates for our 952 cases assembled prior to last year were 65 and 42%, respectively. These results match those of the 16,728 cases assembled by the Japan HCC Research Society, where 63% had a 3-year survival rate and 45% had a 5-year survival rate (Fig. 5). Furthermore, the 3- and 5-year survival rates of our 449 HCC cases with chronic hepatitis and Child A cirrhosis were 75 and

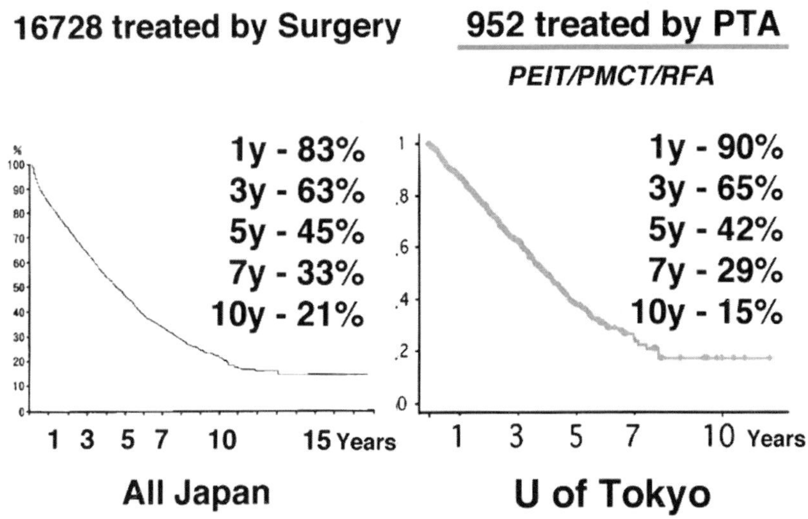

Fig. 5. Comparison of survival rates for PTA treatment (952 cases from University of Tokyo Gastroenterology Department) and surgery from Japan Hepatocellular Carcinoma Research Society.

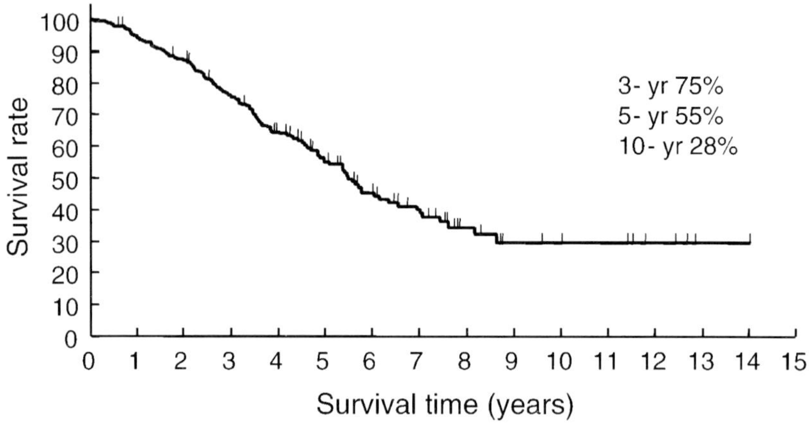

Fig. 6. PTA treatment results (University of Tokyo Gastroenterology Department) 449 cases of hepatocellular carcinoma with chronic hepatitis and Child A cirrhosis.

55%, respectively, which surpasses the results of surgery (Fig. 6). In addition, the recent introduction of radiowave treatment methods, such as radiofrequency ablation (RFA) has further improved percutaneous needle treatment. With the conventional treatment of ethanol injection, three discrete 3-cm foci of tumors, for example, would require hospitalization of 28 days. With RFA treatment, this period is reduced to 7–10 days. Controlled studies of ethanol injection and RFA are currently being conducted, but initial results suggest that RFA may result in an improved prognosis in both the short- and long-term. There is likely to be an increase in the future use of RFA as a treatment modality, which will result in reductions in both the length of hospitalization required as well as treatment costs.

6. PROBLEMS IN MEDICAL CARE FOR HCC NODES

The recurrence of HCC is a major clinical problem. Results indicate that the rate of recurrence of HCC in Type C patients is 10–20% in 1 year, though it climbs to 80% and may reach 100% over a 4–5-year period. These results underscore the author's own experience with cases where HCCs arise in Type C patients with progressive hepatic fibrosis. Even if the HCC nodules are radically cured by surgery or PTA in patients with underlying Type C cirrhosis, the 1–5 mm cirrhotic nodules that follow cannot be prevented from growing to 10 mm and recurring as cancer (in what is known as ectopic recurrence). Accordingly, there are two types of recurrence that are seen with a particularly high frequency in Type C HCC, an insufficiently treated primary lesion and de novo appearance of a new discrete lesion. Measures must be taken with respect to the first persistent carcinoma and the new carcinoma formation that appears ectopically. Type C patients with cirrhosis (F4) have a 7% rate of carcinogenesis and so the rate of recurrence of HCC (15–20% in a year), i.e., including persistent carcinoma and development of new tumors, is likely. It is therefore apparent that a radical cure for HCC cannot be obtained unless the underlying cirrhosis is also addressed and treated. The combination of adequate tumor ablation with anti-fibrotic treatment will be necessary in order to dramatically improve the 5-year survival rate.

7. CURING CIRRHOSIS

Can cirrhosis be cured? As previously outlined, interferon treatment with virus elimination produces a fibrosis progression per year score of −0.28 per year in patients with cirrhosis (F4), which will result in significant amelioration of fibrosis over time [3]. It is, therefore, reasonable that HCC patients with hepatitis Type C should undergo surgery or PTA treatment for the primary tumor together with anti-viral treatment with the aim of virus elimination and amelioration and resolution of fibrosis, i.e., the patient effectively has two diseases that require treatment. Such therapy can match or better the results achieved with a liver transplant since reinfection with the Type C hepatitis virus after transplantation is almost certain to occur. Accordingly, the survival rates with transplant cases steadily fall with the 3-, 5-, and 7-year survival rates publicly cited for transplants, unlike those for patients with non-viral liver diseases, since the latter reach a plateau. The ultimate cure would, therefore, be successful treatment of the HCC nodules coupled with viral elimination. With this in mind, patients for prospective treatment of HCC were divided 6 years ago into either an interferon treatment group ($n = 43$) or a group that received only carcinoma nodule treatment and did not receive interferon ($n = 31$). The 21 patients in whom the virus was eliminated had a 5-year survival rate of 83% while the 31 patients who only received treatment for the primary tumor had a significantly lower 5-year survival rate of 45%. Furthermore, patients with carcinoma nodule treatment where viral elimination was not possible numbered 22 with a 5-year survival rate of 50% These data clearly demonstrate that a radical cure for carcinoma coupled with viral elimination can improve the survival rate.

Viral elimination may take time and it is also possible for cancer to reappear during the process of fibrosis resolution even if the virus can be eliminated. However, it is possible with the combination of proficiency in diagnostic imaging/local treatment and knowledge related to the virus to achieve results equal to or superior to those achieved with transplantation.

8. DELINEATING HIGH-RISK GROUPS FOR HCC

Regarding prognosis, the author would like to emphasize the efforts of primary care physicians, as the results obtained with their cooperation are substantial. For example, when we are choosing between surgery and PTA, we discuss the 5-year survival rate of both treatments although the difference between them is only a few percentage points. Regarding the Type C HCC patients at this facility, the 5-year survival rates for patients with carcinomas discovered during the course of routine out-patient visits was 50% while patients with carcinomas discovered following an acute admission to hospital was significantly lower at 29%. In reality, this 21% difference is critical since even the use of all the current treatments will not produce such a large difference in patient survival. So at present, regular monitoring of out-patients should lead to improvement of the 5-year survival rate. But how is this possible? It is possible with minimal expense and without

TABLE 4

Platelet count at first screening and onset of hepatocellular carcinoma Type C

Platelet count (per mm^3)		Known	At 1st screening	During tracking	Total
21×10^4	($n = 65$)	0			0%
20×10^4	($n = 22$)	2			9%
18×10^4	($n = 42$)	1		+4	12%
16×10^4	($n = 39$)	2		+5	18%
14×10^4	($n = 35$)	6	+1	+1	23%
12×10^4	($n = 32$)	2	+3	+4	28%
10×10^4	($n = 33$)	4		+4	24%
8×10^4	($n = 40$)	6	+3	+8	43%
6×10^4	($n = 23$)	7	+2	+3	52%
4×10^4	($n = 8$)	4			50%
Total	($n = 339$)	34	9	29	72/339 (21%)

'Known' and 'At 1st screening': hepatocellular carcinoma present at first outpatient screening. 'During tracking': hepatocellular carcinoma found during outpatient screening after 1992.

specialized staff to simply pick up high-risk groups for the development of HCC. This delineation can be accomplished with simple measurement of the platelet count which the author has previously stressed [5]. The gene encoding the platelet promoting factor thrombopoietin (TPO) was cloned about 8 years ago. It was noted that 80% of thrombopoietin was produced in the liver. Platelet production may therefore act as an indirect indicator of hepatic status and it is therefore not surprising that the platelet count is empirically lower as hepatic fibrosis worsens. For example, platelet counts for F1, F2, F3 and F4 are 170,000, 150,000, 130,000, and 100,000 per mm^3, respectively. High-risk groups of Type C patients can be established according to the extent of hepatic fibrosis and the use of the platelet count as a surrogate marker for fibrosis is attractive such that initial screening for a reduced platelet count in Type C hepatitis patients may be an efficient means of assessing the risk of subsequent HCC development. At the University of Tokyo's Gastroenterology Department, data have been collected from some 300 patients the author has examined personally, and all of the patients, in attendance as outpatients, were first arranged in accordance with their platelet count upon arrival at the outpatient service. Whether these patients had carcinoma or whether the disease later developed into cancer was documented. Fifty percent of the group with a platelet count below 80,000 developed HCC (Table 4). Approximately 25% of patients with a platelet count between 80,000 and 140,000 developed HCC. These data were compared to those of the Japan Screening Society, which used ultrasound only for the screening of regular citizens. Of over 3,000,000 people randomly surveyed, the detection rate was 315 tumors for every 2,000,000 people. This is an extremely poor detection rate with an efficiency of 0.015%. In contrast, a platelet count can be performed with comparative ease and at little expense. Accordingly, the measurement of the HCV antibody and platelet count was conducted with subsequent effective discernment of HCC risk being possible. The establishment of a high-risk group with a risk of developing HCC of 3%

per year through the use of the combination of the platelet count and HCV antibody would constitute a screening test that is 2000 times more effective than ultrasonography. PIVKAII and fractioning of AFP L3 have recently been introduced as methods to detect the early stages of carcinoma after the establishment of high-risk groups. Measurement of platelet count, anti-HCV antibody titer, and a robust circulating tumor marker can provide an effective means of detection and subsequent effective treatment to facilitate a significant improvement in the 5-year survival rate.

9. FUTURE PERSPECTIVES

Treatment of liver diseases has intensified in Japan where liver diseases due to hepatitis viral infection are frequently observed. There is an effective 'new generation' method of viral hepatitis elimination. Interferon conjugated with polyethylene glycol (PEG interferon) and ribavirin combination therapy is currently considered the best regimen and able to eliminate viral infection in 50% of all Type C hepatitis patients. In addition, we previously reported that elimination of acute Type C hepatitis in about 90% of cases is possible by means of short-term interferon treatment [6]. Although elimination of the Type B hepatitis virus is extremely difficult, a new treatment has been developed involving inhibition of viral reverse transcriptase for long-term 'suppression' of viral proliferation [7–9]. Type C hepatitis gradually proceeds from fibrosis and results in HCC. It seems like 'rain drop break rock in long term'. On the contrary, Type B fulminant hepatitis [10] may take lives in an instant. It seems possible that a deeper understanding of the mechanisms of viral proliferation [9] and potential new agents to suppress the viral proliferation will further aid treatment of patients with Type B fulminant hepatitis [7].

REFERENCES

[1] Chang MH, Chen CJ, Lai MS, Hsu HM, Wu TC, Kong MS, Liang DC, Shau WY, Chen DS. Universal hepatitis B vaccination in Taiwan and the incidence of hepatocellular carcinoma in children. New Engl J Med 1997; 336: 1855–1859.

[2] Yoshida H, Shiratori Y, Moriyama M, Arakawa Y, Ide T, Sata M, Inoue O, Yano M, Tanaka M, Fujiyama S, Nishiguchi S, Kuroki T, Imazeki F, Yokosuka O, Kinoyama S, Yamada G, Omata M. Interferon therapy reduces the risk for hepatocellular carcinoma: national surveillance program of cirrhotic and noncirrhotic patients with chronic hepatitis C in Japan. Ann Intern Med 1999; 131: 174–181.

[3] Shiratori Y, Imazeki F, Moriyama M, Yano M, Arakawa Y, Yokosuka O, Kuroki T, Sata M, Yamada G, Fujiyama S, Yoshida H, Omata M. Histologic improvement of fibrosis in hepatitis C patients with sustained response to interferon therapy. Ann Intern Med 2000; 132: 517–524.

[4] Shiina S, Niwa Y, Omata M. Percutaneous ethanol injection therapy for liver neoplasms. Semin Intervent Radiol 1993; 10: 57–68.

[5] Omata M. Regular medical care for hepatitis within the scope of HCC. Japan Medical Center, 1995; pp. 1–103.

[6] Omata M, Yokosuka O, Takano S, Kato N, Hosoda K, Imazeki F, Tada M, Ito Y, Ohto M. Resolution of acute hepatitis C after therapy with natural beta interferon. Lancet 1991; 338:

914–915.
[7] Omata M. Treatment of chronic hepatitis B infection (Editorial). New Engl J Med 1998; 339: 114–115.
[8] Ono-Nita SK, Kato N, Shiratori Y, Lan KH, Yoshida H, Carrilho FJ, Omata M. Susceptibility of lamivudine-resistant hepatitis B virus to other reverse transcriptase inhibitors. J Clin Invest 1999; 103: 1635–1640.
[9] Yokosuka O, Omata M, Imazeki F, Ito Y, Okuda K. Hepatitis B virus RNA transcripts and DNA in chronic liver disease. New Engl J Med 1986; 315: 1187–1192.
[10] Omata M, Ehata T, Yokosuka O, Hosoda K, Ohto M. Mutations in the precore region of hepatitis B virus DNA in patients with fulminant and severe hepatitis. New Engl J Med 1991; 324: 1699–1704.

Molecular Biology and Immunology in Hepatology
Edited by T. Tsuji, T. Higashi, M. Zeniya and K.-H. Meyer zum Büschenfelde

CHAPTER 11

Gene Expression Profiles in Hepatocellular Carcinoma

Shuichi Kaneko and Kenichi Kobayashi

First Department of Internal Medicine, Kanazawa University School of Medicine, Kanazawa, Japan

INTRODUCTION

Hepatocellular carcinoma (HCC) is an aggressive malignancy with poor prognosis and is one of the most common tumors in the world. To treat this intractable disease, understanding of the genetic abnormalities in HCC is important. Dynamic and closely related changes of gene expression are suspected of being involved in the pathogenesis of HCC. However, only limited numbers of genes have been shown to be associated with the pathogenesis including p53 mutations [1,2], c-myc activation [3,4], β-catenin mutations [5,6], angiopoietin-2 expression [7], and so on. Thus, the simultaneous differences of gene expression in HCC have not been understood using large numbers of genes.

Biomedical research is in the midst of a significant transition that is being driven by two primary factors: the massive increase in the amount of DNA sequence information and the development of technologies to exploit its use. Gene expression profiling methodologies have emerged to make an inventory of transcripts, and several studies have elucidated molecular portraits of human cancer using the serial analysis of gene expression (SAGE) technique, which allows simultaneous monitoring of the expression of tens of thousands of genes in tissue with sequence information [8–11]. With the advent of cDNA microarray technology, genomic-wide expression of hundreds of genes can be simultaneously analyzed, facilitating differential expression monitoring of a large number of activated or suppressed genes under various biological conditions including carcinogenesis [12–18]. In this review, we summarize recent studies of gene expression profiling of HCC using SAGE and cDNA microarray performed in our laboratory, and discuss the possibility of these technologies as a tool for understanding this intractable disease in the field of liver diseases.

1. COMPREHENSIVE GENE EXPRESSION PROFILE OF HCC COMPLICATED IN CHRONIC HEPATITIS

HCC is one of the few human cancers for which an underlying etiology can be identified in most cases, and is almost always associated with chronic liver diseases,

TABLE 1

Characteristics of three libraries of serial gene expression analysis (SAGE)

Histology	Total tags	Unique tags
Normal	30,982	8,596
Chronic hepatitis	31,381	10,172
Hepatocellular carcinoma	32,217	23,372

such as viral hepatitis or cirrhosis. Multistep carcinogenesis is suspected of being involved in hepatocarcinogenesis during chronic liver disease. SAGE was performed in chronic hepatitis C (CHC) and complicated well-differentiated HCC (W-HCC) in a patient, and compared the gene expression profiles of the two samples with that of a normal human liver (NL) by Yamashita et al. [19].

More than 30,000 transcripts were obtained from each of three samples, and a total of over 90,000 transcripts in the three samples were compared (Table 1). Scatter plots of the distribution of all transcripts from CHC and NL were well correlated indicating similar gene expression profiles among two samples. However that from HCC exhibited the existence of many differentially expressed genes compared with those from CHC and NL, whereas abundantly expressed transcripts from W-HCC still showed characteristics of NL. Thus, this study showed that HCC genetically derives from liver, but harbors peculiar gene expression pattern compared with normal liver and background chronically injured liver.

Up-regulation of many interferon-γ inducible genes and oxidative stress-inducible genes were similarly identified in both CHC and W-HCC. W-HCC was characterized by down-regulation of genes associated with xenobiotic catabolism and plasma protein synthesis. Some genes, including unpublished new genes, were specifically up- or down-regulated in W-HCC. Of the representative oncogenes and tumor suppressor genes, the expression levels were low and there were no statistical differences in expression among the three samples. These data demonstrated that the changes in expression of well-known oncogenes and tumor suppressor genes are subtle in W-HCC. However, subtle transcriptional changes in gene expression at low levels may be essentially important in hepatocarcinogenesis.

2. *a*-FETOPROTEIN-PRODUCING HEPATOMA CELL LINES SHARE COMMON EXPRESSION PROFILES

cDNA microarray was used to comprehensively analyze the genetic alterations occurring in hepatoma cell lines and hierarchical clustering algorism which examine the relatedness of gene expression pattern among cell lines as well as genes, was used to address the question if there were some specific subgroups of hepatoma cell lines distinguished by gene expression profiling by Kawai et al. [20].

Among six hepatoma cell lines analyzed, three α-fetoprotein (AFP)-producing hepatoma cell lines (HepG2, HuH7 and Hep3B) were shown to have common gene expression profile compared with those of AFP-negative hepatoma cell lines (HLE,

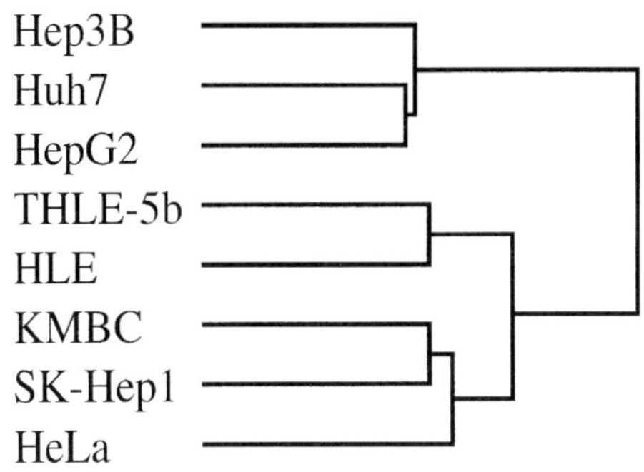

Fig. 1. Hierarchical clustering of gene expression data. The dendrogram shows the relatedness of gene expression profile among cell lines. Cell lines were ordered by the clustering algorithm analysis. The cell lines with the most similar patterns of gene expression are placed adjacent to each other and placed in the same branch of the dendrogram.

THLE-5b and SK-Hep-1) and cancer cell lines of non-hepatocyte origin (HeLa and KMBC) with cDNA microarray (Fig. 1). Analysis of the genes with a common expression profile among the highly AFP-producing cells (HepG2, Huh7 and Hep3B) revealed 254 genes across various categories. Seventy four of the 254 genes were up-regulated, and 180 genes were down-regulated commonly in the three cell lines.

The microarrays used in the study covered only a small portion of genome comprising about 1% of the human total genes; however, the findings suggest that a substantial number of genes associated in various categories shared a common expression profile that was characteristic of AFP-producing cell lines. Clearly, the interpretation of the results using cell lines is limited in the prediction of the behavior of tumors, and it remains to be determined whether the differences in gene expression profiles observed between AFP-producing HCC cells and other cancer cells including AFP-negative HCC can be applied to classify HCC on the basis of gene expression profile in clinical setting in the light of accompanying clinical differences.

3. IDENTIFICATION OF DIFFERENTIALLY EXPRESSED GENES IN HCC

Genes expressed in HCC were analyzed using cDNA microarrays to clarify gene abnormalities in HCC [21]. mRNA was extracted from cancerous and non-cancerous tissues of 10 patients with HCC (Table 2). The mRNA expression rate of each element in HCC was evaluated using the level of mRNA expression in non-cancerous tissue in each patient as a reference.

The expression of 10 genes was enhanced two or more times in HCC cancerous tissue compared with non-cancerous tissue in five or more of the 10 patients (Table 2). In contrast, nine genes were expressed at half the level or less in HCC cancerous tissue compared with non-cancerous tissue. When hierarchical clustering was performed to identify genes related to clinical phenotypes of the patients, 22 genes showed changes associated with the degree of differentiation of HCC (Table 3). Thirteen of these genes were transcriptional factors or tissue-specific expression proteins related to cell

TABLE 2

Characteristics of patients of 10 hepatocellular carcinomas

Case	HBsAg	HCV-Ab	Size of tumor (cm)	Histology
1	−	+	5	Well-differentiated
2	+	−	10	Poorly differentiated
3	+	+	6	Well-differentiated
4	−	+	3	Poorly differentiated
5	−	+	3	Poorly differentiated
6	−	+	14	Poorly differentiated
7	−	+	4	Poorly differentiated
8	−	+	6	Moderately differentiated
9	−	+	4	Moderately differentiated
10	−	+	6	Moderately differentiated

Historical grading of HCCs was decided according to the Classification of Liver Cancer Study Group of Japan.

TABLE 3

Differentially expressed genes in hepatocellular carcinoma compared with the non-cancerous tissue

Gene	No. of genes (Cy5/Cy3 >2.0)	Average (Cy5/Cy)	Gene	No. of genes (Cy5/Cy3 >0.5)	Average (Cy5/Cy)
1	8	2.80	1	9	0.24
2	7	3.47	2	8	0.37
3	6	3.47	3	8	0.34
4	6	5.59	4	7	0.37
5	6	3.70	5	6	0.34
6	5	2.54	6	5	0.46
7	5	2.53	7	5	0.25
8	5	2.57	8	5	0.27
9	5	2.93	9	5	0.44
10	5	4.58			

Commonly expressed genes more than five samples are listed with expression ratio of Cy5 to Cy3 counts. Enhanced expression two or more times, or depressed at half the level or less are listed.

differentiation or development. The number of genes used and functional analysis of the genes detected in this study is still insufficient, and further evaluation is needed. However, all these genes are considered to be genes that characterize HCC and to be useful for not only clarification of the carcinogenic mechanism, but also for establishing diagnostic and therapeutic strategies.

4. MAKING SENSE OF GENOMIC RESULTS FOR HCC

The expression profile or the 'transcriptome', shown in these studies, is a major determinant of cellular phenotype and function. The transcription of genomic DNA to produce mRNA is the first step in the process of protein synthesis, and differences in gene expression are responsible for both morphological and phenotypic differences. In terms of understanding the function of genes, knowing when, where and to what extent a gene is expressed is central to understanding the activity and biological roles of its encoded protein. In addition, changes in the multi-gene patterns of expression can provide clues about regulatory mechanisms and broader cellular functions and biochemical pathways. In the context of human health and treatment, the knowledge gained from these types of measurements can help determine the causes and consequences of disease, how drugs and drug candidates work in cells and organisms, and what gene products might have therapeutic uses themselves or may be appropriate targets for therapeutic intervention.

However, despite impressive and rapidly growing results, gene expression profiling methodologies demonstrated in this summary are in their infancy. Extracting biologically meaningful data is still difficult. Three studies, data for thousands of genes in HCC, clearly show the possibility of these methodologies as a powerful tool to understand genetic abnormalities occurring in HCC. However, there is a need for more sophisticated systems of knowledge representation that organize the data, facts, observations, relationship and even hypotheses that form the basis of our current scientific understanding.

REFERENCES

[1] Watanabe A, Nishimori H, Tsukishiro T, Okada K, Shimizu Y, Nambu S et al. Hepatocellular carcinoma in 13 patients with hepatitis C virus-associated chronic hepatitis. Cancer Res 1994; 54: 231–235.

[2] Rashid A, Wang JS, Qian GS, Lu BX, Hamilton SR, Groopman JD. Genetic alterations in hepatocellular carcinomas: association between loss of chromosome 4q and p53 gene mutations. Br J Cancer 1999; 80: 59–66.

[3] Abou-Elella A, Gramlich T, Fritsch C, Gansler T. C-myc amplification in hepatocellular carcinoma predicts unfavorable prognosis. Mod Pathol 1996; 9: 95–98.

[4] Terada T, Nakanuma Y. Expression of apoptosis, proliferating cell nuclear antigen, and apoptosis-related antigens (bcl-2, c-myc, Fas, Lewis(y) and p53) in human cholangiocarcinomas and hepatocellular carcinomas. Pathol Int 1996; 46: 764–770.

[5] de La Coste A, Romagnolo B, Billuart P, Renard CA, Buendia MA, Soubrane O et al. Somatic mutations of the beta-catenin gene are frequent in mouse and human hepatocellular carcinomas. Proc Natl Acad Sci USA 1998; 95: 8847–8851.

[6] Miyoshi Y, Iwao K, Nagasawa Y, Aihara T, Sasaki Y, Imaoka S et al. Activation of the beta-catenin gene in primary hepatocellular carcinomas by somatic alterations involving exon 3. Cancer Res 1998; 58: 2524–2527.

[7] Tanaka S, Mori M, Sakamoto Y, Makuuchi M, Sugimachi K, Wands JR. Biologic significance of angiopoietin-2 expression in human hepatocellular carcinoma. J Clin Invest 1999; 103: 341–345.

[8] Zhang L, Zhou W, Velculescu VE, Kern SE, Hruban RH, Hamilton SR et al. Gene expression profiles in normal and cancer cells. Science 1997; 276: 1268–1272.

[9] Lal A, Lash AE, Altschul SF, Velculescu V, Zhang L, McLendon R et al. A public database for gene expression in human cancers. Cancer Res 1999; 59: 5403–5407.

[10] Ferguson AT, Evron E, Umbricht CB, Pandita TK, Chan TA, Hermeking H et al. High frequency of hypermethylation at the 14-3-3 sigma locus leads to gene silencing in breast cancer. Proc Natl Acad Sci USA 2000; 97: 6049–6054.
[11] St Croix B, Rago C, Velculescu V, Traverso G, Romans KE, Montgomery E et al. Genes expressed in human tumor endothelium. Science 2000; 289: 1197–1202.
[12] Khan J, Saal LH, Bittner ML, Chen Y, Trent JM, Meltzer PS. Expression profiling in cancer using cDNA microarrays. Electrophoresis 1999; 20: 223–229.
[13] Xu J, Stolk JA, Zhang X, Silva SJ, Houghton RL, Matsumura M et al. Identification of differentially expressed genes in human prostate cancer using subtraction and microarray. Cancer Res 2000; 60: 1677–1682.
[14] Wang T, Hopkins D, Schmidt C, Silva S, Houghton R, Takita H et al. Identification of genes differentially over-expressed in lung squamous cell carcinoma using combination of cDNA subtraction and microarray analysis. Oncogene 2000; 19: 1519–1528.
[15] Villaret DB, Wang T, Dillon D, Xu J, Sivam D, Cheever MA et al. Identification of genes overexpressed in head and neck squamous cell carcinoma using a combination of complementary DNA subtraction and microarray analysis. Laryngoscope 2000; 110: 374–381.
[16] Moch H, Schraml P, Bubendorf L, Mirlacher M, Kononen J, Gasser T et al. High-throughput tissue microarray analysis to evaluate genes uncovered by cDNA microarray screening in renal cell carcinoma. Am J Pathol 1999; 154: 981–986.
[17] Khan J, Simon R, Bittner M, Chen Y, Leighton SB, Pohida T et al. Gene expression profiling of alveolar rhabdomyosarcoma with cDNA microarrays. Cancer Res 1998; 58: 5009–5013.
[18] Honda M, Kaneko S, Kawai H, Shirota Y, Kobayashi K. cDNA microarray analysis reveals differential gene expression between chronic hepatitis B and C hepatic lesions. Gastroenterology 2001; 120: 955–966.
[19] Yamashita T, Kaneko S, Hashimoto S, Sato T, Nagai S, Toyoda N et al. Comprehensive gene expression profile of hepatocellular carcinoma complicated in chronic hepatitis C (manuscript submitted for publication).
[20] Kawai HF, Kaneko S, Honda M, Shirota Y, Kobayashi K. Alpha-fetoprotein producing hepatoma cell lines share common expression profiles of genes in various categories demonstrated by cDNA microarray analysis. Hepatology 2001; 33: 676–691.
[21] Shirota Y, Kaneko S, Honda M, Kawai HF, Kobayashi K. Identification of differentially expressed genes in hepatocellular carcinoma with cDNA microarrays. Hepatology 2001; 33: 832–840.

Molecular Biology and Immunology in Hepatology
Edited by T. Tsuji, T. Higashi, M. Zeniya and K.-H. Meyer zum Büschenfelde

CHAPTER 12

Gene Therapy for Hepatocellular Carcinoma: Recent Advancements and Problems to Overcome

Shigeki kuriyama [1], Hirohisa Tsujinoue [2], Toshiya Nakatani [2], Hitoshi Yoshiji [2] and Hiroshi Fukui [2]

[1] *Third Department of Internal Medicine, Nara Medical University, Nara, Japan*
[2] *Third Department of Internal Medicine, Kagawa Medical University, Kagawa, Japan*

INTRODUCTION

Hepatocellular carcinoma (HCC) is one of the most common human malignancies worldwide and is also one of the most ominous types of cancer [1]. The worldwide annual incidence of HCC has been estimated to be 250,000–1,000,000 with a male–female ratio of approximately 4 : 1 [2]. In the majority of cases, HCC is found in conjunction with cirrhosis of the liver [3,4]. Radical operation is the only curative modality for HCC, but is appropriate in the minority of patients due to their limited hepatic reserves. Therefore, various alternative therapies, such as intra-arterial chemoembolization, percutaneous intratumoral ethanol injection and orthotopic liver transplantation, have been employed, but there is still no satisfactory treatment for HCC [5–7]. Novel approaches need to be developed if the overall survival rate of patients with HCC is to be significantly improved. Recent advances in recombinant DNA and gene delivery technologies suggest that gene therapy may be a promising alternative to explore.

1. GENE THERAPY PROTOCOLS

Gene therapy, the introduction of foreign genetic material into target cells or tissues to collect a disease phenotype, has rapidly been evolving as a new treatment modality against a variety of human diseases. Now there are 409 active clinical gene therapy protocols in the United States and more than 3000 patients have already undergone gene therapy [8]. Among the 409 protocols, 249 (61%) are approaches to the treatment of various types of cancer. Gene therapy strategies can be divide into two categories, namely ex vivo and in vivo gene therapy protocols. Ex vivo gene therapy involves removal of a part of the target tissue surgically from the patient, isolation and growth of the target autologous cells, introduction of a therapeutic gene into cells in vitro. After verification and selection of genetically modified cells, the process is completed by returning the modified cells into the same patient. In vivo gene therapy does not require removal of cells and the process is done by directly delivering a therapeutic gene into the target cells of the patient. Each strategy has its own inherent advantages and disadvantages. For instance, ex vivo gene therapy allows gene delivery to a defined, pre-selected cells and eliminates the potential side effects of gene transfer into undesirable, non-target cells. In addition, high transduction efficiency of a therapeutic gene can be achieved by repeating gene transfer while culturing cells. Because of these practical advantages, most clinical gene therapy protocols to date have employed ex vivo strategies. However, when considering gene therapy for HCC, it should be noted that most HCCs arise from the cirrhotic liver, but not from the normal liver. Therefore, ex vivo gene therapy which requires an invasive partial hepatectomy does not appear to be practical. In vivo gene therapy appears to be much more desirable and practical for the treatment of HCC.

2. GENE DELIVERY SYSTEMS

Gene delivery systems can be divided into two categories, namely viral and non-viral systems. Gene delivery systems are well reviewed elsewhere [9–13]. Recombinant viral vectors are by far the most efficient vehicles for the transfer of genes into target cells. Therefore, they are preferred over non-viral means. Many viruses have evolved specific mechanisms to enter mammalian cells by way of virus-specific or physiological receptors, to exit from endosomal vesicles, to translocate to the nucleus and to express viral genes with or without integration into the host genome. Recombinant viral vectors, which are designed to express a gene of interest but not the viral proteins, are potent vehicles of gene transfer into isolated cells in vitro or into target tissues in vivo. Among viral vectors, recombinant adenovirus is by far the most effective vehicle for in vivo gene transfer into the liver [14,15]. However, the clinical usefulness of current adenoviral vectors may be limited due to their strong immunogenicity [16–20]. Non-viral vector systems include direct injection of DNA, electroporation, particle bombardment, liposomes and DNA–protein complexes. We have shown that particle-mediated gene transfer using gene gun technology induced much stronger transgene expression in the murine liver compared with simple plasmid injection and electroporation-mediated gene transfer [21]. Transduction efficiency induced by non-viral vectors is in general lower than that induced by viral vectors. The duration of transgene expression induced by non-viral systems is transient and usually shorter than that induced by viral vector systems. Non-viral vectors, however, offer some advantages compared with viral vectors. There are no gene size constraints in non-viral vectors. Furthermore, due to the lack of viral antigens, non-viral vector systems are much safer and much less immunogenic than viral vectors, which makes repeated gene transfer possible.

3. HCC-SELECTIVE TRANSGENE EXPRESSION

A critical issue for effective and safe gene therapy, specifically for safe in vivo gene therapy, is to transfer (tissue targeting) and express (transcriptional targeting) a therapeutic gene of interest to tumor tissues without affecting non-cancerous, normal tissues. Since tumor-selective receptor-mediated vector delivery system has not been established, the use of tumor-selective promoters, such as the α-fetoprotein (AFP) promoter and the carcinoembryonic antigen (CEA) promoter, to direct expression of therapeutic genes is the most promising alternative. We have isolated 204- and 419-bp CEA promoter regions from high CEA-producing human colorectal carcinoma, and demonstrated that they could direct 20-fold expression of a luciferase reporter gene in CEA-producing human colorectal carcinoma cells as compared with non-CEA-producing cells [22]. In CEA-producing colorectal carcinoma cells, the CEA promoter regions have been shown to be as active as the simian virus 40 (SV40) early promoter and the Moloney murine leukemia virus long terminal repeat (LTR) enhancer/promoter, which have been used to direct expression of therapeutic genes as general, strong promoters [23,24].

Similarly, usefulness of the AFP promoter for targeting HCC cells has been demonstrated [25–32]. However, in marked contrast to the CEA promoter, the AFP promoter has been shown to be weak [26,33]. It is critical for successful gene therapy to induce strong expression of the exogenous genes used for therapeutic purposes. For instance, we have shown that stronger intratumoral expression of the tumor necrosis factor-α (TNF-α) gene resulted in more effective anti-HCC activity [34]. Therefore, if HCC cell-selective expression of a therapeutic gene is achieved, weak transgene expression may result in insufficient antitumor effects. To enhance the activity of the AFP promoter, the addition of the AFP enhancer to the AFP promoter has been shown to be more effective in gene therapy for AFP-producing HCC than the promoter alone [35]. Alternatively, to enhance the expression level while maintaining the HCC-selectivity, the AFP enhancer was linked to the albumin promoter. When this chimeric transcriptional regulatory element was used to direct the herpes simplex virus thymidine kinase (HSV-tk) gene, ganciclovir (GCV) treatment caused only AFP and albumin-positive HCC cell death, but not non-hepatocyte tumor cells or AFP and albumin-negative hepatic tumor cells [36,37]. We have also shown that the addition of the 5.1-kb 5′-flanking region of the AFP gene to the non-tissue-specific viral promoters, such as the SV40 promoter and the retroviral LTR promoter, resulted in HCC cell-selective expression of the transduced IL-2 and TNF-α genes [38]. Furthermore, the addition of the AFP enhancer region including domains A and B to the non-tissue-specific, housekeeping phosphoglycerate kinase promoter resulted in HCC cell-selective HSV-tk expression [39].

Other options for tumor-selective transgene expression comprise the use of retroviral vector. Retroviruses provide a potential means of selectively infecting tumor cells because they can only integrate into the genome of dividing cells, but not non-dividing cells [40]; most normal cells surrounding tumors are in a quiescent, non-receptive stage of cell growth. We have shown that expression of a *lacZ* reporter gene was achieved solely in HCC cells but not in normal hepatocytes in vivo by use of recombinant retroviruses carrying the reporter gene under the transcriptional control of the albumin enhancer and promoter region [41]. Vile and Hart [42] also reported that direct injection of a heterologous reporter gene directed by the melanocyte-selective tyrosinase promoter could lead to strong, melanoma-selective transgene expression in vivo. There are, however, non-cancerous normal dividing cells in vivo, such as bone marrow cells and intestinal epithelial cells. We have shown that when retroviruses carrying a suicide cytosine deaminase (CD) gene under the control of the non-tissue-selective retroviral LTR promoter were administered into the peritoneally cavity, they infected bone marrow cells and severe bone marrow suppression was caused by the subsequent 5-fluorocytosine (5-FC) treatment. Conversely, significant bone marrow suppression was not induced despite 5-FC treatment when the CD gene was directed by the CEA promoter [23,24,43]. Taken collectively, these results suggest that in the case of retrovirus-mediated in vivo gene transfer, the use of a tissue-selective transcriptional regulatory element can achieve essentially tumor-selective expression of a foreign gene. Although the usefulness of recombinant retroviruses is limited mainly due to their relatively low transduction efficiency, we have improved retroviral vectors and demonstrated the amelioration of retrovirus-mediated gene transfer into HCC cells [44–46].

4. THERAPEUTIC STRATEGIES FOR GENE THERAPY AGAINST HCC

There are numerous gene therapy strategies for the treatment of various types of cancer. They include tumor suppressor gene therapy, genetic immunotherapy, suicide gene therapy, antisense strategies (inhibition of oncogenes), normal tissue protection (transfer of the multidrug-resistance gene) and anti-angiogenesis strategies. General gene therapy strategies against cancer are well reviewed elsewhere [47]. Therefore, we will focus this review on attempts and achievements of gene therapy against HCC.

4.1. Tumor suppressor gene therapy

Introduction of tumor suppressor genes appears to be a promising strategy, specifically in tumors in which specific defects of tumor suppressor genes have been determined. Among a number of tumor suppressor genes, biochemical characterization of p53 has led to the elucidation of several mechanisms by which p53 might exert a tumor suppression effect [48,49]. Loss of wild-type p53 function either by its mutation or inactivation contributes to the development of malignant tumors and enhances tumor cell resistance to a variety of chemotherapeutic agents [50]. Mutations of p53 have been detected in 0–60% of HCC, depending on geographic locations. Mutations of the p53 gene are less frequent in HCC low-incidence areas, such as Europe and United States, and more frequent in HCC high-incidence areas, such as Asia and Africa, in epidemiologic association with hepatitis B infection and dietary aflatoxin B exposure [51,52]. In total, mutations have been detected in 29% of 716 cases in a global database [53].

Because introduction of wild-type p53 may provide an interesting approach to the treatment of cancer, various attempts using the wild-type p53 gene have been made for the treatment of HCC [54,55]. Xu et al. [56] constructed a retroviral vector carrying the wild-type p53 gene under the transcriptional control of the AFP promoter. They have shown that expression of the exogenous wild-type p53 gene from the retroviral vector was limited to AFP-positive HCC cells and markedly inhibited their clonal growth in monolayer and soft agar cultures. Furthermore, retrovirus-mediated introduction of the wild-type p53 gene increased the sensitivity of HCC cells to the chemotherapeutic agent, cisplatin, indicating that restoration of wild-type p53 expression in HCC cells, in combination with chemotherapeutic drugs, may be a promising approach to the treatment of HCC. Anderson et al. [57] have developed a syngeneic rat model using a p53-mutated HCC cell line that resulted in multifocal liver nodules. They have demonstrated that daily hepatic artery dosing of recombinant adenoviruses carrying the wild-type p53 gene suppressed tumor growth when compared with untreated rats or animals treated with recombinant adenoviruses carrying the *lacZ* gene.

However, the low transduction efficiency achieved by currently available gene transfer techniques represents an important limitation of the strategies based on introduction of tumor suppressor genes to treat cancer, because a nearly 100% transduction efficiency of the wild-type p53 gene to all the tumor cells would be required for inhibiting tumor growth completely. In addition, it has been shown in breast and colorectal carcinoma cells that mutations in the exogenously delivered wild-type p53 gene and its excision by cellular enzymes abrogated effectively wild-type p53 function [58]. Furthermore, mutation or inactivation of the wild-type p53 gene may only be one defect that the cell encounters on its development towards the malignant state. Therefore, introduction of the wild-type p53 gene into a tumor cell may be insufficient to collect the malignant phenotype of the tumor cell.

4.2. Genetic immunotherapy

Accumulating evidence suggests that failure of the immune system to eliminate a tumor is due to the inability of tumor antigens to stimulate an effective immune responses [59,60]. A logical approach to the treatment of cancer is the augmentation of the host immune responses against tumor cells by genetic modification and the rationale of such an approach has been discussed at length [61–63]. Studies in animal tumor models have shown that the unfavorable host–tumor relationship was improved by manipulating the host immune mechanism [64–66].

4.2.1. Transduction of HCC cells with cytokine genes

Cytokines play an important role in the regulation of the immune system. Using gene transfer procedures, tumor cells or stroma cells can be modified to produce immunostimulatory cytokines. Many cytokines, such as IL-2, IL-4, IL-6, IL-7, IL-12, interferon-γ (IFN-γ), TNF-α and granulocyte-macrophage colony stimulating factor (GM-CSF), have been employed for stimulation of immune responses against cancer [67,68].

We constructed retroviral vectors carrying the IL-2, IL-3 or TNF-α gene under the transcriptional control of the albumin promoter or the SV40 promoter. We have shown that various HCC cells infected with the retroviruses carrying the cytokine genes directed by the albumin promoter expressed the cytokine genes much more strongly compared with those infected with the retroviruses carrying the cytokine genes directed by the SV40 promoter. Furthermore, infection of retroviruses containing the albumin promoter induced expression of the cytokine genes solely in HCC cell lines, but not in non-HCC cell lines [69]. We have also shown that murine HCC cells infected with retroviruses carrying the TNF-α gene under the control of the albumin promoter lost their tumorigenicity when implanted in syngeneic mice and induced tumor immunity against parental HCC cells. Furthermore, intratumoral administration of the retroviruses showed the antitumor effect against established HCCs, resulting in significantly prolonged survival periods. Most importantly, intratumoral implantation of the retrovirus-producing cells completely abrogated established HCCs in mice [34].

IL-2 is one of the promising cytokines to induce tumor-specific cellular toxicity. Huang et al. [70] implanted a murine HCC cell line into the liver of syngeneic mice. They intratumorally and intraperitoneally injected recombinant adenoviruses carrying the IL-2 gene and demonstrated long-term remission in 75% of animals. The surviving animals developed systemic antitumoral cellular immunity that protected them against challenges of parental HCC cells implanted at distant sites. Bui et al. [71] constructed recombinant adenoviruses carrying the IL-2 gene controlled either by the AFP promoter or by the cytomegalovirus promoter. They produced an animal HCC model by implanting human HCC cells in severe combined immunodeficiency mice. Intratumoral injection of the adenoviruses resulted in growth retardation and regression in a majority of established HCCs, but with a much wider therapeutic index and less systemic toxicity using the adenoviruses with the AFP promoter.

IFNs are cytokines with antitumor activity. The therapeutic effect of the fibroblast-mediated IFN-α gene therapy in combination with IL-2-activated killer cells on nude mice bearing human HCC was investigated by Cao et al. [72]. They have demonstrated that when fibroblasts transduced with the IFN-α gene were intraperitoneally implanted into HCC-bearing nude mice, the growth of HCC was inhibited and the survival time of the mice was extended. The growth of HCC was inhibited more obviously when IL-2-activated killer cells were injected intravenously and IL-2 was injected intraperitoneally after IFN-α gene-transduced fibroblasts had been implanted. IL-12 is also one of the promising cytokines with potent antitumor activity. Usefulness of gene therapy with IL-12 against metastatic liver tumors was demonstrated by using a mouse model, with the outcome of prolongation of median survival time [73–75]. Similarly, usefulness of gene therapy with IL-12 against HCC has been shown elsewhere [76].

4.2.2. Enhancement of tumor immunogenicity

Tumor cells can escape immunological surveillance by several mechanisms including the selective loss of major histocompatibility complex (MHC) class I antigens and β_2-microglobulin and lack of the appropriate costimulatory molecules. Lymphocyte activation requires recognition of a MHC/antigen complex and costimulatory signals. One of the strategies to increase immunogenicity of tumor cells is the transduction of tumor cells with genes coding for MHC class I molecules or members of the B7 family of costimulatory molecules [77]. However, when a T-cell encounters the antigen in the absence of these costimulatory signals, it becomes unresponsive or undergoes apoptotic cell death [78,79]. Therefore, tumor antigens presented in the context of MHC class I proteins alone may fail to stimulate an antitumor effect. The importance of B7 in antitumor immunity has been shown in murine therapeutic models. Chen et al. [80] have shown that immunization of mice with B7-expressing tumor led to regression of established B7-negative tumors. Tatsumi et al. [81,82] have shown that transduction of human HCC cells with the B7-1 gene substantially augmented primary cytolytic activity against parental human HCC cells, resulting in a significant tumor rejection or at least inhibition of tumor growth in a mouse model.

4.2.3. Genetic modification of dendritic cells

Antigen-presenting cells (APCs) are the initiators and modulators of the immune response and play a central role in the generation and regulation of antitumor immunity. Dendritic cells are very potent APCs that express MHC class I and II molecules and costimulatory molecules [83–85]. Dendritic cells can be engineered to present tumor antigens by either pulsing them with tumor peptides or tumor extracts, by fusing them with tumor cells or by introducing genes coding for the relevant tumor antigens and/or cytokines using viral or non-viral vectors. Administration of these engineered dendritic cells can promote potent antitumor immunity [86–88]. Guo et al. [89] have shown that immunization with hybridoma cells produced from fusion of HCC cells with activated B-cells not only induced a protective effect on parental HCC rechallenge, but also cured pre-established HCC tumors in a rat model. Vollmer et al. [90] have shown that dendritic cells engineered to express AFP produced T-cell responses in mice, as evidenced by the generation of AFP-specific cytotoxic T-lymphocytes, cytokine-producing T-cells and protective immunity. AFP plasmid-based immunization was shown to generate less potent responses, supporting a rationale of gene therapy-based strategy for HCC treatment using engineered dendritic cells.

4.3. Suicide gene therapy against HCC

The basic principle underlying suicide gene system is intracellular conversion of a relatively non-toxic prodrug to a highly toxic drug by an enzyme that is not normally present in the cell. Viruses, bacteria and fungi often use unique metabolic pathways not used by mammalian cells, and contain genes for enzymes that perform metabolic conversions that mammalian cells do not perform. Such distinctive enzymes have often been the target of drugs developed for the treatment of infections. Such agents are lethal for the infecting microbe, but do not harm the host cell, because it lacks the enzyme system necessary to activate the drug [91,92]. Likewise, tumor cells modified genetically with a suicide gene can be selectively killed during administration of the appropriate non-toxic prodrug.

4.3.1. HSV-tk gene

The best studied and most widely used suicide gene to date is the HSV-tk gene. HSV-tk enzyme can efficiently phosphorylate nucleoside analogues such as GCV and acyclovir (ACV) into monophosphorylated molecules. They are then converted by cellular phosphokinases into triphosphate substrate, which are incorporated into elongating DNA during cellular division, causing chain termination and selective killing of dividing cells by apoptosis. Thus, the nucleoside analogues are toxic under the dual conditions that target cells are both dividing and expressing HSV-tk. Since GCV and ACV are relatively poor substrates for mammalian thymidine kinases, concentrations can be achieved that are lethal to cells expressing HSV-tk, but are non-toxic to normal mammalian cells. Both GCV and ACV have been clinically used as antiviral chemotherapeutic agents, and detailed information on their safety is available. We have shown that HSV-tk-transduced HCC cells exhibited dose-dependent susceptibility to GCV and ACV. The transduced HCC cells had a more than 1000-fold increase in sensitivity to GCV toxicity as compared with parental HCC cells, but only a 30-fold increase in sensitivity to ACV toxicity [93]. These results demonstrate that the therapeutic index was much higher in GCV treatment than in ACV treatment, indicating that GCV may be preferable to ACV as a prodrug in HSV-tk transduction strategies.

One of most promising aspects of the HSV-tk/GCV system observed in both in vitro and in vivo experiments is that tumor cells not actually expressing the HSV-tk gene, but in proximity to HSV-tk-expressing cells, are killed after exposure to GCV. Such an unexpected phenomenon, the so-called bystander effect, is extremely important for achieving effective therapeutic outcomes against cancer, because it appears impossible to introduce a therapeutic gene into all the cells of a tumor using currently available gene transfer techniques. Although the mechanism mediating the bystander effect is not completely understood, the phenomenon acts either as a result of metabolic cooperation in which toxic metabolites of GCV phosphorylation are passed via gap junctions between neighboring cells or by the exchange of apoptotic vesicles between closely juxtaposed cells [94–96]. We have shown that strong and effective bystander effects on HCC were induced by the HSV-tk/GCV system not only in vitro, but also in vivo [93,97–103].

It has been shown that there is a contribution of the host's immune system to the in vivo bystander effect [104]. We and others have observed that when grafts consisting of HSV-tk-transduced tumor cells were killed in vivo by GCV treatment, antitumor immunity was generated so that a subsequent challenge with untransduced parental tumor cells led to rejection [98–102,105–110]. These results imply that hosts' immune responses play a role in the antitumor effect induced by the HSV-tk/GCV system. To examine the immunological mechanisms involved in cancer gene therapy using the HSV-tk/GCV system, we retrovirally introduced the HSV-tk gene into a murine HCC cell line. When HSV-tk-transduced HCC cells were mixed with parental cells at a 50% ratio and implanted subcutaneously into immunocompetent syngeneic mice, complete inhibition of tumor formation was achieved by GCV treatment. Conversely, no significant inhibitory effects on tumor formation were observed in athymic nude mice. When established HCCs in immunocompetent mice containing HSV-tk-transduced HCC cells at an only 5% ratio were treated with GCV, marked infiltration of lymphocytes, including $CD4^+$ and $CD8^+$, and apoptotic death of HCC cells were induced, and significant reduction or even complete regression of established HCCs was achieved. Furthermore, such cured mice rejected rechallenge with parental HCC cells into the contraflank regions [100,102]. These results indicate that cancer gene therapy with the HSV-tk/GCV system can indeed induce efficient antitumor effects and protective immunity in immunocompetent mice, but not in nude mice, indicating that T-cell-mediated immune responses may be a critical factor for achieving successful gene therapy against cancer using the HSV-tk/GCV system.

Application of the HSV-tk gene transduction system to malignancy was pioneered by Moolten [111], and a number of reports have been published illustrating the efficiency in both in vitro and in vivo tumor models. In the field of gene therapy with the

HSV-tk gene against HCC, Macri and Gordon [112] demonstrated the effectiveness of the HSV-tk/GCV system for the treatment of HCC, using the transgenic mice carrying the HSV-tk gene under the control of the AFP promoter. A number of studies have shown that the HSV-tk/GCV system caused tumor regression in rodent models of HCC. However, it has also been shown that the HSV-tk/GCV system induced significant hepatic damages [113,114]. To avoid the adverse reaction, tumor-selective expression of the HSV-tk gene has been attempted. Several groups have utilized the AFP promoter to direct the HSV-tk gene in retroviral, adenoviral or adeno-associated viral vectors [26–29,31,36,37]. We have used the albumin promoter to control the HSV-tk gene in a retroviral vector and demonstrated that repeated intratumoral injections of HSV-tk-carrying retroviruses and GCV treatment resulted in complete regression of established HCC in all mice used in the experiment. Animals that completely eradicated tumors exhibited protective immunity against wild-type HCC [115]. These results suggest that repeated injections of HSV-tk-carrying retroviruses followed by GCV treatment is a potent modality for the treatment of solid tumors including HCC.

4.3.2. Bacterial CD gene

Another promising suicide gene is the bacterial CD gene. CD is a non-mammalian enzyme found in many bacteria and fungi but absent in eukaryotes, which functions to deaminate cytosine to uracil. It has been shown that through a similar mechanism CD can deaminate the relatively non-toxic 5-FC to the highly toxic 5-fluorouracil (5-FU) [116,117]. Normal mammalian cells do not possess CD and are relatively resistant to 5-FC. Recently, the *Escherichia coli* CD gene was cloned [118,119] and the investigators have established mammalian cell lines that constitutively express CD following transfection of the *E. coli* CD gene [120,121]. Those genetically modified cells were selectively sensitive to 5-FC as compared with unmodified parental cells. An attractive feature of this system is that 5-FC and 5-FU have been already utilized in routine clinical treatment as an antifungal and antitumor agent, respectively, so that extensive pharmacological information is available on both drugs. We have shown that HCC cells transduced with the bacterial CD gene were susceptible to 5-FC toxicity in a dose-dependent manner, while untransduced parental cells exhibited the substantial resistance to 5-FC [122]. CD-transduced HCC cells showed a sensitivity to 5-FU similar to that of parental HCC cells, indicating that there was no significant difference in the inherent sensitivity of the cells to the toxic end product [123].

As well as the HSV-tk/GCV system, the CD/5-FC system can also induce the bystander effect not only in vitro, but also in vivo [122,124,125]. The metabolite of 5-FC, 5-FU, is freely diffusible across the cellular membrane and spreads from CD-transduced cells to adjacent tumor cells that do not express the CD gene. Therefore, unlike the bystander effect induced by the HSV-tk/GCV system which requires cell-to-cell contact and formation of gap junctions, the bystander effect induced by the CD/5-FC system is not dependent on cell-to-cell contact [126,127]. We have shown that CD-transduced HCC cells caused killing of neighboring parental cells in the presence of 5-FC, irrespective of direct cell-to-cell contact [101]. We have also shown that the strength of the bystander effect induced by the CD/5-FC system correlated very well with the levels of 5-FU generated from 5-FC by CD-transduced cells [123].

As well as the HSV-tk/GCV system, the involvement of immunological mechanisms has been demonstrated in the antitumor effect induced by the CD/5-FC system. Consalvo et al. [128] have demonstrated that development of tumors consisting of 100% CD-transduced cells was not suppressed despite 5-FC treatment in $CD8^+$ T-lymphocyte- and granulocyte-depleted mice and that the tumor immunity elicited by the CD/5-FC system was dependent on $CD4^+$ T-lymphocytes. We have also shown that when syngeneic immunocompetent mice were inoculated subcutaneously with parental murine HCC cells containing as little as 5% CD-transduced HCC cells, significant inhibition of tumor formation was induced by 5-FC treatment. Furthermore, established HCC tumors in immunocompetent mice containing only 5% CD-transduced cells were infiltrated markedly with $CD4^+$ and $CD8^+$ T-lymphocytes and macrophages by 5-FC treatment, such that significant reduction or even complete regression of tumors was observed. These tumor-free mice resisted subsequent rechallenge with wild-type tumor. Conversely, when athymic nude mice were inoculated with a cell mixture containing CD-transduced cells and parental HCC cells at a ratio of 40 : 60, all developed tumors despite 5-FC treatment [129]. These results indicate that the host immune responses elicited by the CD/5-FC system, but not the transfer of cytotoxic 5-FU generated by CD-transduced cells, appear to play a critical role in in vivo antitumor effects.

4.4. Antisense strategy

Antisense gene therapy may be a promising approach to genetic modulation that can be used to diminish gene expression by introducing molecules that identify and inactivate specifically targeted mRNA sequences, resulting in suppression of translation. Such antisense molecules include complementary oligonucleotides and antisense DNAs. Antisense gene therapy appears to be particularly useful for the treatment of tumors with overactive oncogenes. In HCC, high expression of the *ras* oncogene family, such as Ha-*ras* and N-*ras*, has been reported [130–133]. Baba et al. [134] have shown that significant inhibition of HCC development was observed in rats treated with Ha-*ras* antisense during exposure to the hepatocarcinogen *N*-nitrosomorpholine. Liao et al. [135] have shown that an antisense Ha-*ras* oligonucleotide was effective for inducing apoptosis of HCC cells in vitro and for retarding tumor growth in vivo. Although antisense gene therapy is an attractive strategy, several factors restrict the practicality of this approach. For instance, to completely block a target oncogene, multiple copies of the antisense molecules need to be introduced into a single tumor cell, which is apparently impossible by using currently available gene transfer techniques. Furthermore, the half-lives of antisense therapeutics are considerably short and allow only transient inhibition of target gene expression. Finally, the presence of multiple oncogenic contributions, which are common in aneuploid human tumors, may be an additional difficulty for successful cancer gene therapy with antisense strategies.

4.5. Antiangiogenesis strategy

The growth of a solid tumor is now widely recognized to depend on the process of neovascularization. Without angiogenesis, tumors cease to grow beyond even a few millimeters in volume. It has been reported that tumor cells secrete angiogenic factors to promote their survival and growth [136–138]. Among these factors, vascular endothelial growth factor (VEGF) is one of the most potent angiogenic factors. We have shown that VEGF plays a critical role in the development of HCC in cooperation with endothelial cells [139]. Two tyrosine kinases, *fms*-like tyrosine kinase (flt-1) and the kinase insert domain-containing receptor/murine homologue, fetal liver kinase-1 (KDR/Flk-1), both of which are type III tyrosine kinase receptors, have been identified as high-affinity VEGF receptors [140]. We have shown that KDR/Flk-1 is a major regulator of VEGF-mediated HCC development and angiogenesis not only at the initial stage, but also after the tumor has fully developed and that KDR/Flk-1 is also a major regulator of malignant ascites formation in a mouse HCC model [141,142]. Although the biological process that underlines VEGF-mediated signaling pathways remains to be elucidated, we recently demonstrated that protein kinase C, especially the β-isoform, is a major regulator of VEGF-mediated HCC development and angiogenesis [143].

Because angiogenesis is a critical process for tumor development, strategies aimed at blocking angiogenic factors are expected to inhibit tumor growth or even to induce tumor regression. Kang et al. [144] have shown that human HCC cells transduced with an antisense-VEGF cDNA exhibited a suppressed synthesis of VEGF protein. When an expression vector bearing the antisense-VEGF cDNA was injected peritumorally by liposomes, growth of HCC formed subcutaneously in nude mice was inhibited. Another strategy explores natural antagonist to angiogenesis, such as angiostatin and endostatin [145,146]. Although gene transfer of angiostatin by retroviral and adenoviral vectors has been used for the treatment of different tumors in animal models [147], usefulness of these anti-angiogenic strategies remains to be examined in HCC models.

5. CLINICAL GENE THERAPY TRIALS AGAINST HCC

To our knowledge, few gene therapy clinical trials for HCC have been published. The only one published report was a phase I study which involved the use of the wild-type p53 gene. Habib and colleagues [55,148] performed a phase I clinical trail, in which eight liver cirrhotic patients with histologically proven HCC due to viral hepatitis were given percutaneous intratumoral injection of plasmid carrying the human wild-type p53 gene. Each patient was injected with 2 mg of naked wild-type p53 plasmid DNA intratumorally under computed tomography scan guidance. Tumor size, serum AFP levels and liver function tests were monitored every month prior to and during the period of the study. Of the eight patients, one had complete response for 19 months, and three had significant reduction in tumor volume. There was evidence for an immune-mediated bystander effect [149]. Adverse reactions of the treatment were minimal. Although the usefulness of this gene therapy strategy has to be estimated in a large number of clinical trials, these results suggest that the intratumoral injection of the wild-type p53 gene is a promising approach to the clinical treatment of HCC. Another clinical gene therapy protocol against HCC using the wild-type p53 gene was directed by Venook and Warren and the review of the protocol by NIH was introduced in a gene therapy journal [8,150]. According to the protocol, recombinant adenoviruses carrying the wild-type p53 gene are infused into HCC through the hepatic artery. Although the protocol was approved on May 15, 1996, the results of the trial are not yet available. The results of a phase I/II trial using the insulin-like growth factor I antisense gene and the B7-1 gene was introduced in a review article by Mitry et al. [151]. As far as we know, there are no other ongoing clinical gene therapy trials against HCC. This may reflect the difficulties of gene therapy against HCC.

6. PROBLEMS TO OVERCOME FOR SUCCESSFUL GENE THERAPY AGAINST HCC

A number of promising gene therapy approaches to the treatment of HCC have been explored and encouraging results have been demonstrated in animal HCC models. It is, however, true that there are a number of problems to overcome for achieving successful clinical outcomes in gene therapy against HCC. Firstly, tumors including HCC are genetically unstable so that they are extraordinarily adaptable to environmental alterations. In addition, tumors are heterogeneous in many aspects, such as malignant grades, genetic mutations, expression of oncogenes and tumor suppressor genes, and immunogenicity. Therefore, tumor cells may acquire resistance to some treatment modalities using gene therapy strategies. Furthermore, multicentric development is common in HCC so that the single liver contains multiclonal HCC. If a successful antitumor effect is induced against a single HCC clone, it may not work against different HCC clones in the same patient. Secondly, as well as multicentric development of HCC, intrahepatic metastasis is also frequently observed in patients with HCC, resulting in multiple HCC lesions in the liver. Therefore, usefulness of local lesional gene therapy may be limited for the treatment of HCC and systemic, or at least whole hepatic, gene therapy is required for successful gene therapy against HCC, which makes successful gene therapy for HCC extremely difficult. Thirdly, the spontaneous behavior of human tumors is somewhat different, not only from that of malignant cells in vitro, but also from that of experimental tumors in animal models. For instance, the study with transgenic mice that develop spontaneous HCC has shown that when HCC cells established from the transgenic mouse were transduced with cytokine genes, they worked as a tumor vaccine and prevented tumor development of parental HCC cells subsequently implanted into non-transgenic counterparts. Conversely, vaccination of pretumoral transgenic animals with various combinations of cytokine gene-transduced HCC cells failed to inhibit tumor onset and progression [152]. These results indicate that an adequate animal model has to be produced for evaluating antitumor effects of gene therapy. Furthermore, most patients with HCC have underlying liver cirrhosis. We have shown that underlying liver cirrhosis is not only a high risk factor for HCC development, but also a substantial promoting factor for HCC invasion and metastasis [153–155]. Therefore, an accurate animal model of HCC should have HCC formed on the liver cirrhosis. Finally and most importantly, a major obstacle for successful gene therapy against cancer is the lack of ideal vector for transferring therapeutic genes. Efficiency of gene transduction into a tumor by currently available vectors is not sufficient at all for inducing successful clinical outcomes against cancer. Furthermore, the diffusion ability of gene therapy vector carrying a therapeutic gene into a target tumor is an extremely important issue. Bao et al. [156] have shown that when recombinant adenoviruses were infused into the animals, the expression of a reporter gene seemed to distribute preferentially at the peripheries of the tumor nodules, and low levels of transgene expression were seen inside the nodules. They have also shown that infusion of recombinant adenoviruses carrying the wild-type p53 gene into the animals did not induce significant suppression of liver tumor development and that exogenous p53 was also expressed at the peripheries of the lesions. It is, therefore, indispensable to develop an improved or new vector that has the ability of high transduction efficiency into tumor cells in vivo. Thus, although there are a number of obstacles for achieving successful gene therapy against cancer including HCC, progress of gene therapy has been rapid and important observations have been emerging, not only from animal studies, but also from ongoing clinical trials. Furthermore, molecular biology and the related technologies have been progressing more quickly than we expected. The future improvement of present vector systems as well as the employment of new vector systems will likely expand the applicability and efficacy of gene therapy. There is no question that gene therapy will have a clinical reality and will be one of the most important treatment modalities for a variety of human diseases, including cancer.

REFERENCES

[1] Cook GC. Hepatocellular carcinoma: one of the world's most common malignancies. Q J Med 1985; 233: 705–708.
[2] Parkin DM, Pisani P, Ferlay J. Estimates of the worldwide incidence of 25 major cancers in 1990. Int J Cancer 1999; 15: 827–841.
[3] Kew MC. Clinical, pathologic, and etiologic heterogeneity in hepatocellular carcinoma: evidence from Southern Africa. Hepatology 1981; 1: 366–369.
[4] Brotodihardjo AE, Tait N, Weltman MD, Liddle C, Little JM, Farrell GC. Hepatocellular carcinoma in western Sydney: aetiology, changes in incidence, and opportunities for better outcomes. Med J Aust 1994; 161: 433–435.
[5] Colombo M. Hepatocellular carcinoma. J Hepatol 1992; 15: 225–236.
[6] Venook AP. Treatment of hepatocellular carcinoma: too many options? J Clin Oncol 1994; 12: 1323–1334.
[7] Farmer DG, Busuttil RW. The role of multimodal therapy in the treatment of hepatocellular carcinoma. Cancer 1994; 73: 2669–2670.
[8] Human gene marker/therapy clinical protocols. Hum Gene Ther 2000; 11: 2543–2617.
[9] Glorioso JC, Naldini L, Kay MA. Viral vectors for gene therapy: the art of turning infectious agents into vehicles of therapeutics. Nat Med 2001; 7: 33–40.
[10] Shetty K, Wu GY, Wu CH. Gene therapy of hepatic diseases: prospects for the new millennium. Gut 2000; 46: 136–139.
[11] Ferry N, Heard JM. Liver-directed gene transfer vectors. Hum Gene Ther 1998; 9: 1975–1981.
[12] Davern TJ II, Scharschmidt BF. Gene therapy for liver disease. Dig Dis 1998; 16: 23–37.
[13] Ghosh SS, Takahashi M, Thummala NR, Parashar B, Chowdhury NR, Chowdhury JR. Liver-directed gene therapy: promises, problems and prospects at the turn of the century. J Hepatol 2000; 32: 238–252.
[14] Nakatani T, Kuriyama S, Tominaga K, Tsujimoto T, Mitoro A, Yamazaki M et al. Assessment of efficiency and safety of adenovirus mediated gene transfer into normal and damaged murine livers. Gut 2000; 47: 563–570.

[15] Tominaga K, Kuriyama S, Okuda H, Tsujinoue H, Nakatani T, Tsujimoto T et al. Adenoviral administration into the biliary tract can induce re-expression of the original gene construct in rat livers without immunosuppressive strategies. Gene Ther (in press).
[16] Kuriyama S, Tominaga K, Kikukawa M, Nakatani T, Tsujinoue H, Yamazaki M et al. Inhibitory effects of human sera on adenovirus-mediated gene transfer into rat liver. Anticancer Res 1998; 18: 2345–2352.
[17] Kuriyama S, Tominaga K, Kikukawa M, Tsujimoto T, Nakatani T, Tsujinoue H et al. Transient cyclophosphamide treatment before intraportal readministration of an adenoviral vector can induce re-expression of the original gene construct in rat liver. Gene Ther 1999; 6: 749–757.
[18] Kuriyama S, Tominaga K, Mitoro A, Tsujinoue H, Nakatani T, Yamazaki M et al. Immunomodulation with FK506 around the time of intravenous re-administration of an adenoviral vector facilitates gene transfer into primed rat liver. Int J Cancer 2000; 85: 839–844.
[19] Nagao S, Kuriyama S, Okuda H, Tominaga K, Nakatani T, Tsujinoue H et al. Adenovirus-mediated gene transfer into tumors: evaluation of direct readministration of an adenoviral vector into subcutaneous tumors of immunocompetent mice. Int J Oncol 2001; 18: 57–65.
[20] Tsujinoue H, Kuriyama S, Tominaga K, Okuda H, Nakatani T, Yoshiji H et al. Intravenous readministration of an adenoviral vector performed long after the initial administration failed to induce re-expression of the original transgene in rats. Int J Oncol 2001; 18; 575–580.
[21] Kuriyama S, Mitoro A, Tsujinoue H, Nakatani T, Yoshiji H, Tsujimoto T et al. Particle-mediated gene transfer into murine livers using a newly developed gene gun. Gene Ther 2000; 7: 1132–1136.
[22] Cao G, Kuriyama S, Gao J, Mitoro A, Cui L, Nakatani T et al. Comparison of carcinoembryonic antigen promoter regions isolated from human colorectal carcinoma and normal adjacent mucosa to induce strong tumor-selective gene expression. Int J Cancer 1998; 78: 242–247.
[23] Cao G, Kuriyama S, Gao J, Kikukawa M, Cui L, Nakatani T et al. Effective and safe gene therapy for colorectal carcinoma using the cytosine deaminase gene directed by the carcinoembryonic antigen promoter. Gene Ther 1999; 6: 83–90.
[24] Cao G, Kuriyama S, Cui L, Nagao S, Pan X, Toyokawa Y et al. Analysis of the human carcinoembryonic antigen promoter core region in colorectal carcinoma-selective cytosine deaminase gene therapy. Cancer Gene Ther 1999; 6: 572–580.
[25] Huber BE, Richards CA, Krenitsky TA. Retroviral-mediated gene therapy for the treatment of hepatocellular carcinoma: an innovative approach for cancer therapy. Proc Natl Acad Sci USA 1991; 88: 8039–8043.
[26] Ido A, Nakata K, Kato Y, Nakao K, Murata K, Fujita M et al. Gene therapy for hepatoma cells using a retrovirus vector carrying herpes simplex virus thymidine kinase gene under the control of human α-fetoprotein gene promoter. Cancer Res 1995; 55: 3105–3109.
[27] Kaneko S, Hallenbeck P, Kotani T, Nakabayashi H, McGarrity G, Tamaoki T et al. Adenovirus-mediated gene therapy of hepatocellular carcinoma using cancer-specific gene expression. Cancer Res 1995; 55: 5283–5287.
[28] Kanai F, Shiratori Y, Yoshida Y, Wakimoto H, Hamada H, Kanegae Y et al. Gene therapy for α-fetoprotein-producing human hepatoma cells by adenovirus-mediated transfer of the herpes simplex virus thymidine kinase gene. Hepatology 1996; 23: 1359–1368.
[29] Kanai F, Lan K-H, Shiratori Y, Tanaka T, Ohashi M, Okudaira T et al. In vivo gene therapy for α-fetoprotein-producing hepatocellular carcinoma by adenovirus-mediated transfer of cytosine deaminase gene. Cancer Res 1997; 57: 461–465.

[30] Arbuthnot P, Bralet MP, Thomassin H, Danan JL, Bréchot C, Ferry N. Hepatoma cell-specific expression of a retrovirally transferred gene is achieved by alpha-fetoprotein but not insulinlike growth factor II regulatory sequences. Hepatology 1995; 22: 1788–1796.

[31] Arbuthnot PB, Bralet MP, Le Jossic C, Dedieu JF, Perricaudet M, Bréchot C et al. In vitro and in vivo hepatoma cell-specific expression of a gene transferred with an adenoviral vector. Hum Gene Ther 1996; 7: 1503–1514.

[32] He P, Tang ZY, Liu BB, Ye SL, Liu YK. The targeted expression of the human interleukin-2/interferon α2b fused gene in α-fetoprotein-expressing hepatocellular carcinoma cells. J Cancer Res Clin Oncol 1999; 125: 77–82.

[33] Watanabe K, Saito A, Tamaoki T. Cell-specific enhancer activity in a far upstream region of the human α-fetoprotein gene. J Biol Chem 1987; 262: 4812–4818.

[34] Cao G, Kuriyama S, Du P, Sakamoto T, Kong X, Masui K et al. Complete regression of established murine hepatocellular carcinoma by in vivo tumor necrosis factor α gene transfer. Gastroenterology 1997; 112: 501–510.

[35] Mawatari F, Tsuruta S, Ido A, Ueki T, Nakao K, Kato Y et al. Retrovirus-mediated gene therapy for hepatocellular carcinoma: selective and enhanced suicide gene expression regulated by human α-fetoprotein enhancer directly linked to its promoter. Cancer Gene Ther 1998; 5: 301–306.

[36] Su H, Chang JC, Xu SM, Kan YW. Selective killing of AFP-positive hepatocellular carcinoma cells by adeno-associated virus transfer of the herpes simplex virus thymidine kinase gene. Hum Gene Ther 1996; 7: 463–470.

[37] Su H, Lu R, Chnag JC, Kan YW. Tissue-specific expression of herpes simplex virus thymidine kinase gene delivered by adeno-associated virus inhibits the growth of human hepatocellular carcinoma in athymic mice. Proc Natl Acad Sci USA 1997; 94: 13891–13896.

[38] Cao G, Kuriyama S, Tsujinoue H, Chen Q, Mitoro A, Qi Z. A novel approach for inducing enhanced and selective transgene expression in hepatocellular-carcinoma cells. Int J Cancer 2000; 87: 247–252.

[39] Cao G, Kuriyama S, Gao J, Nakatani T, Chen Q, Yoshiji H et al. Gene therapy for hepatocellular carcinoma based on tumour-selective suicide gene expression using the alpha-fetoprotein (AFP) enhancer and a housekeeping gene promoter. Eur J Cancer 2001; 37: 140–147.

[40] Miller DG, Adam MA, Miller AD. Gene transfer by retrovirus vectors occurs only in cells that are actively replicating at the time of infection. Mol Cell Biol 1990; 10: 4239–4242.

[41] Kuriyama S, Yoshikawa M, Ishizaka S, Tsujii T, Ikenaka K, Kagawa T et al. A potential approach for gene therapy targeting hepatoma using a liver-specific promoter on a retroviral vector. Cell Struct Funct 1991; 16: 503–510.

[42] Vile RG, Hart IR. Use of tissue-specific expression of the herpes simplex virus thymidine kinase gene to inhibit growth of established murine melanomas following directed intratumoral injection of DNA. Cancer Res 1993; 53: 3860–3864.

[43] Cao G, Kuriyama S, Gao J, Mitoro A, Cui L, Nagao S et al. In vivo gene transfer of a suicide gene under the transcriptional control of the carcinoembryonic antigen promoter results in bone marrow transduction but can avoid bone marrow suppression. Int J Oncol 1999; 15: 107–112.

[44] Kuriyama S, Sakamoto T, Kikukawa M, Nakatani T, Toyokawa Y, Tsujinoue H et al. Expression of a retrovirally transduced gene under control of an internal housekeeping gene promoter does not persist due to methylation and is restored partially by 5-azacytidine treatment. Gene Ther 1998; 5: 1299–1305.

[45] Yoshimatsu T, Tamura M, Kuriyama S, Ikenaka K. Improvement of retroviral packaging cell lines by introducing the polyomavirus early region. Hum Gene Ther 1998; 9: 161–172.
[46] Tsujinoue H, Kuriyama S, Nakatani T, Yoshiji H, Akahane T, Toyokawa Y et al. Amelioration of retrovirus-mediated gene transfer into hepatocellular carcinoma cells. Int J Oncol 2001; 18: 801–807.
[47] Gómez-Navarro J, Curiel DT, Douglas JT. Gene therapy for cancer. Eur J Cancer 1999; 35: 867–885.
[48] Prives C. How loops, beta sheets, and alpha helices help us to understand p53. Cell 1994; 78: 543–546.
[49] Vogelstein B, Kinzler KW. p53 function and dysfunction. Cell 1992; 70: 523–526.
[50] Lowe SW, Ruley HE, Jacks T, Housman DE. p53-dependent apoptosis modulates the cytotoxicity of anticancer agents. Cell 1993; 74: 957–967.
[51] Soussi T, Legros Y, Lubin R, Ory K, Schlichtholz B. Multifactorial analysis of p53 alteration in human cancer: a review. Int J Cancer 1994; 57: 1–9.
[52] Buetow KH, Sheffield VC, Zhu M, Zhou T, Shen FM, Hino O et al. Low frequency of p53 mutations observed in a diverse collection of primary hepatocellular carcinomas. Proc Natl Acad Sci USA 1992; 89: 9622–9626.
[53] Greenblatt MS, Bennett WP, Hollstein M, Harris CC. Mutations in the p53 tumor suppressor gene: clues to cancer etiology and molecular pathogenesis. Cancer Res 1994; 54: 4855–4878.
[54] Bookstein R, Demers W, Gregory R, Maneval D, Park J, Wills K. p53 gene therapy in vivo of hepatocellular and liver metastatic colorectal cancer. Semin Oncol 1996; 23: 66–77.
[55] Habib NA, Mitry RR, Sadri R. p53 and gene therapy for hepatocellular carcinoma. Adv Exp Med Biol 1998; 451: 499–504.
[56] Xu GW, Sun ZT, Forrester K, Wang XW, Coursen J, Harris CC. Tissue-specific growth suppression and chemosensitivity promotion in human hepatocellular carcinoma cells by retroviral-mediated transfer of the wild-type p53 gene. Hepatology 1996; 24: 1264–1268.
[57] Anderson SC, Johnson DE, Harris MP, Engler H, Hancock W, Huang WM et al. p53 gene therapy in a rat model of hepatocellular carcinoma: intra-arterial delivery of a recombinant adenovirus. Clin Cancer Res 1998; 4: 1649–1659.
[58] Vinyals A, Peinado MA, Gonzalez-Garrigues M, Monzo M, Bonfil RD, Fabra A. Failure of wild-type p53 gene therapy in human cancer cells expressing a mutant p53 protein. Gene Ther 1999; 6: 22–33.
[59] Roth C, Rochlitz C, Kourilsky P. Immune response against tumors. Adv Immunol 1994; 57: 281–351.
[60] Chouaib S, Asselin-Paturel C, Mami-Chouaib F, Caignard A, Blay JY. The host–tumor immune conflict: from immunosuppression to resistance and destruction. Immunol Today 1997; 18: 493–497.
[61] Colombo MP, Forni G. Cytokine gene transfer in tumor inhibition and tumor therapy: where are we now? Immunol Today 1994; 15: 48–51.
[62] Parmiani G, Colombo MP, Melani C, Arienti F. Cytokine gene transduction in the immunotherapy of cancer. Adv Pharmacol 1997; 40: 259–307.
[63] Tuting T, Storkus WJ, Lotze MT. Gene-based strategies for the immunotherapy of cancer. J Mol Med 1997; 75: 478–491.
[64] Zier K, Gansbacher B, Salvadori S. Preventing abnormalities in signal transduction of T cells in cancer: the promise of cytokine gene therapy. Immunol Today 1996; 17: 39–45.
[65] Musiani P, Modesti A, Giovarelli M, Cavallo F, Colombo MP, Lollini PL et al. Cytokines, tumor-cell death and immunogenicity: a question of choice. Immunol Today 1997; 18: 32–36.

[66] Schmidt-Wolf GD, Schmidt-Wolf IG. Cytokines and gene therapy. Immunol Today 1995; 16: 173–175.
[67] Tepper RI, Mulé JJ. Experimental and clinical studies of cytokine gene-modified tumor cells. Hum Gene Ther 1994; 5: 153–164.
[68] Miller AR, McBride WH, Hunt K, Economou JS. Cytokine-mediated gene therapy for cancer. Ann Surg Oncol 1994; 1: 436–450.
[69] Cao G, Kuriyama S, Du P, Sakamoto T, Yang W, Masui K. Construction of retroviral vectors to induce strong hepatoma cell-specific expression of cytokine genes. J Gastroenterol Hepatol 1996; 11: 1053–1061.
[70] Huang H, Chen SH, Kosai K, Finegold MJ, Woo SL. Gene therapy for hepatocellular carcinoma: long-term remission of primary and metastatic tumors in mice by interleukin-2 gene therapy in vivo. Gene Ther 1996; 3: 980–987.
[71] Bui LA, Butterfield LH, Kim JY, Ribas A, Seu P, Lau R et al. In vivo therapy of hepatocellular carcinoma with a tumor-specific adenoviral vector expressing interleukin-2. Hum Gene Ther 1997; 8: 2173–2182.
[72] Cao X, Wang J, Zhang W, Chen G, Kong X, Tani K. Treatment of human hepatocellular carcinoma by fibroblast-mediated human interferon alpha gene therapy in combination with adoptive chemoimmunotherapy. J Cancer Res Clin Oncol 1995; 121: 457–462.
[73] Caruso M, Pham-Nguyen K, Kwong YL, Xu B, Kosai KI, Finegold M et al. Adenovirus-mediated interleukin-12 gene therapy for metastatic colon carcinoma. Proc Natl Acad Sci USA 1996; 93: 11302–11306.
[74] Siders WM, Wright PW, Hixon JA, Alvord WG, Back TC, Wiltrout RH et al. T cell and NK cell-independent inhibition of hepatic metastases by systemic administration of an IL-12-expressing recombinant adenovirus. J Immunol 1998; 160: 5465–5474.
[75] Hirschowitz EA, Naama HA, Evoy D, Lieberman MD, Daly J, Crystal RG. Regional treatment of hepatic micrometastasis by adenovirus vector-mediated delivery of interleukin-2 and interleukin-12 cDNAs to the hepatic parenchyma. Cancer Gene Ther 1999; 6: 491–498.
[76] Weber SM, Shi F, Heise C, Warner T, Mahvi DM. Interleukin-12 gene transfer results in CD8-dependent regression of murine CT26 liver tumors. Ann Surg Oncol 1999; 6: 186–194.
[77] Galea-Lauri J, Farzaneh F, Garken J. Novel costimulators in the immune gene therapy of cancer. Cancer Gene Ther 1996; 3: 202–214.
[78] Schwartz RH. Costimulation of T lymphocytes: the role of CD28, CTLA-4, and B7/BB1 in interleukin-2 production and immunotherapy. Cell 1992; 71: 1065–1068.
[79] June CH, Bluestone JA, Nadler LM, Thompson CB. The B7 and CD28 receptor families. Immunol Today 1994; 15: 321–331.
[80] Chen L, Ashe S, Brady WA, Hellstrom I, Hellstrom KE, Ledbetter JA et al. Costimulation of antitumor immunity by the B7 counterreceptor for the T lymphocyte molecules CD28 and CTLA-4. Cell 1992; 71: 1093–1102.
[81] Tatsumi T, Takehara T, Katayama K, Mochizuki K, Yamamoto M, Kanto T et al. Expression of costimulatory molecules B7-1 (CD80) and B7-2 (CD86) on human hepatocellular carcinoma. Hepatology 1997; 25: 1108–1114.
[82] Tatsumi T, Takehara T, Kanto T, Kuzushita N, Ito A, Kasahara A et al. B7-1 (CD80)-gene transfer combined with interleukin-12 administration elicits protective and therapeutic immunity against mouse hepatocellular carcinoma. Hepatology 1999; 30: 422–429.
[83] Banchereau J, Steinman RM. Dendritic cells and the control of immunity. Nature 1998; 392: 245–252.
[84] Grabbe S, Beissert S, Schwarz T, Granstein RD. Dendritic cells as initiators of tumor

immune responses: a possible strategy for tumor immunotherapy. Immunol Today 1995; 16: 117–121.

[85] Girolomoni G, Ricciardi-Castagnoli P. Dendritic cells hold promise for immunotherapy. Immunol Today 1997; 18: 102–104.

[86] Hsu FJ, Benike C, Fagnoni F, Liles TM, Czerwinski D, Taidi B et al. Vaccination of patients with B-cell lymphoma using autologous antigen-pulsed dendritic cells. Nat Med 1996; 2: 52–58.

[87] Specht JM, Wang G, Do MT, Lam JS, Royal RE, Reeves ME et al. Dendritic cells retrovirally transduced with a model antigen gene are therapeutically effective against established pulmonary metastases. J Exp Med 1997; 186: 1213–1221.

[88] Wan Y, Bramson J, Carter R, Graham F, Gauldie J. Dendritic cells transduced with an adenoviral vector encoding a model tumor-associated antigen for tumor vaccination. Hum Gene Ther 1997; 8: 1355–1363.

[89] Guo Y, Wu M, Chen H, Wang X, Liu G, Li G et al. Effective tumor vaccine generated by fusion of hepatoma cells with activated B cells. Science 1994; 263: 518–520.

[90] Vollmer CM Jr., Eiber FC, Butterfield LH, Ribas A, Dissette VB, Koh A et al. Alpha-fetoprotein-specific genetic immunotherapy for hepatocellular carcinoma. Cancer Res 1999; 59: 3064–3067.

[91] Moolten FL. Drug sensitivity ('suicide') genes for selective cancer chemotherapy. Cancer Gene Ther 1994; 1: 279–287.

[92] Mullen CA. Metabolic suicide genes in gene therapy. Pharmacol Ther 1994; 63: 199–207.

[93] Kuriyama S, Nakatani T, Masui K, Sakamoto T, Tominaga K, Yoshikawa M et al. Evaluation of prodrugs ability to induce effective ablation of cells transduced with viral thymidine kinase gene. Anticancer Res 1996; 16: 2623–2628.

[94] Freeman SM, Abbound CN, Whatenby KA, Packman CH, Koeplin DS, Moolten FL. The 'bystander effect': tumor regression when a fraction of the tumor mass is genetically modified. Cancer Res 1993; 53: 5274–5283.

[95] Fick J, Barker FG II, Dazin P, Westphale EM, Beyer EC, Israel MA. The extent of heterocellular communication mediated by gap junctions is predictive of bystander tumor cytotoxicity in vitro. Proc Natl Acad Sci USA 1995; 92: 11071–11075.

[96] Bi WL, Parysek LM, Warnick R, Stambrook PJ. In vitro evidence that metabolic cooperation is responsible for the bystander effect observed with HSV-tk retroviral gene therapy. Hum Gene Ther 1993; 4: 725–731.

[97] Kuriyama S, Yoshikawa M, Tominaga K, Nakatani T, Sakamoto T, Fukui H et al. Gene therapy for the treatment of hepatoma by retroviral-mediated gene transfer of the herpes simplex virus thymidine kinase. Int Hepatol Commun 1993; 1: 253–259.

[98] Kuriyama S, Nakatani T, Masui K, Sakamoto T, Tominaga K, Yoshikawa M et al. Bystander effect caused by suicide gene expression indicates the feasibility of gene therapy for hepatocellular carcinoma. Hepatology 1995; 22: 1838–1846.

[99] Kuriyama S, Sakamoto T, Masui K, Nakatani T, Tominaga K, Kikukawa M et al. Tissue-specific expression of HSV-tk gene can induce efficient antitumor effect and protective immunity to wild-type hepatocellular carcinoma. Int J Cancer 1997; 71: 470–475.

[100] Kuriyama S, Kikukawa M, Masui K, Okuda H, Nakatani T, Akahane T et al. Cancer gene therapy with HSV-tk/GCV system depends on T-cell-mediated immune responses and causes apoptotic death of tumor cells in vivo. Int J Cancer 1999; 83: 374–380.

[101] Kuriyama S, Mitoro A, Yamazaki M, Tsujinoue H, Nakatani T, Akahane T et al. Comparison of gene therapy with the herpes simplex virus thymidine kinase gene and the

bacterial cytosine deaminase gene for the treatment of hepatocellular carcinoma. Scand J Gastroenterol 1999; 34: 1033–1041.

[102] Kuriyama S, Tsujinoue H, Nakatani T, Mitoro A, Akahane T, Okuda H et al. Gene therapy for hepatocellular carcinoma. In: Niho Y, editor. Molecular Target for Hematological Malignancies and Cancer. Fukuoka: Kyushu University Press, 2000; pp. 29–37.

[103] Toyokawa Y, Kuriyama S, Tsujinoue H, Nakatani T, Mitoro A, Yoshiji H et al. Retrovirus-mediated in vivo gene therapy using the herpes simplex virus thymidine kinase gene against carcinomatous peritonitis. Scand J Gastroenterol 2000; 35: 852–860.

[104] Paillard F. Bystander effects in enzyme/prodrug gene therapy. Hum Gene Ther 1997; 8: 1733–1735.

[105] Barba D, Hardin J, Sadelain M, Gage FH. Development of anti-tumor immunity following thymidine kinase-mediated killing of experimental brain tumors. Proc Natl Acad Sci USA 1994; 91: 4348–4352.

[106] Caruso M, Panis Y, Gagandeep S, Houssin D, Salzmann JL, Klatzmann D. Regression of established macroscopic liver metastases after in situ transduction of a suicide gene. Proc Natl Acad Sci USA 1993; 90: 7024–7028.

[107] Gagandeep S, Brew R, Green B, Christmas SE, Klatzmann D, Poston GJ et al. Prodrug-activated gene therapy: involvement of an immunological component in the 'bystander effect'. Cancer Gene Ther 1996; 3: 83–88.

[108] Vile RG, Nelson JA, Castleden S, Chong H, Hart IR. Systemic gene therapy of murine melanoma using tissue specific expression of the HSVtk gene involves an immune component. Cancer Res 1994; 54: 6228–6234.

[109] Vile RG, Castleden S, Marshall J, Camplejohn R, Upton C, Chong H. Generation of an anti-tumour immune response in a non-immunogenic tumour: HSVtk killing in vivo stimulates a mononuclear cell infiltrate and a Th1-like profile of intratumoral cytokine expression. Int J Cancer 1997; 71: 267–274.

[110] Kianmanesh AR, Perrin H, Panis Y, Fabre M, Nagy HJ, Houssin D et al. A 'distant' bystander effect of suicide gene therapy: regression of nontransduced tumors together with a distant transduced tumor. Hum Gene Ther 1997; 8: 1807–1814.

[111] Moolten FL. Tumor chemosensitivity conferred by inserted herpes thymidine kinase genes: paradigm for a prospective cancer control strategy. Cancer Res 1986; 46: 5276–5281.

[112] Macri P, Gordon JW. Delayed morbidity and mortality of albumin/SV40 T-antigen transgenic mice after insertion of an α-fetoprotein/herpes virus thymidine kinase transgene and treatment with ganciclovir. Hum Gene Ther 1994; 5: 175–182.

[113] van der Eb MM, Cramer SJ, Vergouwe Y, Schagen FHE, van Krieken JHJM, van der Eb AJ et al. Severe hepatic dysfunction after adenovirus-mediated transfer of the herpes simplex virus thymidine kinase gene and ganciclovir administration. Gene Ther 1998; 5: 451–458.

[114] Brand K, Arnold W, Bartels T, Lieber A, Kay MA, Strauss M et al. Liver-associated toxicity of the HSV-tk/GCV approach and adenoviral vectors. Cancer Gene Ther 1997; 4: 9–16.

[115] Kuriyama S, Masui K, Kikukawa M, Sakamoto T, Nakatani T, Nagao S et al. Complete cure of established murine hepatocellular carcinoma is achievable by repeated injections of retroviruses carrying the herpes simplex virus thymidine kinase gene. Gene Ther 1999; 6: 525–533.

[116] Kilstrup M, Meng LM, Neuhard J, Nygaard P. Genetic evidence for a repressor of synthesis of cytosine deaminase and purine biosynthesis enzymes in *Escherichia coli*. J Bacteriol 1989; 171: 2124–2127.

[117] Anderson L, Kilstrup M, Neuhard J. Pyrimidine, purine and nitrogen control of cytosine

deaminase synthesis in *Escherichia coli* K12. Involvement of the glnLG and purR genes in the regulation of codA expression. Arch Microbiol 1989; 152: 115–118.
[118] Danielsen S, Kilstrup M, Barilla K, Jochimsen B, Neuhard J. Characterization of the *Escherichia coli* codBA operon encoding cytosine permease and cytosine deaminase. Mol Microbiol 1992; 6: 1335–1344.
[119] Austin EA, Huber BE. A first step in the development of gene therapy for colorectal carcinoma: cloning, sequencing, and expression of *Escherichia coli* cytosine deaminase. Mol Phrmacol 1993; 43: 380–387.
[120] Mullen CA, Kilstrup M, Blaese RM. Transfer of the bacterial gene for cytosine deaminase to mammalian cells confers lethal sensitivity to 5-fluorocytosine: a negative selection system. Proc Natl Acad Sci USA 1992; 89: 33–37.
[121] Huber BE, Austin EA, Good SS, Knick VC, Tibbels S, Richards CA. In vivo antitumor activity of 5-fluorocytosine on human colorectal carcinoma cells genetically modified to express cytosine deaminase. Cancer Res 1993; 53: 4619–4626.
[122] Kuriyama S, Masui K, Sakamoto T, Nakatani T, Tominaga K, Fukui H et al. Bacterial cytosine deaminase suicide gene transduction renders hepatocellular carcinoma sensitive to the prodrug 5-fluorocytosine. Int Hepatol Commun 1995; 4: 72–79.
[123] Kuriyama S, Masui K, Sakamoto T, Nakatani T, Kikukawa M, Tsujinoue H et al. Bystander effect caused by cytosine deaminase gene and 5-fluorocytosine in vitro is substantially mediated by generated 5-fluorouracil. Anticancer Res 1998; 18: 3399–3406.
[124] Huber BE, Austin EA, Richards CA, Davis ST, Good SS. Metabolism of 5-fluorocytosine to 5-fluorouracil in human colorectal tumor cells transduced with the cytosine deaminase gene: significant antitumor effects when only a small percentage of tumor cells express cytosine deaminase. Proc Natl Acad Sci USA 1994; 91: 8302–8306.
[125] Rowley S, Lindauer M, Gebert JF, Haberkorn U, Oberdorfer F, Moebius U et al. Cytosine deaminase gene as a potential tool for the genetic therapy of colorectal cancer. J Surg Oncol 1996; 61: 42–48.
[126] Hirschowitz EA, Ohwada A, Pascal WR, Russi TJ, Crystal RG. In vivo adenovirus-mediated gene transfer of the *Escherichia coli* cytosine deaminase gene to human colon carcinoma-derived tumors induces chemosensitivity to 5-fluorocytosine. Hum Gene Ther 1995; 6: 1055–1063.
[127] Dong Y, Wen P, Manome Y, Parr M, Hirshowitz A, Chen L et al. In vivo replication-deficient adenovirus vector-mediated transduction of the cytosine deaminase gene sensitizes glioma cells to 5-fluorocytosine. Hum Gene Ther 1996; 7: 713–720.
[128] Consalvo M, Mullen CA, Modesti A, Musiani P, Allione A, Cavallo F et al. 5-fluorocytosine-induced eradication of murine adenocarcinomas engineered to express the cytosine deaminase suicide gene requires host immune competence and leaves an efficient memory. J Immunol 1995; 154: 5302–5312.
[129] Kuriyama S, Kikukawa M, Masui K, Okuda H, Nakatani T, Sakamoto T et al. Cytosine deaminase/5-fluorocytosine gene therapy can induce efficient anti-tumor effects and protective immunity in immunocompetent mice but not in athymic nude mice. Int J Cancer 1999; 81: 592–597.
[130] Hu LF, Wang LP, Ju LW, Huang LH, Li XL, Li XZ et al. Expression of N-ras gene in human primary hepatocarcinoma. Sci Sin [B] 1986: 29: 181–186.
[131] Himeno Y, Fukuda Y, Hatanaka M, Imura H. Expression of oncogenes in human liver disease. Liver 1998; 8: 208–212.
[132] Tashiro F, Morimura S, Hayashi K, Makino R, Kawamura H, Horikoshi N et al. Expression of the c-Ha-ras and c-myc genes in aflatoxin B1-induced hepatocellular carcinomas. Biochem Biophys Res Commun 1986; 138: 858–864.

[133] Zhang XK, Huang DP, Chiu DK, Chiu JF. The expression of oncogenes in human developing liver and hepatomas. Biochem Biophys Res Commun 1987; 142: 932–938.
[134] Baba M, Yamamoto R, Ishii H, Tatsuta M. Ha-*ras* mutations in N-nitrosomorpholine-induced lesions and inhibition of hepatocarcinogenesis by antisense sequences in rat liver. Int J Cancer 1997; 72: 815–820.
[135] Liao Y, Tang ZY, Liu KD, Ye SL, Huang Z. Apoptosis of human BEL-7402 hepatocellular carcinoma cells released by antisense H-ras DNA — in vitro and in vivo studies. J Cancer Res Clin Oncol 1997; 123: 25–33.
[136] Folkman J. Angiogenesis in cancer, vascular, rheumatoid and other disease. Nat Med 1995; 1: 27–31.
[137] Fidler IJ, Ellis LM. The implications of angiogenesis for the biology and therapy of cancer metastasis. Cell 1994; 79: 185–188.
[138] Fox SB, Gatter KC, Harris AL. Tumour angiogenesis. J Pathol 1996; 179: 232–237.
[139] Yoshiji H, Kuriyama S, Yoshii J, Yamazaki M, Kikukawa M, Tsujinoue H et al. Vascular endothelial growth factor tightly regulates in vivo development of murine hepatocellular carcinoma cells. Hepatology 1998; 28: 1489–1496.
[140] Shibuya M. Role of VEGF-flt receptor system in normal and tumor angiogenesis. Adv Cancer Res 1995; 67: 281–316.
[141] Yoshiji H, Kuriyama S, Hicklin DJ, Huber J, Yoshii J, Miyamoto Y et al. KDR/Flk-1 is a major regulator of vascular endothelial growth factor-induced tumor development and angiogenesis in murine hepatocellular carcinoma cells. Hepatology 1999; 30: 1179–1186.
[142] Yoshiji H, Kuriyama S, Hicklin DJ, Huber J, Yoshii J, Ikenaka Y et al. The vascular endothelial growth factor receptor KDR/Flk-1 is a major regulator of malignant ascites formation in the mouse hepatocellular carcinoma model. Hepatology 2001; 33: 841–847.
[143] Yoshiji H, Kuriyama S, Ways DK, Yoshii J, Miyamoto Y, Kawata M et al. Protein kinase C lies on the signaling pathway for vascular endothelial growth factor-mediated tumor development and angiogenesis. Cancer Res 1999; 59: 4413–4418.
[144] Kang MA, Kim KY, Seol JY, Kim KC, Nam MJ. The growth inhibition of hepatoma by gene transfer of antisense vascular endothelial growth factor. J Gene Med 2000; 2: 289–296.
[145] O'Reilly MS, Holmgren L, Chen C, Folkman J. Angiostatin induces and sustains dormancy of human primary tumors in mice. Nat Med 1996; 2: 689–692.
[146] O'Reilly MS, Boehm T, Shing Y, Fukai N, Vasios G, Lane WS et al. Endostatin: an endogenous inhibitor of angiogenesis and tumor growth. Cell 1997; 88: 277–285.
[147] Griscelli F, Li H, Bennaceur-Griscelli A, Soria J, Opolon P, Soria C et al. Angiostatin gene transfer: inhibition of tumor growth in vivo by blockage of endothelial cell proliferation associated with a mitosis arrest. Proc Natl Acad Sci USA 1998; 95: 6367–6372.
[148] Habib NA, Ding SF, el-Masry R, Mitry RR, Honda K, Michail NE et al. Preliminary report: the short-term effects of direct p53 DNA injection in primary hepatocellular carcinomas. Cancer Detect Prev 1996; 20: 103–107.
[149] Farzaneh F, Trefzer U, Sterry W, Walden P. Gene therapy of cancer. Immunol Today 1998; 19: 294–296.
[150] Regulatory issues. Hum Gene Ther 1995; 6: 1086–1090.
[151] Mitry RR, Mansour MR, Havlík R, Habib NA. Gene therapy for liver tumours. Adv Exp Med Biol 2000; 465: 193–205.
[152] Morel A, de La Coste A, Fernandez N, Berson A, Kaybanda M, Molina T et al. Does preventive vaccination with engineered tumor cells work in cancer-prone transgenic mice? Cancer Gene Ther 1998; 5: 92–100.
[153] Kuriyama S, Yamazaki M, Mitoro A, Tsujimoto T, Kikukawa M, Okuda H et al. Analysis

of intrahepatic invasion of hepatocellular carcinoma using fluorescent dye-labeled cells in mice. Anticancer Res 1998; 18: 4181–4188.

[154] Kuriyama S, Yamazaki M, Mitoro A, Tsujimoto T, Kikukawa M, Tsujinoue H et al. Hepatocellular carcinoma in an orthotopic mouse model metastasizes intrahepatically in cirrhotic but not in normal liver. Int J Cancer 1999; 80: 471–476.

[155] Tsujimoto T, Kuriyama S, Yamazaki M, Nakatani Y, Okuda H, Yoshiji H et al. Augmented hepatocellular carcinoma progression and depressed Kupffer cell activity in rat cirrhotic livers. Int J Oncol 2001; 18: 41–47.

[156] Bao JJ, Zhang WW, Kuo MT. Adenoviral delivery of recombinant DNA into transgenic mice bearing hepatocellular carcinomas. Hum Gene Ther 1996; 7: 355–365.

Molecular Biology and Immunology in Hepatology
Edited by T. Tsuji, T. Higashi, M. Zeniya and K.-H. Meyer zum Büschenfelde

CHAPTER 13

Novel Immunological Approach for the Treatment of Hepatocellular Carcinoma

Toshihiro Higashi [1], Kazuhiro Nouso [2], Masayuki Uemura [2], Shin-ichiro Nakamura [2] and Yoshiyuki Kobayashi [2]

[1] *Okayama Citizen's Hospital, Okayama, Japan*
[2] *Department of Medicine and Medical Science, Okayama University Graduate School of Medicine and Dentistry, Okayama, Japan*

INTRODUCTION

Hepatocellular carcinoma (HCC) is one of the most prevalent malignancies in East Asia, including within Japan [1]. A computer cohort simulation carried out in the USA has predicted that approximately 27,000 deaths will result from HCC just in the years 2010–2019 in the USA [2]. The data suggest that hepatitis C virus (HCV)-related HCC will be one of the most challenging diseases worldwide during the first and second decades of the 21st century. Almost all HCCs occur from chronic viral-related liver injuries, and especially from liver cirrhosis. Presently, medical interventions include surgical resection, chemoembolization, percutaneous ethanol injection, percutaneous microwave coagulation therapy and/or radio-frequency ablation. However, the prognosis is still poor due to the high reoccurrence rate of multicentric tumor development and intrahepatic metastasis via the portal vein. New strategies for HCC treatment have been recommended in order to achieve a better prognosis.

Since Rosenberg demonstrated that lymphokine-activated killer (LAK) cells could be safely administered to humans with advanced cancer [3], LAK cells have received particular attention as a potential mechanism of adoptive immunotherapy. However, preparation for adoptive immunotherapy with LAK cells in combination with recombinant (r) interleukin (IL)-2 is time-consuming, and complete recoveries appear to be infrequent [4]. Therefore, established papers describing the availability of adoptive immunotherapy for advanced cancer appear to be on the decline as of the middle of the last decade. Recently, however, T cell-mediated immunotherapies targeting cancer-testis antigens or melanocyte differentiation antigens have been attempted in melanoma patients, and some trials have been reported to be clinically effective [5–7]. In this chapter, the results of human HCC adoptive immunotherapy studies and trials are summarized, and the future perspectives for vaccine immunotherapy in patients with HCC are discussed.

1. ADOPTIVE IMMUNOTHERAPY USING LAK CELLS IN HUMAN HCC

In 1984, it was reported that non-specific, sensitized LAK cells could be generated by incubating fresh murine or human lymphocytes with IL-2, and following systemic administration of these cells, the growth of established pulmonary metastasis could be reduced in animal models [3]. In a follow-up study, Rosenberg also reported that for advanced human tumors, treatment with LAK cells and IL-2 could lead to tumor regression by more than 50% of the volume in 11 of 25 patients [8]. This effect was superior to that of treatment with high-dose IL-2 alone in patients with advanced melanoma; however, a significant difference was not observed in patients with advanced renal cell carcinoma [9]. Sequential tumor biopsies from patients who received an infusion of LAK cells with or without IL-2 showed increased infiltration of T cells, consisting mainly of $CD8^{+}$ T cells, in addition to augmentation of HLA-DR expression by the tumor cells [10]. Although LAK cell adoptive immunotherapy with IL-2 was shown to be effective in some patients with advanced tumors, adverse effects including fluid retention or capillary leak syndrome, hypotension, multiorgan failure and cardiac events due to high-dose administration of IL-2 remain to be resolved [4].

With respect to adoptive immunotherapy for HCC, experimental and clinical studies have been vigorously conducted. In 1986, Okuno et al. first reported that serum alpha-fetal protein was markedly decreased and ascitic fluid retention was transiently reduced by the adoptive transfer of LAK cells into an HCC patient [11]. The effectiveness of infusion of LAK cells combined with rIL-2 via a percutaneously placed hepatic arterial catheter was also documented in five patients with advanced HCC [12]. Marked reduction of tumor size and disappearance of portal thrombi following administration of this therapy were documented in one patient, whereas neither clinical improvement nor severe adverse effects were observed in two patients who received rIL-2 alone. One randomized study using spleen-derived LAK cells activated with rIL-2 revealed a lower reoccurrence rate in the LAK-treated group [13]. Another randomized trial also mentioned that the 2-year cumulative disease-free rate in the adoptive immunotherapy group was significantly higher than that in the chemotherapy group when the subjects were restricted to patients who had previously undergone hepatic resection with a negative margin [14]. To date, Takayama et al. have reported the most attractive result in adoptive immunotherapy for HCC [15]. They conducted a randomized trial to assess the efficacy of immunotherapy in 150 HCC patients who had received curative resection. The immunotherapy group showed significantly longer recurrence-free and disease-specific survival rates than did the control group, although the overall survival was not different between the groups. Taken together, these studies support adoptive immunotherapy in combination with rIL-2 as effective in some HCC patients as observed by a decreased rate of reoccurrence. However, it has also been established that complete remission of HCC is not achieved by adoptive immunotherapy alone, and therefore, new strategies for HCC treatment have been recommended.

2. IMMUNOTHERAPY TARGETING TUMOR-SPECIFIC ANTIGEN

Since the discovery of the gene MAGE-1, which encodes an antigen recognized by autologous cytotoxic lymphocytes in an HLA class-I restricted fashion in melanoma cells [16], vaccine therapy targeting tumor-specific antigens has been vigorously studied. Clinical vaccine trials using dendritic cells pulsed with tumor-specific antigenic peptides in patients with various malignant tumors other than melanoma have also been attempted, e.g., HER-2/neu or MUC1 in breast cancer [17], prostate-specific membrane antigen in prostate cancer [18] and MAGE-3 for bladder carcinoma [19] (Table 1). All these trials have revealed that cytotoxic T lymphocyte (CTL) activity was elicited against administered antigens concomitantly with tumor regression using dendritic cell vaccinations. Further recent developments in vaccination for malignant melanoma have been described in detail [20].

In general, immunotherapy is classified into two categories: undefined tumor antigens or defined tumor antigens used for immunization. In addition, active and passive immunization methods are available in each category. In instances where tumor-specific antigens are not defined, T lymphocytes that have been stimulated in vitro with tumor cells or tumor antigens may be used for infusion. For active immunization a number of options are available. Antigen-stimulated tumor cells may be given in combination with various cytokines [21], or antigen-presenting cells (APCs), such as dendritic cells stimulated either with peptides derived from tumor HLAs [22] or transfected with tumor-derived RNA [23] may be given, or heat shock proteins bound to tumor-derived peptides [24] can be used for immunization. However, since the stimuli of each antigenic peptide may be too small to elicit an immune response and reciprocal inhibition between each peptide may occur, it is uncertain whether the antigenicity in these strategies is efficient or not.

In contrast, in cases where tumor-specific antigens are well defined, adoptive immunotherapy using in vitro stimulated tumor-specific T lymphocytes can be performed as a form of passive immunization. For active immunization, vaccinations with anti-

TABLE 1

Clinical vaccine trials using dendritic cells pulsed with tumor-specific antigenic peptides

Tumor antigen	Cancer
Tissue-specific protein	
gp100, Mart-I/Melan-A, tyrosinase	Melanoma
Prostatic-specific membrane protein	Prostate cancer
Cancer-testis antigen	
MAGE-1, MAGE-3, NY-ESO-1	Melanoma
MAGE-3	Bladder carcinoma
Oncogene product	
HER2/neu	Breast cancer
Others	
MUC1	Breast cancer

TABLE 2

Vaccine therapy in cases where tumor-specific antigens are defined

Passive immunization
T cells reactive against tumor cells elicited by stimulation with antigenic peptides in vitro
Active immunization
Antigenic proteins or peptides
Antigen presenting cells such as dendritic cells pulsed with synthesized peptides or antigenic gene transfected
Tumor-specific gene DNA
Tumor-specific genes cloned into either viral or bacterial vectors
Cytokines such as IL-2, IL-12, GM-WF, IFN-γ

genic proteins or peptides, such as HLA class-I, adjuvant or heat shock proteins, or DNA encoding tumor-specific antigens, high affinity T cell responses are expected. The most attractive method for immunization, which has been attempted clinically, is the re-infusion of APCs, specifically dendritic cells, following in vitro stimulation with tumor-specific antigens. Various cytokines, such as IL-2, IL-12, IFN-γ, and GM-CSF, are clinically and experimentally used for augmentation of antigen presentation [25–28]. In the future, vaccination with tumor-specific genes cloned into either viral or bacterial vectors will be possible (Table 2).

3. IMMUNOTHERAPY FOR HUMAN HCC IN PROSPECT

Our laboratory has analyzed the cancer-testis antigen gene expression in human HCC samples. The mRNA expression rates of MAGE-1, -3, GAGE, BAGE and NY-ESO-1 were 67, 39, 36, 21 and 30% in HCC tissues, respectively [29]. Expression of these genes was not detectable in the corresponding non-HCC samples (Fig. 1). We also examined the expression of MAGE-1 and -3 gene products in human HCC samples by immunohistochemical and Western blot analysis. Both proteins were expressed in 80 and 60% of HCC samples, respectively [30] (Fig. 2 and Table 3). These results suggest that peptides derived from MAGE-1 or -3 might be suitable targets for immunotherapy in human HCC.

Since MAGE-3 peptides can elicit cytotoxic activity in an HLA-A1 and -A2 restricted fashion [16,31], and the frequencies of the HLA-A2 haplotype in Japanese and Caucasians are 44 and 49%, respectively [32], MAGE-3-derived peptides which bind to HLA-A2 are suggested to be favorite candidates for immunotherapy in Japanese HCC patients. We have performed CTL assays using MAGE-3-derived peptides in HLA-A2-positive healthy volunteers or HCC patients. The CTL activity was examined by either ^{51}Cr release or ELISPOT assays. The effector cells were either peripheral mononuclear cells (PBMC) pulsed with MAGE-3 peptide or PBMC after co-culture with MAGE-3 peptide-pulsed dendritic cells. The target cells were either peptide-pulsed T2 cells or established HCC culture cells, which were positive for HLA-A2 and MAGE-3 gene expression. However, a MAGE-3-derived peptide-specific CTL response was not elicited in either the ^{51}Cr release assay or in the ELISPOT assay. Immune

TABLE 3

Positivity of mRNA and protein of MAGE-1 and -3

	MAGE-1			MAGE-3		
	mRNA	Immunoblot	Staining	mRNA	Immunoblot	Staining
Histology						
Well-differentiated HCC	5/8	4/5	1/12	2/7	4/5	1/11
Moderately differentiated HCC	15/17	7/8	4/19	8/17	4/8	1/16
Poorly differentiated HCC	1/2	1/2	1/2	1/2	1/2	0/2
Stage						
I	6/8	2/3	0/9	1/7	2/3	0/7
II	7/8	4/5	3/11	4/8	2/5	0/10
III	5/6	4/4	2/8	4/6	3/4	2/7
IVA	1/3	2/3	1/3	1/3	2/3	0/3
IVB	2/2	n.d.	0/2	1/2	n.d.	0/2
Total	21/27 (78%)	12/15 (80%)	6/33 (18%)	11/26 (42%)	9/15 (60%)	2/29 (7%)

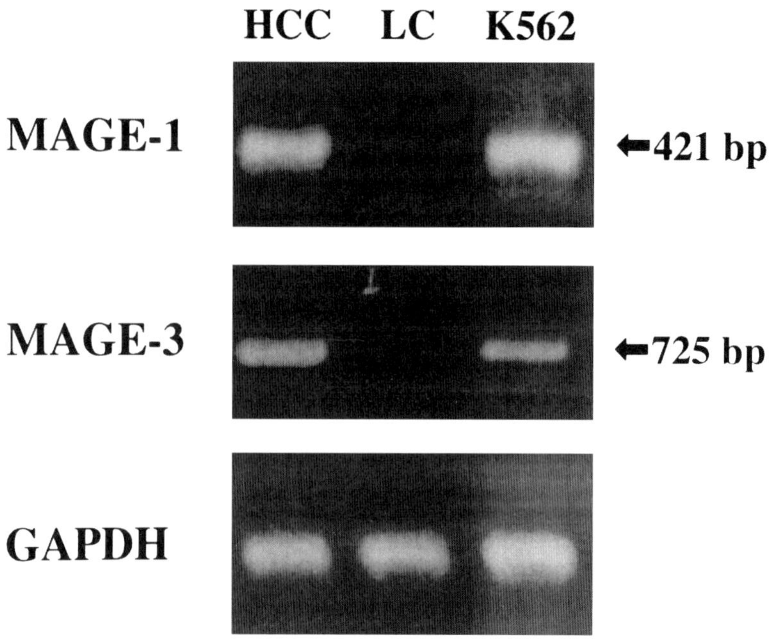

Fig. 1. RT-PCR for MAGE-1 and MAGE-3 mRNAs. The expected products of 421 and 725 bp which corresponded to MAGE-1 and MAGE-3 gene, respectively, were detected in the HCC and K563 cells, but not in liver cirrhosis sample.

responses against MAGE antigens were not frequently observed even in melanoma patients after immunization [33]. In contrast, NY-ESO-1, which was cloned as one of the cancer-testis antigens in an esophageal cancer [34], is the most immunogenic antigen known to date. A clinical trial of vaccine therapy using NY-ESO-1-derived peptides has been attempted in melanoma patients. Tumor regression or stabilization was recognized in some patients [35]. Since the NY-ESO-1 gene is expressed in a significant proportion of HCC patients as described above, NY-ESO-1 peptides seem to be a more favored candidate than MAGE-3 for vaccine therapy in HCC patients.

Most malignant tumors, however, escape immune surveillance. We have analyzed the expression of antigen-processing and -presenting molecules in human HCC samples to further elucidate the mechanisms of immune escape. Our results demonstrated that the expression of the co-stimulatory molecules B7-1 and B7-2 was decreased in HCC samples as compared to the corresponding non-HCC tissues, and HLA class-I expression was also diminished in HCC, but less frequently than the co-stimulatory molecules. These results suggest a potential role of the reduced expression of these molecules in facilitating HCC escape from immune surveillance. The functional importance of B7 molecules in eliciting CTL responses has been mentioned [36]. In an experimental study, tumor rejection was observed in implanted HCC cells transfected with the B7-1 molecule [37]. Since the antigen-presenting function of dendritic cells has been reported

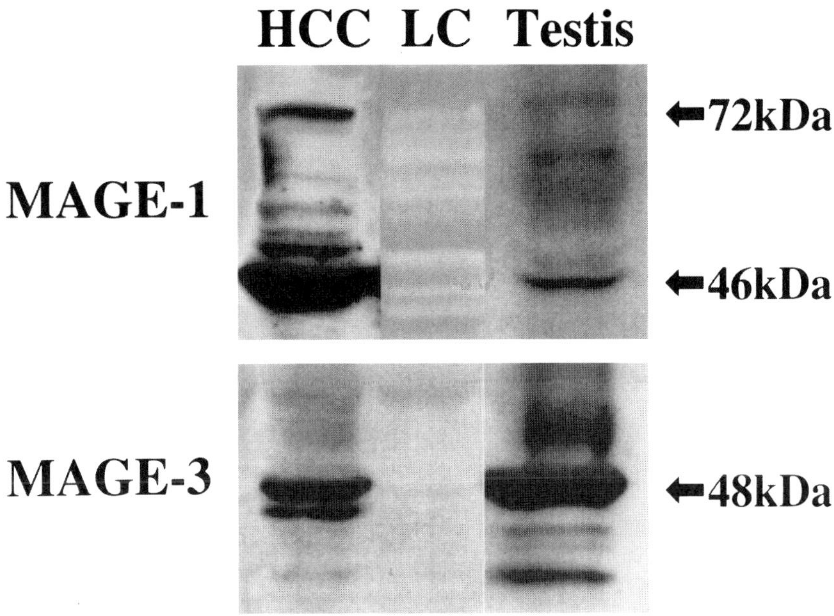

Fig. 2. Expression of MAGE-1 and MAGE-3 gene products by Western blot analysis using monoclonal antibodies, 77B for MAGE-1 and 57B for MAGE-3. The molecular weight of MAGE-1 was 46 kDa and that of MAGE-3 protein was 48 kDa, respectively. These protein were exclusively observed in HCC and the testicular tissue.

to be diminished in patients with HCV-related chronic liver diseases as compared to controls [38], augmentation of B7 expression by gene transfer in HCC patients might be beneficial. Furthermore, vaccination with dendritic cells that have engulfed killed tumor cells or those that have fused with cultured tumor cells has also been attempted for enhancement of tumor-specific antigen presentation in experimental models [39]. In addition, facilitating the expression of antigen-presenting molecules with various cytokines, such as IL-2, IL-12 or IFN-γ, also appears to be necessary to elicit CTL responses.

We have reported one case where primary lesions of HCC and pulmonary metastasis had naturally disappeared [40]. Therefore, vaccine therapy seems to be a rational approach if we can identify more immunogenic HCC-specific antigens for immunization and if we can properly manipulate their presentation on the APC surface. Additionally, enhancement of the interaction between tumor cells and CTLs, and between APCs and CTLs would be beneficial. It has been observed that CTL responses against the NY-ESO-1 protein are associated with the development of specific serum IgG antibodies in melanoma patients [41]. Therefore, we propose that an effort should be made to find new antigenic molecules specific for HCC by the SEREX method [42], which is an excellent strategy for screening antibody production against autologous tumor-specific antigens.

CONCLUSIONS

Natural regression of HCC is experienced in very few clinical cases and the precise mechanism remains unclear. However, this phenomenon suggests that there are active immune responses against HCC. Although tumor-specific antigens that can elicit significant CTL responses have not been defined in HCC as of yet, NY-ESO-1 is the most attractive immunogenic antigen for HCC found to date. Once the immune response against NY-ESO-1 is proved, clinical application of vaccine immunotherapy with NY-ESO-1-derived peptides in HLA-A2-positive HCC patients will be possible. Subsequently, immunotherapy may become a modality for patients with HCC, in which the recurrence rate is very high due to multicentric development and early intrahepatic metastasis, and where a complete cure is very difficult to achieve.

REFERENCES

[1] Okuda K. Hepatocellular carcinoma: recent progress. Hepatology 1992; 15: 948–963.

[2] Wong JB, McQuillan GM, McHutchison JG, Poynard T. Estimating future hepatitis C morbidity, mortality, and costs in the United States. Am J Public Health 2000; 90: 1562–1569.

[3] Rosenberg SA. Immunotherapy of cancer by systemic administration of lymphoid cells plus interleukin-2. J Biol Response Mod 1984; 3: 501–511.

[4] Dutcher JP, Creekmore S, Weiss GR, Margolin K, Markowitz AB, Roper M, Parkinson D, Ciobanu N, Fisher RI, Boldt DH et al. A phase II study of interleukin-2 and lymphokine-activated killer cells in patients with metastatic malignant melanoma. J Clin Oncol 1989; 7: 477–485.

[5] Nestle FO, Alijagic S, Gilliet M, Sun Y, Grabbe S, Dummer R, Burg G, Schadendorf D. Vaccination of melanoma patients with peptide- or tumor lysate-pulsed dendritic cells. Nat Med 1998; 4: 328–332.

[6] Reynolds SR, Celis E, Sette A, Oratz R, Shapiro RL, Johnston D, Fotino M, Bystryn JC. HLA-independent heterogeneity of $CD8^+$ T cell responses to MAGE-3, Melan- A/MART-1, gp100, tyrosinase, MC1R, and TRP-2 in vaccine-treated melanoma patients. J Immunol 1998; 161: 6970–6976.

[7] Mackensen A, Herbst B, Chen JL, Kohler G, Noppen C, Herr W, Spagnoli GC, Cerundolo V, Lindemann A. Phase I study in melanoma patients of a vaccine with peptide-pulsed dendritic cells generated in vitro from CD34(+) hematopoietic progenitor cells. Int J Cancer 2000; 86: 385–392.

[8] Rosenberg SA, Lotze MT, Muul LM, Leitman S, Chang AE, Ettinghausen SE, Matory YL, Skibber JM, Shiloni E, Vetto JT et al. Observations on the systemic administration of autologous lymphokine-activated killer cells and recombinant interleukin-2 to patients with metastatic cancer. New Engl J Med 1985; 313: 1485–1492.

[9] Rosenberg SA, Lotze MT, Yang JC, Topalian SL, Chang AE, Schwartzentruber DJ, Aebersold P, Leitman S, Linehan WM, Seipp CA et al. Prospective randomized trial of high-dose interleukin-2 alone or in conjunction with lymphokine-activated killer cells for the treatment of patients with advanced cancer. J Natl Cancer Inst 1993; 85: 622–632.

[10] Cohen PJ, Lotze MT, Roberts JR, Rosenberg SA, Jaffe ES. The immunopathology of sequential tumor biopsies in patients treated with interleukin-2. Correlation of response with T-cell infiltration and HLA-DR expression. Am J Pathol 1987; 129: 208–216.

[11] Okuno K, Takagi H, Nakamura T, Nakamura Y, Iwasa Z, Yasutomi M. Treatment for unresectable hepatoma via selective hepatic arterial infusion of lymphokine-activated killer cells generated from autologous spleen cells. Cancer 1986; 58: 1001–1006.
[12] Ishikawa T, Imawari M, Moriyama T, Ohnishi S, Matsuhashi N, Suzuki G, Takaku F. Immunotherapy of hepatocellular carcinoma with autologous lymphokine-activated killer cells and/or recombinant interleukin-2. J Cancer Res Clin Oncol 1988; 114: 283–290.
[13] Uchino J, Une Y, Kawata A, Wakisaka Y, Hosokawa M. Postoperative chemoimmunotherapy for the treatment of liver cancer. Semin Surg Oncol 1993; 9: 332–336.
[14] Kawata A, Une Y, Hosokawa M, Wakizaka Y, Namieno T, Uchino J, Kobayashi H. Adjuvant chemoimmunotherapy for hepatocellular carcinoma patients. Adriamycin, interleukin-2, and lymphokine-activated killer cells versus adriamycin alone. Am J Clin Oncol 1995; 18: 257–262.
[15] Takayama T, Sekine T, Makuuchi M, Yamasaki S, Kosuge T, Yamamoto J, Shimada K, Sakamoto M, Hirohashi S, Ohashi Y, Kakizoe T. Adoptive immunotherapy to lower postsurgical recurrence rates of hepatocellular carcinoma: a randomised trial [see comments]. Lancet 2000; 356: 802–807.
[16] van der Bruggen P, Traversari C, Chomez P, Lurquin C, De Plaen E, Van den Eynde B, Knuth A, Boon T. A gene encoding an antigen recognized by cytolytic T lymphocytes on a human melanoma. Science 1991; 254: 1643–1647.
[17] Brossart P, Wirths S, Stuhler G, Reichardt VL, Kanz L, Brugger W. Induction of cytotoxic T-lymphocyte responses in vivo after vaccinations with peptide-pulsed dendritic cells [In Process Citation]. Blood 2000; 96: 3102–3108.
[18] Murphy G, Tjoa B, Ragde H, Kenny G, Boynton A. Phase I clinical trial: T-cell therapy for prostate cancer using autologous dendritic cells pulsed with HLA-A0201-specific peptides from prostate-specific membrane antigen. Prostate 1996; 29: 371–380.
[19] Nishiyama T, Tachibana M, Horiguchi Y, Nakamura K, Ikeda Y, Takesako K, Murai M. Immunotherapy of bladder cancer using autologous dendritic cells pulsed with human lymphocyte antigen-A24-specific MAGE-3 peptide. Clin Cancer Res 2001; 7: 23–31.
[20] Jager D, Jager E, Knuth A. Vaccination for malignant melanoma: recent developments. Oncology 2001; 60: 1–7.
[21] Guo YJ, Che XY, Shen F, Xie TP, Ma J, Wang XN, Wu SG, Anthony DD, Wu MC. Effective tumor vaccines generated by in vitro modification of tumor cells with cytokines and bispecific monoclonal antibodies. Nat Med 1997; 3: 451–455.
[22] Griffiths E, Ong H, Soloski MJ, Bachmann MF, Ohashi PS, Speiser DE. Tumor defense by murine cytotoxic T cells specific for peptide bound to nonclassical MHC class I. Cancer Res 1998; 58: 4682–4687.
[23] Gilboa E, Nair SK, Lyerly HK. Immunotherapy of cancer with dendritic-cell-based vaccines. Cancer Immunol Immunother 1998; 46: 82–87.
[24] Srivastava PK, Udono H. Heat shock protein–peptide complexes in cancer immunotherapy. Curr Opin Immunol 1994; 6: 728–732.
[25] Bulfone-Paus S, von Bernuth H, Ruckert R, Wachtlin J, Ungureanu D, Notter M, Krause H, Pohl T, Paus R, Kunzendorf U. Vaccination with tumor cells engineered to secrete interleukin 2-immunoglobulin G fusion protein induces tumor rejection. Cancer Res 1998; 58: 2707–2710.
[26] Bianch R, Grohmann U, Bellaonna ML, Silla S, Ffallarino F, Ayroldi E, Fioretti MC, Puccetti P. IL-12 is both required and sufficient for initiating T cell reactivity to a class I-restricted tumor peptide (P815AB) following transfer of P815AB-pulsed dendritic cells. J Immunol 1996; 157: 1589–1597.

[27] Traversari C, Meazza R, Coppolecchia M, Basso S, Verrecchia A, van der Bruggen P, Ardizzoni A, Gaggero A, Ferrini S. IFN-gamma gene transfer restores HLA-class I expression and MAGE-3 antigen presentation to CTL in HLA-deficient small cell lung cancer. Gene Ther 1997; 4: 1029–1035.
[28] Jager E, Ringhoffer M, Dienes HP, Arand M, Karbach J, Jager D, Ilsemann C, Hagedorn M, Oesch F, Knuth A. Granulocyte-macrophage-colony-stimulating factor enhances immune responses to melanoma-associated peptides in vivo. Int J Cancer 1996; 67: 54–62.
[29] Kobayashi Y, Higashi T, Nouso K, Nakatsukasa H, Ishizaki M, Kaneyoshi T, Toshikuni N, Kariyama K, Nakayama E, Tsuji T. Expression of MAGE, GAGE and BAGE genes in human liver diseases: utility as molecular markers for hepatocellular carcinoma. J Hepatol 2000; 32: 612–617.
[30] Kariyama K, Higashi T, Kobayashi Y, Nouso K, Nakatsukasa H, Yamano T, Ishizaki M, Kaneyoshi T, Toshikuni N, Ohnishi T, Fujiwara K, Nakayama E, Terracciano L, Spagnoli GC, Tsuji T. Expression of MAGE-1 and -3 genes and gene products in human hepatocellular carcinoma. Br J Cancer 1999; 81: 1080–1087.
[31] Gaugler B, Van den Eynde B, van der Bruggen P, Romero P, Gaforio JJ, De Plaen E, Lethe B, Brasseur F, Boon T. Human gene MAGE-3 codes for an antigen recognized on a melanoma by autologous cytolytic T lymphocytes. J Exp Med 1994; 179: 921–930.
[32] Imanishi T, Akaza T, Kimura A, Tokunaga K, Gojobori T. Allele and haplotype frequencies for HLA and complement loci in various ethnic groups. In: Tsuji K, Aizawa M, Sasazuki T, editors. HLA 1991. Proceedings of the Eleventh International Histocompatibility Workshop and Conference. Oxford, Great Britain: Oxford University Press, 1992; pp. 1065–1068.
[33] Marchand M, Weynants P, Rankin E, Arienti F, Belli F, Parmiani G, Cascinelli N, Bourlond A, Vanwijck R, Humblet Y et al. Tumor regression responses in melanoma patients treated with a peptide encoded by gene MAGE-3. Int J Cancer 1995; 63: 883–885.
[34] Chen YT, Boyer AD, Viars CS, Tsang S, Old LJ, Arden KC. Genomic cloning and localization of CTAG, a gene encoding an autoimmunogenic cancer-testis antigen NY-ESO-1, to human chromosome Xq28. Cytogenet Cell Genet 1997; 79: 237–240.
[35] Jager E, Gnjatic S, Nagata Y, Stockert E, Jager D, Karbach J, Neumann A, Rieckenberg J, Chen YT, Ritter G, Hoffman E, Arand M, Old LJ, Knuth A. Induction of primary NY-ESO-1 immunity: $CD8^+$ T lymphocyte and antibody responses in peptide-vaccinated patients with NY-ESO-1+ cancers. Proc Natl Acad Sci USA 2000; 97: 12198–12203.
[36] Jung D, Jaeger E, Cayeux S, Blankenstein T, Hilmes C, Karbach J, Moebius U, Knuth A, Huber C, Seliger B. Strong immunogenic potential of a B7 retroviral expression vector' generation of HLA-B7-restricted CTL response against selectable marker genes. Hum Gene Ther 1998; 9: 53–62.
[37] Tatsumi T, Takehara T, Kanto T, Kuzushita N, Ito A, Kasahara A, Sasaki Y, Hori M, Hayashi N. B7-1 (CD80)-gene transfer combined with interleukin-12 administration elicits protective and therapeutic immunity against mouse hepatocellular carcinoma. Hepatology 1999; 30: 422–429.
[38] Hiasa Y, Horiike N, Akbar SM, Saito I, Miyamura T, Matsuura Y, Onji M. Low stimulatory capacity of lymphoid dendritic cells expressing hepatitis C virus genes. Biochem Biophys Res Commun 1998; 249: 90–95.
[39] Nouri-Shirazi M, Banchereau J, Bell D, Burkeholder S, Kraus ET, Davoust J, Palucka KA. Dendritic cells capture killed tumor cells and present their antigens to elicit tumor-specific immune responses. J Immunol 2000; 165: 3797–3803.
[40] Hino N, Higashi T, Ueki T, Nakatsukasa H, Ooguchi S, Ashida K, Fujio K, Takaki A, Yonei T, Hasui T et al. Disappearance of pulmonary metastases by OK-432 treatment in a case of hepatocellular carcinoma. Acta Med Okayama 1993; 47: 289–292.

[41] Jager E, Nagata Y, Gnjatic S, Wada H, Stockert E, Karbach J, Dunbar PR, Lee SY, Jungbluth A, Jager D, Arand M, Ritter G, Cerundolo V, Dupont B, Chen YT, Old LJ, Knuth A. Monitoring CD8 T cell responses to NY-ESO-1: correlation of humoral and cellular immune responses. Proc Natl Acad Sci USA 2000; 97: 4760–4765.
[42] Sahin U, Tureci O, Schmitt H, Cochlovius B, Johannes T, Schmits R, Stenner F, Luo G, Schobert I, Pfreundschuh M. Human neoplasms elicit multiple specific immune responses in the autologous host. Proc Natl Acad Sci USA 1995; 92: 11810–11813.

Alcoholic Liver Injury

Molecular Biology and Immunology in Hepatology
Edited by T. Tsuji, T. Higashi, M. Zeniya and K.-H. Meyer zum Büschenfelde

CHAPTER 14

Assessment of the Reversibility and Treatments of Alcoholic Liver Disease

J. Christian Bode

Department of Internal Medicine I, Robert-Bosch-Hospital, Teaching Hospital, University of Tuebingen, Tuebingen, Germany

INTRODUCTION

The results of many epidemiologic studies clearly demonstrate that excessive use of alcohol remains the most important cause of cirrhosis in the Western world and a leading cause of mortality during mid-life, especially in males [1–3]. In most countries for which reliable epidemiologic data over the course of several decades are available, there is a close correlation between the growth of average aggregate alcohol consumption and mortality from cirrhosis. In many studies a highly significant positive correlation was found between both, the magnitude and duration of alcohol abuse and the risk of developing cirrhosis [1,2]. However, the variability in expression and extent of liver injury is underlined by the fact that according to data from clinical studies and autopsy studies, only 20 to 30% of alcoholics develop cirrhosis [2,4].

To discuss the treatment of patients with alcoholic liver disease (ALD) it has to be considered that alcohol abuse produces manifold metabolic derangements and leads to a multitude of functional disturbances and other organ injuries. The high prevalence of extrahepatic diseases associated with heavy use of alcohol markedly influences the morbidity and mortality of patients with ALD [5–7]. Quantitative and/or qualitative malnutrition with varying degrees of vitamin and trace element deficiencies increases the complexity of alcohol-related illnesses and adds to the difficulties in the evaluation of therapeutical trials [8].

Further factors which can markedly influence the results of such therapeutical trials in patients with ALD and which have to be kept in mind in their interpretation are:

(a) The broad spectrum of clinical manifestations of alcoholic liver disease ranging from uncomplicated fatty liver to life-threatening fulminant liver injury (see Section 1).

(b) Despite major advances in the elucidation of the manifold direct and indirect metabolic and potentially toxic effects of alcohol on parenchymal and non-parenchymal cells in the liver the pathogenesis of the progressive type of ALD (alcoholic hepatitis, fibrosis and finally cirrhosis) in man has not been clarified (see Section 2).

(c) Trials including patients with ALD have serious methodological problems since alcoholics are often non-compliant for intake of drugs, control visits and, especially, for being abstinent or reporting alcohol intake.

(d) An important aim in all therapeutical studies is to achieve abstinence or, at least, to reduce alcohol intake. Because of the distinct benefit of abstinence on most stages of ALD (see Section 3.1) it may become difficult or impossible to proof the efficacy of any therapeutic measure such as drugs or nutritional supplements.

(e) Until recently, no adequate animal model for the type of alcoholic liver observed in humans was available. The only exception was the liver injury observed following chronic alcohol administration to baboons [10]. Many so-called 'hepatoprotective' drugs have been introduced in the treatment of ALD on the basis of certain effects of these compounds on alcohol-induced metabolic alterations in the liver of experimental animals, mainly rodents. Since these rodent models did not develop the classical pattern characteristic for ALD in humans, the assumption that such biochemical effects are relevant for the treatment of ALD in man remained speculative. The liver injury of rodents fed ethanol intragastrically in the Tsukamoto–French model of ALD seems to resemble more closely that seen in ALD in humans [9,11]. Whether or not this model is more appropriate to test therapeutic agents remains to be seen.

1. SPECTRUM OF ALCOHOLIC LIVER DISEASE

Chronic alcohol abuse may cause a wide spectrum of liver pathology. The histological spectrum of ALD extends from uncomplicated fatty liver over various degrees of alcoholic hepatitis (AH) and hepatic fibrosis to ultimately cirrhosis [12–14] (Fig. 1). Correspondingly, the clinical picture varies greatly; the extreme on the one hand is the patient without any complaints or symptoms in whom routine check-up reveals an enlarged liver and/or abnormal liver tests. The other extreme is represented by the patient with decompensated cirrhosis with jaundice, ascites, bleeding esophageal varices, and hepatic encephalopathy (details in [12–14]). As schematically shown in Fig. 1, the development of the more advanced stages of liver disease usually takes many years of alcohol abuse. There is convincing evidence that females develop cirrhosis at a reduced cumulative ethanol dose compared with males [15].

The natural history of ALD without treatment has been intensively investigated in earlier studies. Details of the results of these studies are beyond the scope of this article; they have been reviewed elsewhere [16,17]. Regarding any type of treatment, it is important to emphasize that the prognosis of ALD is variable among individuals within its different clinical and histological stages. For example, the mortality rate in patient hospitalized for an acute episode of alcoholic hepatitis varies between 5 and 100% [18,19]. The prognosis of patients with alcoholic hepatitis without cirrhosis seems to be remarkably better than that of patients in whom an acute episode of alcoholic hepatitis is superimposed on complete cirrhosis [16,17,20–22] (Table 1). Other factors which are of prognostic value for patients with alcoholic hepatitis are: presence of encephalopathy, presence of ascites, initial serum bilirubin > 15 mg/dl, prothrombin time prolonged (>6 s), renal failure (creatinine clearance < 50 ml/min) [16,17]. To assess the prognosis of

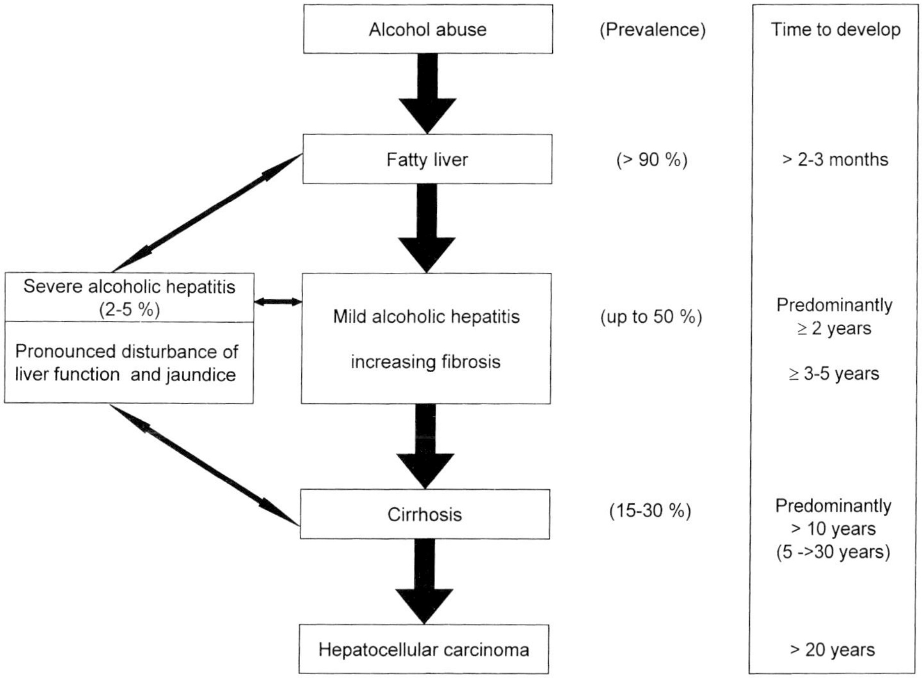

Fig. 1. Schematic representation of the development of the main types of alcoholic liver disease.

TABLE 1

Short-term mortality in patients with alcoholic hepatitis (AH) with and without cirrhosis

Selection of patients	Cirrhosis	*n*	Mortality (%)	Reference
Severe AH				
Combined data from 15 studies	yes	121	70	[21]
	no	42	24	
All patients admitted because of AH	yes	118	31.4	[22]
	no	61	6.6	

individual patients with ALD complex severity scores have been developed to improve the assessment of new treatments for ALD [23].

The superimposition of some other disease process may influence the worsening of ALD, a fact that has been elucidated in recent years. The influence of chronic viral hepatitis on the course of ALD has been extensively studied. While the evidence for a synergistic role of hepatitis B virus and alcohol in the development of cirrhosis remains controversial [24], there is substantial evidence that chronic HCV infection accelerates the progression of liver injury in chronic alcohol abusers [25,26]. In subjects with high alcohol intake the coexistence of HCV infection multiplies the alcohol-associated risk of cirrhosis [27].

2. TREATMENT

This review will focus on general measures for treatment of ALD, including abstinence from alcohol, nutritive support, relief of vitamin and trace element deficiencies and, in more detail, specific pharmacotherapy. The therapy of alcohol dependence and of complications of advanced stages of alcoholic liver disease, such as ascites, encephalopathy, spontaneous bacterial peritonitis, and bleeding from esophageal varices will not be discussed here.

2.1. Abstinence and reversibility of ALD

The main goal in the treatment of all patients with ALD is abstinence from alcohol [14,28–31]. The prognosis for patients at most stages of ALD is markedly improved by abstinence.

Alcoholic fatty liver is completely reversed when alcohol ingestion is stopped. Hepatomegaly, the main clinical finding in patients with uncomplicated fatty liver, will return to normal within a month or two following cessation of the toxin.

Moderately severe *alcoholic hepatitis* is also largely reversible once alcohol ceases [16,17,22]. If alcoholic hepatitis coexists with fibrosis or cirrhosis, the morphological sequelae will persist [17,32]. Many reports indicate that clinical overt alcoholic hepatitis often proves fatal. However, the prognosis of patients with moderate/severe alcoholic hepatitis without cirrhosis seems to be remarkably better [20,22] than that of patients in whom an acute episode of severe alcoholic hepatitis is superimposed on complete cirrhosis [17,42] (Table 1). This may at least partly explain the marked differences in the early mortality in the placebo groups of placebo-controlled treatment trials (see Section 2.4).

Alcoholic cirrhosis also tends to improve in patients who stop drinking. In several studies on the natural history of the disease the overall 5-year survival rate was statistically better in the non-drinking groups [16,17,21]. In one study [32] the death rate after 5 years was almost twice as high in cirrhotics who continued to drink as for those who stopped (56% versus 32%). Abstinence seems to have little or no effect on the survival of patients who have developed complications of cirrhosis [33].

Although abstinence is the preferred goal, complete and permanent abstinence is not always achieved in alcohol abusing patients. However, the results of the available treatment approaches for managing alcohol dependence, including new pharmacologic treatments to prevent relapse, have improved markedly [34,35]. Up to 60% of middle-class alcoholics maintain abstinence for at least a year, many for lifetime. Therefore, the physician who treats patients with alcoholic liver disease has an important role to play in referring these patients to appropriate rehabilitation programs and helping them develop and maintain a high level of motivation towards abstinence.

A good example of how important regular interactions of physicians in caring for patients with alcohol problems are, are the results of a placebo-controlled study on

TABLE 2

Effect of a controlled clinical trial of 6 months on mean alcohol consumption and abstinence in patients with alcoholic hepatitis (data from [36])

	Groups according to specific treatment		
	placebo	prednisolone	oxandrolone
Alcohol consumption (g/day; mean ± SD)			
When entering the trial	250 ± 141	271 ± 114	200 ± 153
After 6 months	40 ± 70	40 ± 70	35 ± 74
Abstinence at the end of the trial (after 6 months)	57%	58%	62%

the therapeutic effects of oxandrolone or prednisolone in patients with ALD [36] (see Section 3.3.2). As can be seen in the data summarized in Table 2, the follow-up at monthly intervals led to a pronounced decrease in mean daily alcohol consumption in all three treatment groups. After completing the 6-months treatment period about 60% of the patients were abstinent. This beneficial 'side effect' of the study was much more impressive than that obtained by the drug treatments!

2.2. *Nutritional therapy*

It is generally accepted that chronic alcohol consumption per se is the major cause of ALD [4,13,37]. However, most authorities agree that malnutrition, especially protein–calorie malnutrition, is a common finding in advanced ALD and influences the course of the disease [8,37,39]. On the other side, the nutritional status of many alcohol abusing patients in industrialized countries ('middle-class' alcoholics) with fatty liver or mild stages of alcoholic hepatitis is reported to be adequate with the exception of some deficiencies of vitamins and/or trace elements [40,41].

There is general agreement that a nutritionally balanced diet is advisable for patients with alcoholic liver disease. Overweight should be avoided since excess weight has been found to be an independent risk factor for developing ALD [42]. Dietary habits which may also be important may be the preference of certain meat products. The results obtained in an epidemiologic study [43] and in a more recent case-control study [44] support the assumption that the consumption of pork is closely associated with the development of more severe ALD and cirrhosis mortality. From data obtained in animal experiments it was postulated that the type of fat in this meat influences the rate of progression of ALD [45].

No supplementary nutritional therapy is necessary in most patients with mild to moderate ALD, unless there is evidence for malnutrition. The place of nutritional support in patients with more severe ALD with or without cirrhosis has been more controversial for many years [30,38,39]. On the basis of more recent data nutrition therapy is recommended in all patients with ALD and evidence of malnutrition [29,30].

2.2.1. Protein–calorie supplementation

More than 20 controlled prospective trials on the effect of protein–calorie supplementation on the course and mortality of patients with severe alcoholic hepatitis and/or cirrhosis have been published (for review see [29,38,39,46]). Despite marked differences between most of these studies regarding design, quality, severity of disease, type and amount of nutritional support, etc., it can be concluded that enteral or parenteral protein–calorie supplementation tends to speed recovery of nutritional status and of liver function as measured by usual tests (bilirubin, albumin). In general, the supplements are tolerated and do not exacerbate encephalopathy. However, in most of the studies, the nutritional supplements did not influence the survival rate. A lower mortality in the supplemented group was reported in two earlier short-term studies, one using parenteral supplementation in patients with alcoholic hepatitis [46] and the other using total enteral nutrition in severely malnourished cirrhotics [47]. In a long-term study to evaluate efficacy of oxandrolone (see below) in combination with an oral nutritional support, a significant improvement in survival rate by the nutritional supplementation was found in moderately malnourished patients with ALD, but not in patients with severe malnutrition [48]. In a more recent randomized trial, comparing the short- and long-term effects of total enteral nutrition or steroids in severe alcoholic hepatitis (80% cirrhotic) mortality during treatment was similar in both groups but occurred earlier with enteral feeding [49].

Although it remains uncertain whether or not nutritional supplementation improves short-term or long-term survival it has been concluded that protein–calorie supplementation is of sufficient benefit and necessary in these patients [29]. The main points of guidelines for daily dietary feeding in such patients have been suggested [29,50,51]: calories should provide 1.2 to 1.4 times the required resting energy expenditure (minimum 30 kcal/kg b.w.; 50–55% as carbohydrate, 30–35% as fat) and protein 1.0–1.5 g/kg b.w. Nutrition should be given entirely by voluntary oral intake and/or by small-bore feeding tube, parenteral nutrition should be second choice. Branched-chain amino acids should be reserved for patients who cannot tolerate the necessary amount of standard amino acids without precipitating encephalopathy (for further details see [29,50]).

2.2.2. Vitamins and trace elements

Deficiencies of vitamins and trace elements are frequent findings in patients with ALD, even if they do not suffer from protein–calorie malnutrition [52–55]. The deficiencies of these micronutrients are caused by decreased intake and/or absorption as well as increased turnover and/or urinary excretion [54,56]. The deficiency in the different vitamins and trace elements are of importance for the development of many functional disturbances and organ injuries in alcoholics. To improve these disturbances and organ injuries, the supplementation of the lacking vitamins and trace elements is clearly indicated in these patients. However, until now, there is no evidence that the development and course of ALD itself is significantly influenced by the supplementation of single or a combination of several of these micronutrients [29,30,52].

B vitamins. Folate deficiency is common in patients with ALD. Important consequences are macrocytic anemia with megaloblastic bone marrow changes, intestinal malabsorption and diarrhea and increased serum concentrations of homocysteine [60]. Deficiency of the two B vitamins thiamine and pyridoxine are also frequently found in patients with ALD. Pronounced thiamine deficiency leads to Wernicke's encephalopathy and deficiency of both vitamins will contribute to the development of peripheral neuropathy [57]. Deficiency of riboflavin is less frequently found in patients with ALD. However, the results of a recent epidemiologic study suggest that riboflavin might have a protective effect on the development of cirrhosis [58]. Vitamin B12 is of great importance for the transfer of methyl groups. Even subclinical deficiency of this vitamin, folate and pyridoxine which is a common finding in chronic alcoholics leads to decreased methylation of DNA [59] and correlates with hyperhomocystinemia [60]. Liberal supplementation of the above mentioned B-vitamins and also of vitamin C is recommended in addition to the protein- and calorie-rich diet [29,53].

Fat-soluble vitamins. ALD is associated with marked disturbances in vitamin A metabolism. Depletion of hepatic vitamin A stores is found even when liver injury is moderate [52]. Symptoms associated with ALD, such as night blindness and azoospermia, may be secondary to vitamin A depletion and its consequences for retinol metabolism. Hepatic vitamin A depletion plays also an important role in hepatic fibrosis. Paradoxically, however, vitamin A excess may also promote fibrosis [52,61]. Supplements of vitamin A in patients with ALD, therefore, must carefully respect the resulting narrow therapeutic window.

Vitamin E (alpha-tocopherol) is part of the antioxidant defense system. Chronic alcohol abuse per se was found to be associated with normal levels of alpha-tocopherol [62]. However, decreased levels have been found in cirrhotics [63] and in animal experiments [52]. Thus, a supplementation of vitamin E has been recommended in excessive alcohol abuse, especially in patients with advanced ALD.

Zinc. Zinc deficiency is common in alcoholics, especially in patients with ALD [55]. In addition to low serum zinc levels depressed zinc concentrations have been reported in liver tissue of patients with various stags of ALD [64] and in other tissues [55]. The main cause of zinc depletion by alcohol abuse is increased urinary zinc loss [55]. Important consequences of zinc deficiency in ALD are depressed immune function, hypogonadism, mental changes (predisposition to hepatic encephalopathy), diarrhea, acrodermatitis and impaired night vision [55]. Because of its important role in many metabolic pathways and clear evidence that zinc plays a role in hepatocellular protection against a variety of toxins and in liver regeneration, supplementation of zinc in patients with ALD is indicated (cave renal insufficiency!).

Selenium. In patients with ALD blood selenium levels and hepatic selenium content is decreased [64,65]. Selenium is an essential component of the glutathione peroxidase, a key enzyme in the elimination of free radicals and an important part of the antioxidant defense system. Because of toxicity of excessive intake of selenium supplementation of this trace element in patients with ALD should be performed only carefully controlled.

2.3. Drug treatment

Intensive research into the mechanisms of ALD during the last decades has identified several potentially important pathogenic factors. Despite this progress our understanding of the pathogenesis of ALD, especially the type of alcoholic hepatitis observed in humans, is still incomplete, a fact that has made it difficult to develop effective drugs to prevent or treat this type of chronic liver disease. What has emerged from the plethora of clinical and experimental research is that the pathogenesis of ALD is certainly a multifactorial process, where both the insults inflicted by alcohol and its metabolism and constitutional factors are important [14,52,61].

A detailed discussion of the present knowledge of the pathogenesis of ALD is beyond the scope of this chapter. Some of the mechanisms that are assumed to be of major importance in the pathogenesis of ALD are the

- hepatotoxicity of acetaldehyde (promotion of lipid peroxidation, formation of acetaldehyde–protein and –DNA adducts) [66],
- oxidative stress (increased formation of reactive oxygen species, reduced antioxidative capacity) [61,67,68],
- gut-derived bacterial toxins, especially endotoxins [68,69],
- activation of Kupffer cells,
- polymorphonuclear leukocytes [68–71],
- increased production of proinflammatory cytokines and other mediators [68,69,72],
- CYP2E1 polymorphism and induction [52,61,67].

The interaction of the aforementioned mechanisms and some additional factors which are assumed to play a role in the development of ALD are summarized in Fig. 2. More detailed aspects of the pathophysiology of ALD are reviewed elsewhere [61,66–70,72].

In the following sections predominantly those drugs will be discussed for which efficacy has been documented in randomized controlled trials. For the judgement of the results of many of these trials it should be stressed that the criteria for the selection of patients varied greatly from one study to another and that in many instances the stage and severity of the disease were not exactly defined. In severely ill patients in whom alcohol has affected many organs, death results frequently from causes other than liver failure. Therefore, in many instances it is difficult to distinguish clearly between death from liver disease or its complications (coma, hemorrhage, hepatic or renal failure) and death from other causes unrelated to ALD. Further, it should be emphasized that many of the studies excluded patients with active infection, pancreatitis, gastrointestinal bleeding, renal failure or other complications. This means that the efficacy of the drugs studied in severe ALD with these complications has not been well studied.

2.3.1. Glucocorticoids

Rationale. Glucocorticoids have been proposed predominantly because of increasing evidence that immunological abnormalities are implicated in the pathogenesis and perpetuation of ALD [18,19,52] and since glucocorticoids may inhibit the overproduction of proinflammatory cytokines [69,72] (Fig. 2). Further, glucocorticoids might be helpful because of the effect in increasing serum albumin and to compensate insufficient stress-induced cortisol production in severely ill alcoholics [28].

Clinical efficacy. Glucocorticoids are the most extensively studied drugs to treat patients with severe ALD, especially alcoholic hepatitis. Between 1971 and 1989 the results of 12 randomized controlled clinical trials on the effect of short-term treatment in patients with severe alcoholic hepatitis have been published (reviewed in [9,18,29,73]).

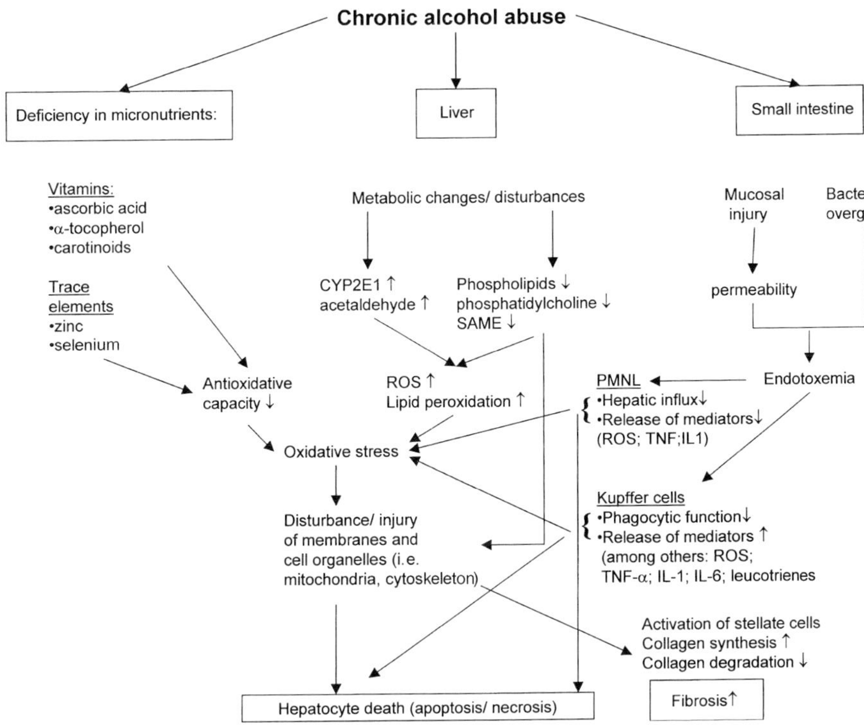

Fig. 2. Schematic representation of important factors involved in the pathophysiology of alcoholic liver disease.

The results were conflicting: five of these trials showed that the glucocorticoid treatment significantly reduced short-term mortality, whereas the other seven studies showed no difference compared with the groups receiving placebo. Because of the inconsistency of the results and the fact that disease severity varied markedly among the different studies, three meta-analysis of the 12 randomized trials were performed. The results of two of the meta-analysis showed a beneficial effect of glucocorticoid treatment [18,73]. In a subgroup of patients with hepatic encephalopathy glucocorticoids reduced short-term mortality by 27–28% [18,73]. No beneficial effect of glucocorticoid treatment was obtained in the third meta-analysis [19,74]. This latter meta-analysis has been criticized because of inadequate statistical analysis [29,75]. In a more recent study glucocorticoid treatment for 1 month in patients with severe alcoholic hepatitis improved the survival at 1 year but not at 2 years [76]. In addition to improved survival prognostic factors were found which help to identify patients who will have distinctly more benefit from glucocorticoid treatment: first, marked liver polymorphonuclear infiltrates in the liver, and, second, increased polymorphonuclear counts in the blood [76].

On the basis of the combined data, treatment of patients with severe alcoholic hepatitis (as defined by the presence of hepatic encephalopathy and/or a Maddrey discriminant function > 32 [77]) is recommended [29]. Prednisolone (40 mg for 4 weeks, followed by a taper) should be used in favor of prednisone [29].

Long-term treatment with glucocorticoids in patients with alcoholic hepatitis with or without cirrhosis has no beneficial effect on the survival rate or may even adversely affect the prognosis and should therefore be avoided [78,79].

2.3.2. Propylthiouracil (PTU)

Rationale. In animal experiments and in human studies it was shown that chronic alcohol feeding/alcohol abuse leads to a 'hypermetabolic' state with increased rates of hepatic oxygen consumption leading to liver damage in oxygen-poor pericentral regions of the liver lobule [29,67,80]. PTU was shown to decrease cellular metabolism and oxygen consumption thereby reducing the risk of hepatocellular necrosis.

Clinical efficacy. Two double-blind controlled trials of short-term PTU treatment in patients with ALD lead to conflicting results (for review see [28,29]).

The long-term treatment of patients with ALD has been studied in one double-blind, randomized, controlled trial involving 310 compliant patients [81]. Treatment with PTU ($n = 157$) at a dose of 150 mg b.i.d. for 2 years reduced the mortality rate significantly from 25% in the placebo group to 13% in the PTU group. The protective effect was mainly observed in a subgroup of severely ill patients (mortality rate PTU 25% vs. 55% in the placebo group). Furthermore, the beneficial effect from PTU therapy was observed most clearly in those patients who continued moderate but not heavy alcohol consumption. Several statistical and other concerns were raised regarding the validity of this study (reviewed in [82]). These concerns have been addressed adequately in a subsequent publication [82]. From the published data it can be concluded that the beneficial effect of PTU may be limited to long-term treatment in patients with more severe ALD who continue to drink moderate amounts of alcohol. The only two randomized, controlled, double-blind studies investigating short-term PTU in acute episodes of alcoholic hepatitis have led to conflicting results (reviewed in [28,29]). According to recently published practice guidelines for the management of ALD, PTU, therefore, should not be used routinely for alcoholic hepatitis until further information is obtained [29]. However, it was stated that the relative safety of this drug allows the clinician to consider its usage for long-term treatment on a 'case by case basis' [29].

2.3.3. Anabolic steroids

Rationale. Androgenic steroids have been shown to reduce or prevent experimental liver injury with several toxic chemicals, to enhance the removal of excess hepatic fat and to accelerate liver regeneration after partial hepatectomy [36]. In patients with ALD marked disturbances in the metabolism of androgenic steroids leading to decreased production and reduced blood levels of testosterone are frequently found [83].

Clinical efficacy. In two earlier controlled studies in small groups of patients with advanced ALD short-term treatment with anabolic steroids had no positive effect on mortality (reviewed in [36]). In a consecutive multi-center study, 36 days of oxandrolone therapy was compared with prednisolone or placebo in patients with moderate or severe alcoholic hepatitis [36]. In a subgroup of patients who survived 2 months after the start of the treatment the conditional 6-months death rate was significantly lower in the group receiving oxandrolone compared to the placebo group. The difference between the two groups levelled off after additional 4 months [36]. When dietary intake was analyzed retrospectively short-term survival did not differ between the groups of the latter study but oxandrolone had a beneficial effect on long-term survival in moderately malnourished patients with vigorous protein–calorie supplementation [84].

In two earlier controlled long-term studies of treatment with testosterone in patients with cirrhosis a significant reduction in mortality after treatment periods of 1.5 years [85] and 4 years [86] was found. However, in these earlier trials patients with different or even unknown etiology of the cirrhosis were included. In a more recent placebo-controlled multi-center trial in men with alcoholic cirrhosis oral testosterone treatment (median treatment period = 28 months) had no beneficial effect on survival and liver biochemistry [87]. From the available data it can be concluded that the use of anabolic steroids (testosterone, oxandrolone) cannot be recommended in patients with ALD until more data are available [29].

2.3.4. Colchicine

Rationale. Colchicine inhibits collagen production and enhances hepatic collagenase activity. In addition, it may inhibit inflammation and associated fibroblast proliferation [88,89].

Clinical efficacy. In two randomized placebo-controlled trials in patients with severe alcoholic hepatitis short-term treatment with colchicine (1 mg/day) did not improve the survival rate [90,91]. Because of its antifibrotic effects, a double-blind controlled trial of colchicine treatment (1 mg/day) was performed in 43 patients with cirrhosis of different etiology [92]. After treatment for up to 4 years there was no significant difference in mortality between the two treatment groups. However, the colchicine group had a greater clinical improvement and a reduction of fibrosis in histology. In an extended placebo-controlled double-blind trial the same authors followed 100 cirrhotic patients (45% in whom alcohol was the etiology) for up to 14 years [93]. The median survival rate was improved from 3.5 years in the placebo group to 11 years in the colchicine group. The study has been criticized because of a variety of problems in the study design and in the evaluation and interpretation of the results. Despite the encouraging results, the efficacy of colchicine in ALD has been judged to remain uncertain [29].

2.3.5. Flavonoids

Two bioflavonoids, silymarin (silibinin) and (+)-cyanidanol-3 have been proposed to treat ALD. They differ distinctly concerning the chemical structure [28].

Rationale. Both compounds have been shown to have marked hepatoprotective effects against several types of experimental liver injury, e.g., that caused by carbon tetrachloride, thioacetamide, phalloidin, and galactosamine (reviewed in [28,94]). Both flavonoids act as radical scavengers and have been reported to stabilize cell membranes. Both flavonoids exert the beneficial effects on experimental liver injury only when they are administered before the toxins.

Clinical efficacy: Silymarin (silibinin). Two short-term trials have claimed that silymarin improves a number of laboratory parameters in patients with mild to moderate ALD but both trials had several flaws in the design and execution of the study (reviewed in [28]). Three long-term double-blind placebo-controlled trials using silymarin have been performed. In the first trial 170 cirrhotics (61% with alcohol abuse) received either 420 mg silymarin/day or placebo [95]. Silymarin treatment improved the 4-years survival rate significantly (silymarin 58% vs. 39% in the placebo group). Further analysis of the data showed that only patients with Child A classification and those with alcoholic cirrhosis had a significant benefit from silymarin treatment. In the second published multi-center trial in patients with biopsy-proven alcoholic cirrhosis, silymarin (450 mg/day) for 2 years had no effect on survival or the course of the disease [96]. Preliminary results of a multi-center German double-blind placebo-controlled 4-years study with silymarin in patients with ALD did not show any effect of the drug on survival (H.K. Seitz, personal communication). In conclusion, until now, the use of the drug cannot be recommended for treatment of patients with ALD.

Clinical efficacy: (+)-cyanidanol-3. The results of four controlled trials on the effect of cyanidanol treatment on the course of the disease in patients with alcoholic hepatitis or cirrhosis have been published (reviewed in [28]). In three short-term studies (up to 3 months) no beneficial effect of the drug was seen. In one study, in which cyanidanol treatment lasted for 5 months, some improvement was reported in clinical symptoms and in a number of liver function tests but no effect on survival was observed [28]. Because of side effects (autoimmune hemolytic anemia) the drug has been withdrawn from the market in Germany.

2.3.6. Polyunsaturated phosphatydylcholine (PPC)

Rationale. The development of ALD has been shown to be associated with marked changes in hepatic phospholipid metabolism resulting in decreased content of phospholipids and especially of PPC [52,61]. PPC has been shown to protect against immune mediated hepatocyte damage [97], to restore several metabolic abnormalities associated with experimental ALD [37,61] and, more recently, to selectively modulate lipopolysaccharide-induced Kupffer cell activation [98]. In addition, PPC was shown to reverse alcohol-induced increase in gut permeability in rats [99]. In a baboon model of ALD the feeding of a mixture of PPC extracted from soybeans, especially rich in dilinoleoyl phosphatydylcholine, which has a high bioavailability, exerted a pronounced protection against alcohol-induced fibrosis and cirrhosis [100].

Clinical efficacy. PPC was assessed in a double-blind placebo-controlled trial over 2 years in 104 patients with alcoholic hepatitis [101]. There was a notable trend for improved survival in the PPC group compared with placebos (69% vs. 49%, respectively) but the difference was not statistically significant ($p = 0.11$). The greatest tendency towards improved survival was observed in a subgroup of patients with moderately severe disease [101]. On the basis of the experimental and these clinical data a large, placebo-controlled, double-blind multi-center trial is presently ongoing in the US.

2.3.7. S-adenosyl-methionine (SAM)

Rationale. SAM is the most important methylating agent in various transmethylation reactions that are important to synthesis of nucleic acids and proteins. Chronic alcohol consumption has been shown to lead to a depletion of hepatic SAM. SAM depletion may have a number of adverse effects, such as reduced synthesis of glutathione, polyamines and phosphatidylcholine (reviewed in [61,102]). These disturbances are likely to influence the integrity of membrane functions and to reduce the antioxidative capacity. Supplementation with SAM was shown to attenuate ALD in the baboon (reviewed in [61,102]).

Clinical efficacy. SAM treatment has been shown to be beneficial in several types of nonalcoholic intrahepatic cholestasis [102]. Recently, the results of the first long-term randomized placebo-controlled double-blind, multi-center trial of SAM in 123 patients with alcoholic cirrhosis have been published [103]. Most of the patients (93.5%) were in Child class A or class B. They were treated with SAM (1200 mg/day orally) or placebo for 2 years. The overall mortality or liver transplantation at the end of the trial decreased from 30% in the placebo group to 16% in the SAM group but the difference was not statistically significant ($p = 0.077$). When only the results of patients with Child class A and B were included in the analysis, the overall mortality or liver transplantation was significantly greater in the placebo group (29% vs. 12%, $p = 0.025$) [103]. Although this beneficial effect of SAM therapy needs to be confirmed in additional controlled clinical trials in ALD, the safety of this drug documented in several clinical trials in patients with intrahepatic cholestasis [102] allow the clinician to consider its usage on a case by case basis.

2.3.8. Malotilate

Rationale. Malotilate reduces some of the pathologic features of experimental ALD, such as steatosis and fibroneogenesis [104], and reverses the inhibition of ethanol on hepatocyte regeneration in partially hepatectomized rats [105].

Clinical efficacy. Malotilate had no significant effect on survival in earlier clinical trials in alcoholic hepatitis [106]. In a multi-center European randomized placebo-controlled trial 407 patients with various stages of ALD received either malotilate 1500 mg/day, malotilate 750 mg/day or placebo for 1–4 years [107]. Survival assessed by the conventional log-rank tests was slightly better in the 750 mg/day group than in the two other treatment groups ($p = 0.06$). Based on the present data the efficacy of malotilate in ALD remains uncertain and its use cannot be recommended until more data are available.

2.3.9. Pentoxifylline (POF)

Rationale. Increased production of TNFα and other proinflammatory cytokines by Kupffer cells and monocytes are important factors in the pathophysiology of ALD in man and in experimental animals (Fig. 2). Excess formation of TNFα can cause hepatocyte injury and TNFα-receptor knockout mice were resistant to ALD [108,109]. POF has been shown to inhibit TNFα production [108].

Clinical efficacy. In a placebo-controlled, double-blind trial patients with severe alcoholic hepatitis were treated with POF (3×400 mg/day; $n = 49$) or placebo ($n = 52$) for 4 weeks [108]. The short-term mortality was significantly reduced in the group receiving POF compared to placebo (24.5% vs. 46.1%; $p = 0.037$). The improved survival rate was associated with a pronounced and highly significant decrease in the development of the hepato-renal syndrome as cause of death [108]. On the basis of these results and because of only little side effects of the drug POF has become a promising candidate for the treatment of patients with severe alcoholic hepatitis but confirmatory studies are needed before POF can be generally recommended for this type of liver disease.

2.3.10. Miscellaneous

Insulin + glucagon. The combined infusion of insulin and glucagon has been shown to enhance hepatocellular regeneration [28]. Full details of four controlled clinical trials in patients with alcoholic hepatitis have been published. Using daily 12 h infusions of insulin and glucagon for 3 weeks resulted in two trials in no benefit and in two other trials in a significant difference or a trend for improved survival (reviewed in [29]). Until now, this therapy has not received general acceptance [29].

D-Penicillamine (100 mg/day for 2 months) had no significant effect on the course of 40 patients with moderately severe alcoholic hepatitis [110].

Thioctic acid was proposed for therapy of ALD because of its antioxidant properties. However, one randomized, double-blind study of 300 mg thioctic acid versus placebo in patients with moderately severe ALD for 6 months did not have any beneficial effect on the course of the disease [111].

Broad spectrum antibiotics to prevent endotoxemia. The results of various experimental and clinical studies support the hypothesis that gut-derived endotoxins play a significant role in the development and progression of ALD by enhancing the release of potentially toxic mediators by phagocytes and neutrophil leukocytes (Fig. 2) [68–70]. In animal experiments long-term administration of nonabsorbable antibiotics prevented hepatic injury and the development of liver fibrosis in rats receiving a cirrhogenic diet [69]. More recently it was shown that intestinal sterilization using two antibiotics prevented alcohol-induced liver injury in rats on the Tsukamoto–French protocol [112]. In a randomized, placebo-controlled double-blind trial in 50 patients with ALD paromomycin sulfate treatment for 3 weeks did not significantly influence endotoxin concentration in the blood [113]. However, treatment with a combination of polymyxin B and neomycin in a small group of cirrhotics resulted in a marked decrease in plasma endotoxin concentration [114]. Further studies in this area are needed to clarify whether blocking of endotoxin production by intestinal sterilization has a beneficial effect on the course of ALD, especially severe alcoholic hepatitis.

2.4. Liver transplantation

Alcoholic cirrhosis has been a controversial indication for liver transplantation until the early nineties, mainly because of ethical considerations related to the shortage of donor livers [115–117]. During the last decade liver transplantation has become a generally accepted option for patients with end-stage alcoholic cirrhosis in whom life-threatening complications develop despite abstinence from alcohol. The data of more recent studies indicate that liver transplantation increases the 5-years survival of patients with severe alcoholic cirrhosis [117,118]. Further, it has been shown that this type of treatment is justified for alcoholic cirrhosis even in cases of recidivism, which obviously hardly affect survival and compliance with the immunosuppressive regimen [119]. 1-year survival is approximately 80% [117,119] and does not differ from survival rates of patients transplanted for nonalcoholic liver disease. Overall relapse rates have been reported between 11 and 32% [116,117,119]. In one recent series recovery of employment was the only significantly different variable between alcoholic (30%) and nonalcoholic patients (60%) [119].

REFERENCES

[1] Lelbach WK. Cirrhosis in the alcoholic and its relation to the volume of alcohol abuse. Ann NY Acad Sci 1975; 252: 85–105.

[2] Smart RG, Mann RE. Recent liver cirrhosis declines: estimates of the impact of alcohol abuse treatment and alcoholics anonymous. Addiction 1993; 88(2): 193–198.

[3] Lelbach WK. Epidemiologie des Alkoholismus und alkoholassoziierter Organschäden. In: Seitz HK, Lieber CS, Simanowski UA, editors. Handbuch Alkohol, Alkoholismus, alkoholbedingte Organschäden. Heidelberg: JA Barth, 2000; pp. 9–54.

[4] Schenker S, Montalvo R. Alcoholic liver disease. Gastroenterology 1997; 13: 237–247.

[5] Adrian M, Layne N. Alcohol-associated morbidity. In: Carmi A, Schneider S, editors. Drugs and alcohol. Heidelberg: Springer, 1987; pp. 166–183.

[6] Gerke P, Hapke U, Rumpf HJ, John U. Alcohol-related diseases in general hospital patients. Alcohol Alcohol 1997; 32: 179–184.

[7] Sjogren H, Eriksson A, Brostrom G, Ahlm K. Quantification of alcohol-related mortality in Sweden. Alcohol Alcohol 2000; 35: 601–611.

[8] Odeleye OE, Watson RR. Alcohol-related nutritional derangements: implications for nutritional support. In: Watson RR, Watzel B, editors. Nutrition and alcohol. Boca Raton, FL: CRC Press, 1992; pp. 1–38.

[9] Hall P de la M, Lieber CS, DeCarli LM, French SW, Lindros KO, Jarvelainen H et al. Models of alcoholic liver disease in rodents: a critical evaluation. Alcohol Clin Exp Res 2001; 25: 254S–261S.

[10] Lieber CS, Robins SJ, Li JJ, DeCarli LM, Mak KM, Fasulo JM et al. Phosphatidylcholine protects against fibrosis and cirrhosis in the baboon. Gastroenterology 1994; 106: 152–159.

[11] Tsukamoto H, French SW, Benson N, Delgado G, Rao GA, Larkin EC et al. Severe and progressive steatosis and focal necrosis in rat liver induced by continuous intragastric infusion of ethanol and low fat diet. Hepatology 1985; 5(2): 224–232.

[12] Maddrey WC. Alcohol and the liver: an overview. In: Hall P, editor. Alcoholic liver disease, pathology and pathogenesis, 2nd ed. London: E Arnold, 1995; pp. 3–13.

[13] Bode JC. Alcoholic liver disease. In: Porro GB, Cremer M, Krejs G, Ramadori G, Rask-Madsen J, editors. Gastroenterology and hepatology. London: McGraw-Hill, 1999; pp. 511–522.

[14] Bode JC. Klinik und Therapie alkoholischer Leberschäden In: Seitz HK, Lieber CS, Simanowski UA, editors. Handbuch Alkohol, Alkoholismus, alkoholbedingte Organschäden. Heidelberg: JA Barth, 2000; pp. 275–298.

[15] Gavaler JS, Arria AM. Increased susceptibility of woman to alcoholic liver disease: artifactual or real? In: Hall P, editor. Alcoholic liver disease, pathology and pathogenesis, 2nd ed. London: E Arnold, 1995; pp. 123–133.

[16] Galambos JT. Alcoholic hepatitis. In: Schaffner F, Sherlock S, Levy CM, editors. The liver and its diseases. Stuttgart: Thieme, 1974; pp. 255–267.

[17] Schenker S. Alcoholic liver disease: evaluation of natural history and prognostic factors. Hepatology 1984; 4: 36S–43S.

[18] Reynold TB, Benhamou JP, Blake J, Naccarato R, Orrego H. Treatment of acute alcoholic hepatitis. Gastroenterol Int 1989; 2: 208–216.

[19] Christensen E, Gluud C. Glucocorticosteroids are not effective in alcoholic hepatitis. Am J Gastroenterol 1999; 94: 3065–3066.
[20] Klatskin G. Alcoholic hepatitis. In: Gerok W, Sickinger K, Hennekeuser HH, editors. Alcohol and the liver. Stuttgart: Schattauer, 1971; pp. 282–287.
[21] Theodossi A, Eddleston AL, Williams R. Controlled trial of methylprednisolone therapy in severe acute alcoholic hepatitis. Gut 1982; 23: 75–79.
[22] Bode JC, Kruse G, Mexas P, Martini GA. Alcoholic fatty liver, alcoholic hepatitis and alcoholic cirrhosis. Drinking behavior and incidence of clinical, clinico-chemical and histological findings in 282 patients. Dtsch Med Wochenschr 1984; 109: 1516–1521.
[23] Orrego H, Israel Y, Blake JE, Medline A. Assessment of prognostic factors in alcoholic liver disease: toward a global quantitative expression of severity. Hepatology 1983; 3: 896–905.
[24] Okuda K, Ohnishi K. The role of viral infections in alcoholic liver disease. In: Hall P, editor. Alcoholic liver disease, pathology and pathogenesis, 2nd ed. London: E Arnold, 1995; pp. 147–159.
[25] Grellier LF, Dusheiko GM. The role of hepatitis C virus in alcoholic liver disease. Alcohol Alcohol 1997; 32: 103–111.
[26] Schiff ER. Hepatitis C and alcohol. Hepatology 1997; 26: 39S–42S.
[27] Corrao G, Arico S. Independent and combined action of hepatitis C virus infection and alcohol consumption on the risk of symptomatic liver cirrhosis. Hepatology 1998; 27: 914–919.
[28] Bode JC. Drug therapy for alcoholic liver disease. In: Okolicsanyi L, Csomos G, Crepaldi G, editors. Assessment and management of hepatobiliary disease. Heidelberg: Springer, 1987; pp. 365–376.
[29] McCullough AJ, O'Connor JFB. Alcoholic liver disease: proposed recommendations for the American College of Gastroenterology. Am J Gastroenterol 1998; 93: 2022–2036.
[30] Schenker S, Martin RR. Treatment of alcoholic liver disease. In: Arroyo V, Bosch J, Bruguera M, Rodes J, Sanchez Topias JM, editors. Treatment of liver diseases. Barcelona: Masson SA, 1999; pp. 207–219.
[31] Powell WJ Jr, Klatskin G. Duration of survival in patients with Laennec's cirrhosis. Influence of alcohol withdrawal, and possible effects of recent changes in general management of the disease. Am J Med 1968; 44: 406–420.
[32] Pares A, Caballeria J, Bruguera M, Torres M, Rodes J. Histological course of alcoholic hepatitis. Influence of abstinence, sex and extent of hepatic damage. J Hepatol 1986; 2(1): 33–42.
[33] McCormick PA, Morgan MY, Phillips A et al. The effects of alcohol use on rebleeding and mortality in patients with alcoholic cirrhosis following variceal hemorrhage. J Hepatol 1992; 14: 99–103.
[34] Garbutt JC, West SL, Carey TS, Lohr KN, Crews FT. Pharmacological treatment of alcohol dependence: a review of the evidence. JAMA 1999; 281(14): 1318–1325.
[35] O'Connor PG, Schottenfeld RS. Patients with alcohol problems. N Engl J Med 1998; 338(9): 592–602.
[36] Mendenhall CL, Anderson S, Garcia-Pont P, Goldberg S, Kiernan T, Seeff LB et al. Short-term and long-term survival in patients with alcoholic hepatitis treated with oxandrolone and prednisolone. N Engl J Med 1984; 311(23): 1461–1479.
[37] Lieber CS. Alcohol and the liver: 1994 update. Gastroenterology 1994; 106: 1085–1105.
[38] Archard JL. Malnutrition and the role of nutritional support in alcoholic liver disease. Am J Gastroenterol 1987; 82(1): 1–7.

[39] Schenker S, Halff GA. Nutritional therapy in alcoholic liver disease. Semin Liver Dis 1993; 13: 196–129.

[40] Wheeler, EF. The effect of alcohol abuse on energy and nutrient intake. Eur J Gastroenterol Hepatol 1990; 2: 395–398.

[41] Salaspuro M. Nutrition status of alcoholics from different social groups. In: Watson RR, Watzel B, editors. Nutrition and alcohol. Boca Raton, FL: CRC Press, 1992; pp. 65–74.

[42] Naveau S, Giraud V, Borotto E, Aubert A, Capron F, Chaput JC. Excess weight risk factor for alcoholic liver disease. Hepatology 1997; 25(1): 108–111.

[43] Nanji AA, French SW. Relationship between pork consumption and cirrhosis. Lancet 1985; 1(8430): 681–683.

[44] Bode C, Bode JC, Erhardt JG, French BA, French SW. Effect of the type of beverage and meat consumed by alcoholics with alcoholic liver disease. Alcohol Clin Exp Res 1998; 22(8): 1803–1805.

[45] Nanji AA, Mendenhall CL, French SW. Beef fat prevents alcoholic liver disease in the rat. Alcohol Clin Exp Res 1989; 13(1): 15–19.

[46] Nasrallah SM, Galambos JT. Aminoacid therapy of alcoholic hepatitis. Lancet 1980; 2(8207): 1276–1277.

[47] Cabre E, Gonzalez-Huix F, Abad-Lacruz A, Esteve M, Acero D, Fernandez-Banares F et al. Effect of total enteral nutrition on the short-term outcome of severely malnourished cirrhotics. A randomized controlled trial. Gastroenterology 1990; 98(3): 715–720.

[48] Mendenhall CL, Moritz TE, Roselle GA, Morgan TR, Nemchausky BA, Tamburro CH et al. A study of oral nutritional support with oxandrolone in malnourished patients with alcoholic hepatitis: results of a Department of Veterans Affairs cooperative study. Hepatology 1993; 17(4): 564–576.

[49] Cabre E, Rodriguez-Iglesias P, Caballeria J, Quer JC, Sanchez-Lombrana JL, Pares A et al. Short- and long-term outcome of severe alcohol-induced hepatitis treated with steroids or enteral nutrition: a multicenter randomized trial. Hepatology 2000; 32(1): 36–42.

[50] Nompleggi DJ, Bonkovsky HL. Nutritional supplementation in chronic liver disease: an analytical review. Hepatology 1994; 19(2): 518–533.

[51] Kondrup J, Muller MJ. Energy and protein requirements of patients with chronic liver disease. J Hepatol 1997; 27(1): 239–247.

[52] Lieber CS. Hepatic, metabolic and toxic effects of ethanol: 1991 update. Alcohol Clin Exp Res 1991; 15(4): 573–592.

[53] Halsted CH, Keen CL. Alcoholism and micronutrient metabolism and deficiencies. Eur J Gastroenterol Hepatol 1990; 2: 399–405.

[54] Thomson AD, Pratt OE. Interaction of nutrients and alcohol: Absorption, transport, utilization and metabolism. In: Watson RR, Watzel B, editors. Nutrition and alcohol. Boca Raton, FL: CRC Press, 1992; pp. 75–100.

[55] McClain CJ, Kasarskis EJ. Zinc and alcohol. In: Watson RR, Watzel B, editors. Nutrition and alcohol. Boca Raton, FL: CRC Press, 1992; pp. 281–308.

[56] Bode JC, Bode C. Alcohol malnutrition and the gastrointestinal tract. In: Watson RR, Watzel B, editors. Nutrition and alcohol. Boca Raton, FL: CRC Press, 1992; pp. 423–428.

[57] Butterworth RF, D'amour M, Bruneau J, Heroux M, Brissette. Role of thiamine deficiency in the pathogenesis of alcohol peripheral neuropathy and the Wernicke–Korsakoff syndrome: An update. In: Palmer TN, editor. Alcoholism: A molecular perspective. New York, NY: Plenum Press, 1991; pp. 269–273.

[58] Corrao G, Torchio P, Zambon A, D'Amicis A, Lepore AR, di Orio F. Alcohol consumption and micronutrient intake as risk factors for liver cirrhosis: a case-control study. The

Provincial Group for the study of Chronic Liver Disease. Ann Epidemiol 1998; 8(3): 154–159.
[59] Cravo M, Camilo ME, Resende M, Cardoso JN, Leitao CN, Mira FC. DNA-methylation and subclinical vitamin deficiency of folate, pyridoxal phosphate and vitamin B12 in chronic alcoholics. Clin Nutr 1997; 16: 29–35.
[60] Cravo ML, Gloria LM, Selhub J, Nadeau MR, Camilo ME, Resende MP et al. Hyperhomocysteinemia in chronic alcoholism: correlation with folate, vitamin B-12, and vitamin B-6 status. Am J Clin Nutr 1996; 63(2): 220–222.
[61] Lieber CS. Alcoholic liver disease: new insights in pathogenesis lead to new treatments. J Hepatol 2000; 32(1 Suppl.): 113–128.
[62] Fernandez-Sola J, Villegas E, Nicolas JM, Deulofeu R, Antunez E, Sacanella E et al. Alcohol Clin Exp Res 1998; 22(2): 422–427.
[63] Rocchi E, Borghi A, Paolillo F, Pradelli M, Casalgrandi G. Carotenoids and liposoluble vitamins in liver cirrhosis. J Lab Clin Med 1991; 118(2): 176–185.
[64] Bode JC, Hanisch P, Henning H, Koenig W, Richter FW, Bode C. Hepatic zinc content in patients with various stages of alcoholic liver disease and in patients with chronic active and chronic persistent hepatitis. Hepatology 1988; 8(6): 1605–1609.
[65] Dworkin BM, Rosenthal WS, Stahl RE, Panesar NK. Decreased hepatic selenium content in alcoholic cirrhosis. Dig Dis Sci 1988; 33: 1213–1217.
[66] Jokelainen K. Acetaldehyde and liver disease. In: Agarwal DP, Seitz HK, editors. Alcohol in health and disease. New York: Marcel Dekker, 2001; pp. 387–406.
[67] Lindros KO. Alcoholic liver disease: pathobiological aspects. J Hepatol 1995; 23(Suppl. 1): 7–15.
[68] Thurman RG, Bradford BU, Knecht KT, Iimuro Y, Arteel GE, Yin M et al. Endotoxin, Kupffer cells and alcoholic liver injury. In Blum HE, Bode JC, Bode C, Sartor, editors. Gut and the liver. London: Kluwer Academic Publishers, 1998; pp. 222–240.
[69] Bode JC, Parlesak A, Bode C. Gut-derived bacterial toxins (endotoxin) and alcoholic liver disease. In: Agarwal DP, Seitz HK, editors. Alcohol in health and disease. New York: Marcel Dekker, 2001; pp. 369–386.
[70] Oneta C. The role of Kupffer cells in alcoholic liver disease. In: Agarwal DP, Seitz HK, editors. Alcohol in health and disease. New York: Marcel Dekker, 2001; pp. 407–426.
[71] Spitzer, JA. Acute and chronic endotoxaemia: effects on hepatic neutrophil influx and respiratory burst. In: Blum HE, Bode JC, Bode C, Sartor RB, editors. Gut and the liver. Dordrecht: Kluwer Academic Publishers, 1998; pp. 195–202.
[72] McClain CJ, Barve S, Deaciuc I, Hill DB. Tumor necrosis factor and alcoholic liver disease. Alcohol Clin Exp Res 1998; 22: 248S–252S.
[73] Imperiale TF, McCullough AJ. Do corticosteroids reduce mortality from alcoholic hepatitis? A meta-analysis of the randomized trials. Ann Intern Med 1990; 113(4): 299–307.
[74] Christensen E, Gluud C. Glucocorticosteroids are not effective in alcoholic hepatitis. Am J Gastroenterol 1999; 94(10): 3065–3066.
[75] Imperiale TF, O'Connor JB, McCullough AJ. Corticosteroids are effective in patients with severe alcoholic hepatitis. Am J Gastroenterol 1999; 94(10): 3066–3068.
[76] Mathurin P, Duchatelle V, Ramond MJ, Degott C, Bedossa P, Erlinger S et al. Survival and prognostic factors in patients with severe alcoholic hepatitis treated with prednisolone. Gastroenterology 1996; 110(6): 1847–1853.
[77] Maddrey WC, Boitnott JK, Bedine MS, Weber FL Jr, Mezey E, White RI Jr. Corticosteroid therapy of alcoholic hepatitis. Gastroenterology 1978; 75(2): 193–199.
[78] Tygstrup N, Juhl E and the Copenhagen study group for liver diseases. The treatment of alcoholic cirrhosis. The effect of continued drinking and prednisone on survival. In:

Sickinger GW, Hennekeuser HH, editors. Alcohol and the liver. Stuttgart: Schattauer, 1971; pp. 519–526.
[79] Schlichting P, Juhl E, Poulsen H, Winkel P. Alcoholic hepatitis superimposed on cirrhosis. Clinical significance and effect of long-term prednisone treatment. Scand J Gastroenterol 1976; 11(3): 305–312.
[80] Arteel GE, Iimuro Y, Yin M, Raleigh JA, Thurman RG. Chronic enteral ethanol treatment causes hypoxia in rat liver tissue in vivo. Hepatology 1997; 25(4): 920–926.
[81] Orrego H, Blake JE, Blendis LM, Compton KV, Israel Y. Long-term treatment of alcoholic liver disease with propylthiouracil. N Engl J Med 1987; 317(23): 1421–1427.
[82] Orrego H, Blake JE, Blendis LM, Compton KV, Volpe R, Israel Y. Long-term treatment of alcoholic liver disease with propylthiouracil. Part 2: Influence of drop-out rates and of continued alcohol consumption in a clinical trial. J Hepatol 1994; 20(3): 343–349.
[83] Van Thiel DH, Gavaler JS. Endocrine consequences of alcohol abuse. Alcohol Alcohol 1990; 25(4): 341–344.
[84] Mendenhall CL, Moritz TE, Roselle GA, Morgan TR, Nemchausky BA, Tamburro CH et al. A study of oral nutritional support with oxandrolone in malnourished patients with alcoholic hepatitis: results of a Department of Veterans Affairs cooperative study. Hepatology 1993; 17(4): 564–576.
[85] Wells R. Prednisolone and testosterone proprionate in cirrhosis of the liver. A controlled trial. Lancet 1969; 1: 1416–1419.
[86] Islam N, Islam A. Testosterone propionate in cirrhosis of the liver. Br J Clin Pract 1973; 27(4): 125–128.
[87] The Copenhagen Study Group. Testosterone treatment of men with alcoholic cirrhosis: A double-blind study. Hepatology 1986; 6(5): 807–813.
[88] Rojkind M. Fibrosis and cirrhosis. In: Arias IM, Frenkel M, Wilson JHP, editors. The liver annual 1. Amsterdam: Elsevier, 1981; pp. 126–148.
[89] Tanner MS, Jackson D, Mowat AP. Hepatic collagen synthesis in a rat model of cirrhosis, and its modification by colchicine. J Pathol 1981; 135(3): 179–187.
[90] Akriviadis EA, Steindel H, Pinto PC, Fong TL, Kanel G, Reynolds TB et al. Failure of colchicine to improve short-term survival in patients with alcoholic hepatitis. Gastroenterology 1990; 99(3): 811–818.
[91] Trinchet JC, Beaugrand M, Callard P, Hartmann DJ, Gotheil C, Nusgens BV et al. Treatment of alcoholic hepatitis with colchicine. Results of a randomized double blind trial. Gastroenterol Clin Biol 1989; 13(6–7): 551–555.
[92] Kershenobich D, Uribe M, Suarez GI, Mata JM, Perez-Tamayo R, Rojkind M. Treatment of cirrhosis with colchicine. A double-blind randomized trial. Gastroenterology 1979; 77(3): 532–536.
[93] Kershenobich D, Vargas F, Garcia-Tsao G, Perez Tamayo R, Gent M, Rojkind M. Colchicine in the treatment of cirrhosis of the liver. N Engl J Med 1988; 318(26): 1709–1713.
[94] Flora K, Hahn M, Rosen H, Benner K. Milk thistle (*Silybum marianum*) for the therapy of liver disease. Am J Gastroenterol 1998; 93(2): 139–143.
[95] Ferenci P, Dragosics B, Dittrich H, Frank H, Benda L, Lochs H et al. Randomized controlled trial of silymarin treatment in patients with cirrhosis of the liver. J Hepatol 1989; 9(1): 105–113.
[96] Pares A, Planas R, Torres M, Caballeria J, Viver JM, Acero D et al. Effects of silymarin in alcoholic patients with cirrhosis of the liver: results of a controlled, double-blind, randomized and multicenter trial. J Hepatol 1998; 28(4): 615–621.

[97] Neuberger J, Hegarty JE, Eddleston AL, Williams R. Effect of polyunsaturated phosphatidylcholine on immune mediated hepatocyte damage. Gut 1983; 24(8): 751–755.

[98] Oneta CM, Mak KM, Lieber CS. Dilinoleoylphosphatidylcholine selectively modulates lipopolysaccharide-induced Kupffer cell activation. J Lab Clin Med 1999; 134(5): 466–470.

[99] Bode C, Vollmer E, Hug J, Bode JC. Increased permeability of the gut to polyethylene glycol and dextran in rats fed alcohol. Ann NY Acad Sci 1991; 625: 837–840.

[100] Lieber CS, Robins SJ, Li J, DeCarli LM, Mak KM, Fasulo JM, Leo MA. Phosphatidylcholine protects against fibrosis and cirrhosis in the baboon. Gastroenterology 1994; 106(1): 152–159.

[101] Panos MZ, Polson R, Johnson R, Portmann B, Williams R. Polyunsaturated phosphatidyl choline for acute alcoholic hepatitis: a double-blind, randomized, placebo-controlled trial. Eur J Gastroenterol Hepatol 1990; 2(5): 351–355.

[102] Lieber CS. Role of *S*-adenosyl-L-methionine in the treatment of liver diseases. J Hepatol 1999; 30(6): 1155–1159.

[103] Mato JM, Camara J, Fernandez de Paz J, Caballeria L, Coll S, Caballero et al. *S*-adenosylmethionine in alcoholic liver cirrhosis: a randomized, placebo-controlled, double-blind, multicenter clinical trial. J Hepatol 1999; 30(6): 1081–1089.

[104] Monna T. Effect of malotilate on experimental liver fibrosis (cirrhosis) induced by carbon tetrachloride or egg yolk sensitization. In: Oda T, Tygstrup N, editors. Hematotrophic agent malotilate. Tokyo: Excerpta Medica, 1982; pp. 44–53.

[105] Takada A, Nei J, Tamino H, Takase S. Effects of malotilate on ethanol-inhibited hepatocyte regeneration in rats. J Hepatol 1987; 5(3): 336–343.

[106] Mutimer D, Brunner H, Berthelot, Portmann B, James O. Malotilate in alcoholic hepatitis — lessons from 3 European controlled trials. Hepatology 1988; 8: 1411.

[107] Keiding S, Badsberg JH, Becker U, Bentsen KD, Bonnevie O, Caballeria J et al. The prognosis of patients with alcoholic liver disease. An international randomized, placebo-controlled trial on the effect of malotilate on survival. J Hepatol 1994; 20(4): 454–460.

[108] Akriviadis E, Botla R, Briggs W, Han S, Reynolds T, Shakil O. Pentoxifylline improves short-term survival in severe acute alcoholic hepatitis: a double-blind, placebo-controlled trial. Gastroenterology 2000; 119(6): 1637–1648.

[109] Morgan TR, McClain CJ. Pentoxifylline and alcoholic hepatitis. Gastroenterology 2000; 119(6): 1787–1791.

[110] Resnick RH, Boitnott J, Iber FL, Makopour H, Cerda JJ. Preliminary observations of d-penicillamine therapy in acute alcoholic liver disease. Digestion 1974; 11: 257–265.

[111] Marshall AW, Graul RS, Morgan MY, Sherlock S. Treatment of alcohol-related liver disease with thioctic acid: a six month randomised double-blind trial. Gut 1982; 23(12): 1088–1093.

[112] Adachi Y, Moore LE, Bradford BU, Gao W, Thurman RG. Antibiotics prevent liver injury in rats following long-term exposure to ethanol. Gastroenterology 1995; 108(1): 218–224.

[113] Bode C, Schaefer C, Fukui H, Bode JC. Effect of treatment with paromomycin on endotoxemia in patients with alcoholic liver disease — a double-blind, placebo-controlled trial. Alcohol Clin Exp Res 1997; 21(8): 1367–1373.

[114] Ferro D, Quintarelli C, Lattuada A, Leo R, Alessandroni M, Mannucci PM et al. High plasma levels of von Willebrand factor as a marker of endothelial perturbation in cirrhosis: relationship to endotoxemia. Hepatology 1996; 23(6): 1377–1383.

[115] Schenker S, Perkins HS, Sorelli MF. Should patients with end-stage alcoholic liver disease have a new liver. Liver transplantation in alcoholics. Hepatology 1990; 11(2): 314–319.

[116] Lucey MR, Beresford TP. Alcoholic liver disease: to transplant or not to transplant? Alcohol Alcohol 1992; 27(2): 103–108.

[117] Krom RA. Liver transplantation and alcohol: who should get transplants? Hepatology 1994; 20(1 Pt 2): 28S–32S.

[118] Poynard T, Naveau S, Doffoel M, Boudjema K, Vanlemmens C, Mantion G et al. Evaluation of efficacy of liver transplantation in alcoholic cirrhosis using matched and simulated controls: 5-year survival. Multi-centre group. J Hepatol 1999; 30(6): 1130–1137.

[119] Pageaux GP, Michel J, Coste V, Perney P, Possoz P, Perrigault PF et al. Alcoholic cirrhosis is a good indication for liver transplantation, even for cases of recidivism. Gut 1999; 45(3): 421–426.

Autoimmune Liver Diseases

Molecular Biology and Immunology in Hepatology
Edited by T. Tsuji, T. Higashi, M. Zeniya and K.-H. Meyer zum Büschenfelde

CHAPTER 15

Molecular Mechanisms of Autoimmune Hepatitis

Arndt Vogel and Michael P. Manns

Department of Gastroenterology, Hepatology and Endocrinology, Hannover Medical School, Hannover, Germany

INTRODUCTION

Autoimmune diseases are chronic inflammatory conditions characterized by a loss of immunological tolerance to self-antigens. The pathogenic mechanisms leading to human autoimmunity are poorly understood. Most autoimmune diseases will not have a single cause and it has been postulated that both genetic factors and environmental triggers determine the initiation and progression of autoimmunity. Autoimmune hepatitis (AIH) is a chronic, mainly periportal hepatitis associated with hypergammaglobulinemia and circulating autoantibodies, which, in most cases, responds to immunosuppressive treatment [1]. The disease is most prevalent among females, displays an immunogenetic association with the HLA A1-B8-DR3 or DR4 haplotype [2], and the presence of extrahepatic syndromes [3]. The multifactorial definition of AIH illustrates that a single cause or a single test for the accurate diagnosis of AIH is not available. Therefore, the diagnosis is based upon a number of diagnostic criteria, as recently defined by the International Autoimmune Hepatitis Group, and upon the exclusion of other causes of chronic hepatitis [4]. The combination of seroimmunologic and molecular biologic tests [5] permits a precise discrimination between autoimmune hepatitis and other causes of chronic hepatitis. The exclusion of replicating hepatitis virus infection together with the presence of female sex, hypergammaglobulinemia, and response to immunosuppressive treatment are the key components of an accurate diagnosis.

Autoantibodies are a diagnostic hallmark of AIH detectable by serological in vitro assays. Autoantibody profiles have been utilized as a means of subclassification of AIH. According to this approach, AIH type 1 is characterized by the presence of antinuclear antibodies (ANA) and/or anti-smooth muscle antibodies (SMA), AIH type 2 is characterized by anti-liver–kidney microsomal autoantibodies (LKM-1) directed against cytochrome P450 (CYP) 2D6 [6] and with lower frequency against UDP-glucuronosyltransferases (UGT) [7] and AIH type 3 is characterized by autoantibodies against soluble liver antigens (SLA/LP) [8,9]. Clinically, AIH type 2 shows earlier age of onset than AIH type 1 and AIH type 3, a higher inflammatory activity and more frequent relapses and progression to cirrhosis under immunosuppressive treatment.

1. AUTOIMMUNE HEPATITIS AND GENETIC FACTORS

Genetic factors appear to be involved in the pathogenesis of AIH. However, a conclusive role of a single genetic locus capable of explaining the etiology of AIH has not been identified thus far, and the genetic background is therefore considered to be polygenic. The most conclusive association with autoimmune hepatitis is that related to the major histocompatibility complex. The significance of HLA polymorphisms in terms of disease susceptibility and severity lies in the observation that most autoimmune T cell dependent and all T cell-mediated responses are MHC restricted. Interestingly, the majority of genetic variations between alleles are concentrated in regions of the gene, which encode the floor and the lip of the antigen-binding groove. Polymorphisms within this region may affect predisposition to autoimmune diseases by several mechanisms including, for example, shaping of the T cell repertoire, peptide selection and presentation, and peptide transport. In European patients, several studies suggested that there is a strong genetic association with the HLA haplotype A1-B8-DRB1*0301 and the DRB*0401 antigen [10–12]. Analysis of the clinical course of patients with HLA A1-B8-DRB1*0301 haplotype revealed that they develop AIH at a significantly younger age, relapse more frequently under immunosuppressive treatment and are more frequently referred for liver transplantation [13]. Subsequent investigations of the encoding HLA alleles identified that genetic susceptibility to AIH type 1 is related to the six amino acid sequence LLEQKR at position 67–72 of the DRB1 polypeptide, which are located on the edge of the α-helix, and that the critical amino acid is lysine at position 71 (Fig. 1). Analysis of MHC genes in different population of AIH patients revealed that the immunogenetic associations with AIH vary regionally. In Japan, the A1-B8-DR3 haplotype is almost absent, and a typical association with HLA DRB1*0405 has been found [14]. Argentinean adults with AIH have an increased frequency of HLA DRB1*0405 and Mexicans of HLA DRB1*0404 [15,16]. These findings are likely to be influenced by genetic heterogeneity that exists in evolutionary divergent populations. On the other hand, they may reflect different underlying etiologies in terms of initiating events, such as different viral triggers. Regardless of the mechanisms, it is apparent that the MHC locus per se is insufficient for the development of autoimmune diseases, as shown by the decrease of autoimmune disease concordance rate of siblings in comparison with that of monozygotic twins. Therefore, several studies have focused on other non-MHC genes, and variations in a number of genes that are important in the regulation of immune responses have been associated with the development of autoimmune hepatitis.

Activation of the complement system by foreign cells produces powerfully immunogenic costimuli [17]. Complement components C1, C2, C4 and the CR1/2 complement receptors are also important for delivering tolerogenic signals, since inherited deficiencies of these elements in human beings are associated with susceptibility to autoimmune diseases [18]. Early studies showed that AIH type 1 was frequently associated with persistently low serum complement levels. C4 phenotyping revealed an association of

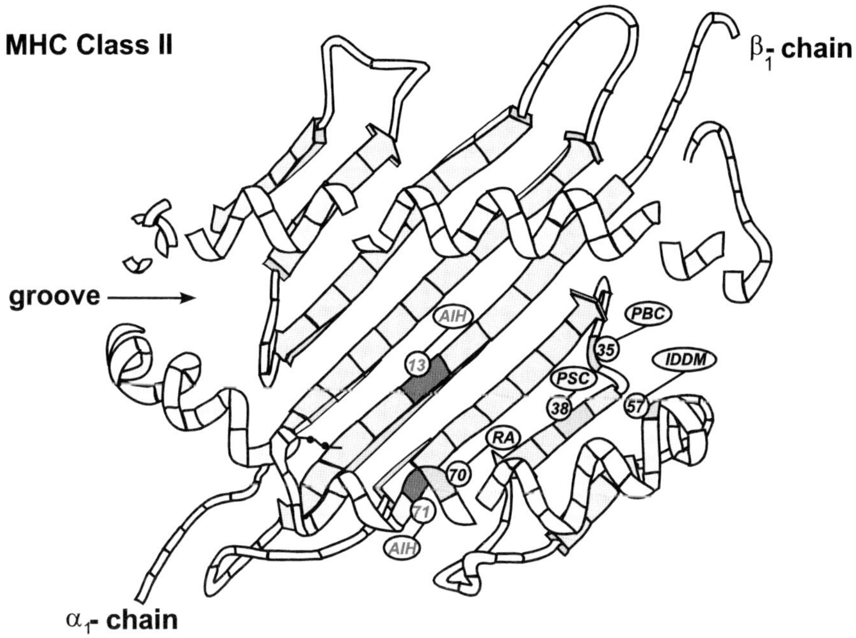

Fig. 1. Structure of the MHC complex and positions of amino acids that correlate with an increased risk for autoimmune hepatitis (AIH), primary biliary cirrhosis (PBC) and primary biliary cholangitis (PSC) [2].

null allotypes at the *C4A* or the *C4B* loci with AIH type 1 and that serum C4 levels are indeed lower in patients with C4A. Furthermore, *C4A* deletions are associated with increased mortality and a higher tendency to relapse during immunosuppressive treatment. Homozygosity for C4A deletion correlated with a much stronger increase in the relative risk for hepatitis (RR = 18.1) than did a single deletion (RR = 3.3). While the increased risk for AIH type 1 in patients with single gene deletion may be the result of a strong linkage disequilibrium with HLA B3*0101, the strong increase in risk in homozygous patients suggests an additional role for C4 in disease susceptibility [19].

Since immune responses are regulated by multiple cytokines, polymorphisms in the induction of cytokine responses might exert profound effects on autoimmune responses. Tumor necrosis factor α (TNFα) has diverse effects on immune responses and inflammatory cells [20,21]. In some contexts, TNFα promotes self-tolerance and T cell deletion, whereas, in others, TNFα promotes T cell activation and autoimmune diseases [22]. Interestingly, a polymorphism in the promoter region of TNFα, a -380A allele, was associated with the risk of developing AIH and with an unfavorable clinical course. This polymorphism results in an increased transcription of TNFα. However, TNFα exhibits a strong linkage disequilibrium with the HLA A1-B8-DR3 haplotype and stratification analysis indicates that the association with the TNF*2 promoter polymorphism is interdependent with DRB1*0301 [23,24].

Cell surface proteins of the B7 family, displayed on antigen-presenting cells, deliver immunogenic costimuli to T cells by signaling through CD28 and inducible costimulator

(ICOS) receptors [25–27]. The B7 proteins are induced on antigen presenting cells by other immunogenic stimuli such as necrotic cells and antigen receptor signals in B cells. In other contexts, B7/CD28 costimuli are tolerogenic, notably in immature thymocytes where they enhance clonal deletion and in regulatory $CD4^+/CD25^+$ T cells, where they might be required for peripheral tolerance [28]. B7 proteins also transmit tolerogenic signals to T cells by engaging another receptor, cytotoxic T lymphocyte antigen 4 (CTLA-4), that is present at very low levels in resting T cells and increased by chronic antigen signals [29]. CTLA-4 is therefore believed to play an important role in the maintenance of peripheral tolerance by modulation of T cell immune responses. Agarwal et al. investigated the role of CTLA-4 polymorphisms in AIH and were able to associate an A to G substitution at position 49 with an increased susceptibility for AIH. However, the relevance of this finding remains unclear, since this substitution results in a Ser to Ala substitution in the leader sequence of this protein, which theoretically should have little effect on posttranslational processing or protein localization. This Thr/Ala polymorphism is also in strong linkage with a downstream $(AT)_n$ repeat, which may affect RNA stability [30].

Recent data have indicated immunomodulatory capabilities of 1,25-dihydroxy-vitamin D_3. A role of vitamin D in autoimmune disease has also been suggested by in vivo experiments. It has been demonstrated that 1,25-dihydroxyvitamin D_3 administration is capable of preventing the development of autoimmune diseases in animal models of multiple sclerosis and diabetes mellitus [31,32]. 1,25-Dihydroxyvitamin D_3 exerts its biological effects through the vitamin D receptors (VDR), which are intracellular polypeptides. There are several polymorphisms within the VDR gene, which were first identified to be associated with bone turnover and bone density. However, analyses of autoimmune diseases have led to the discovery of an association with different autoimmune diseases. Vogel et al. demonstrated that polymorphisms in the vitamin D receptor gene are not only associated with primary biliary cirrhosis, but also with autoimmune hepatitis [33]. However, further studies are needed to elucidate the mechanisms by which the vitamin D receptor contributes to the development of human autoimmune diseases.

2. AUTOIMMUNE HEPATITIS IN APECED

Autoimmune polyendocrinopathy-candidiasis-ectodermal dystrophy (APECED) is a rare autosomal recessive disorder, which is characterized by an immune-mediated destruction of endocrine tissues, chronic candidiasis and additional ectodermal disorders [34,35]. Typically, the disease presentation includes candidiasis, hypoparathroidism and adrenocortical failure. The spectrum of associated clinical disease components includes insulin-dependent diabetes mellitus, autoimmune thyroid disease, pernicious anemia and chronic active hepatitis. In contrast to many other autoimmune diseases, APECED is associated with mutations of a single gene, designated autoimmune regulator (*AIRE*) [36]. The *AIRE* gene has been mapped to chromosome 21q22.3, spans approximately 13 kb and consists of 14 exons, which encode a predicted protein of 545 amino acids. The AIRE protein has several domains indicative of a transcriptional regulator protein, which has recently been demonstrated by Pitkänen et al. [37,38]. Sequence comparisons

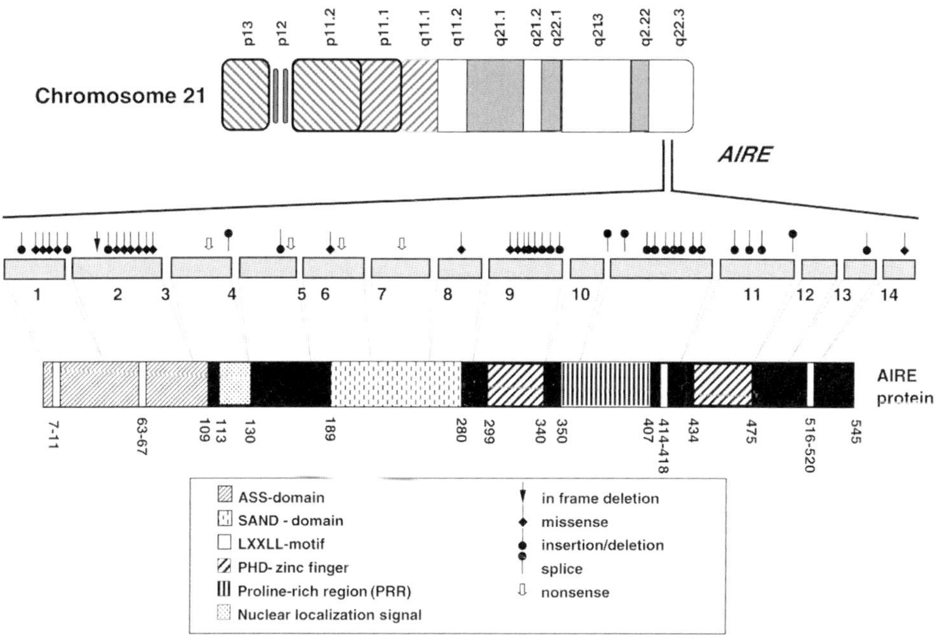

Fig. 2. Schematic presentation of the *AIRE* gene locus on chromosome 21 and the position of known mutations on different exons and on the AIRE protein [40].

have identified two PHD-zinc fingers, LXXLL motifs, and a Sand domain [36]. *AIRE* is not expressed in the target tissues of autoimmune destruction in APECED. However, expression has been shown in medullary epithelial cells and in monocyte-derived cells of the thymus, and in cells of lymph nodes, the spleen and in fetal liver [39]. This expression pattern and the predicted protein function may indicate that AIRE is capable of playing a role in the induction and maintenance of immune tolerance. So far, 45 different mutations of the *AIRE* gene have been identified and are distributed throughout the entire coding region (Fig. 2) [36,44,60–66]. Several of the *AIRE* mutations predict the transcription and translation of a truncated protein, which may be non-functional [41]. However, a conclusive correlation between *AIRE* mutations and the clinical APECED presentation has not yet been elucidated [42–44].

The variety of autoimmune diseases seen in APECED patients suggests that *AIRE* may contribute to the etiology of other autoimmune disorders. However, recent findings have indicated that common mutations in the *AIRE* gene do not play a mayor role in sporadic autoimmune diseases, such as autoimmune thyroid disease, diabetes mellitus type 1, Addison's disease and autoimmune liver diseases, and are therefore a unique feature of APECED [45–48]. In spite of these differences, the *AIRE* gene defect will help to identify biochemical and immunological pathways important in the establishment and maintenance of tolerance. Most likely along these pathways further gene defects and polymorphisms will be found, which play an etiological role in the development of organ-specific autoimmune diseases.

3. AUTOIMMUNITY AND VIRUSES

Historically, infectious agents have often been cited as triggers of autoimmune diseases. However, in most cases, there is still no firm evidence that a particular infectious agent is associated with the onset of disease. The difficult distinction is whether pathological immunity is truly directed against self and not against infectious non-self. To understand how infectious agents might induce autoimmunity, it has to be considered that all individuals harbor potentially autoreactive cells and that these cells remain harmless until they are somehow activated. Potential mechanisms linking infections to autoimmune diseases fall into two categories: direct effects, i.e. molecular mimicry and indirect effects, i.e. bystander activation and superantigen-mediated activation of autoreactive T cells and B cells.

3.1. Molecular mimicry

Molecular mimicry is one of the favored, yet still controversial theories by which infectious agents may activate these cells against self-antigens. During the last two decades, hundreds of articles focused on epitope mimicry and provided many arguments supporting this hypothesis but failed to prove it so far. According to the hypothesis, a susceptible individual acquires an infection with an agent that has antigens that are immunologically similar to the host antigens but can induce an immune response when presented to T cells. As a result, the immune response that is generated cross reacts with host tissues leading to tissue destruction. These cross-reacting immune responses can either be on the humeral (antibody) or T cell mediated level or both. Several criteria should be fulfilled to establish evidence that molecular mimicry is involved in the pathogenesis of autoimmune diseases [49]: (1) There has to be an association between the infection and the autoimmune disease, which has to persist in the absence of the initiating microbe. (2) The cross-reacting epitopes should be identified and the corresponding immunological cells such as antigen-presenting cells and effector cells like T cells has to be determined during the infection and the autoimmune diseases. (3) It should be demonstrated that both the critical epiptopes and the corresponding T cells are required and necessary to provoke the autoimmune disease.

3.2. Bystander activation

In several animal models of autoimmune diseases, molecular mimicry was supposed to initiate the autoimmune injury; however, critical re-evaluation revealed that rather another mechanism was involved grouped under the term bystander activation. In the process of an infection, tissue damage and necrosis may uncover cryptic autoantigens and formerly quiescent autoreactive T cells and B cells may become activated due to a local production of cytokines [50]. Additionally, in the course of an infection, antigen-presenting cells might be induced to up-regulate MHC molecules and appropriate costimulatory molecules, which subsequently enable the activation autoreactive cells.

3.3. Superantigens

Superantigens are peptides, which are produced by many different pathogens including bacteria, mycoplasmas and viruses. They are not MHC restricted and activate T cells by laterally binding to the outer surface of class II MHC molecules on antigen presenting cells and the relatively non-polymorphic variable Vβ chain of the T cell receptor, without being processed previously. In the presence of inflammatory cytokines, these reactions may overshoot a critical threshold and activate autoreactive T cells and B cells. In humans, oligoclonal TCR Vβ expression has been detected in lesions of multiple sclerosis, rheumatic arthritis and diabetes mellitus and the expression of a superantigen has been suggested in these tissues [51]. Another mechanism by which virus could influence superantigen-mediated autoimmune disease was proposed by Mitchell et al. Normal T cell activated by superantigens in uninfected mice died as a result of their activation, whereas T cells that were activated during a viral infection survived longer in vivo and in culture [52]. This bystander effect may contribute to the ability of viral infection and superantigens to induce autoimmunity.

3.4. Autoimmune hepatitis and viruses

Various viruses have long been assumed to be causative agents of autoimmune hepatitis. However, for most viruses, no conclusive concept has been demonstrated. Some reports have suggested that measles or Epstein–Barr virus infection could trigger the autoimmune process; others have implicated hepatitis viruses as initiators of the disease [53–58]. In one instance, molecular mimicry was assumed. It was shown that the B cell epitope of cytochrome P450, which is targeted by LKM-1 autoantibodies in AIH-2, displays homology with the immediate early antigen IE 175 of herpes simplex virus. One case has been reported, in which the only differences in HLA identical twins with discordant manifestation of AIH was exposure to HSV [6,59].

4. AUTOIMMUNE HEPATITIS AND DRUGS

AIH-2 is characterized by anti-liver/kidney microsomal (anti-LKM) autoantibodies, which are directed against CYP2D6, an enzyme, which metabolizes more than 40 different drugs. In about 10% of AIH patients, in addition, autoantibodies directed against enzymes of phase 2 of drug metabolism, namely UDP-glucuronosyltransferases, are found [7]. Similar autoantibodies are also autoantigens in drug-induced hepatitis. The LKM-2 autoantibody, directed CYP2C9 is detected in ticrynafen-induced hepatitis. The liver microsomal (LM) autoantibody, directed against CYP1A2 is found in patients with dihydralazine hepatitis.

Drug-induced hepatitis is a rare event of severe, often life-threatening hepatitis after prolonged treatment with a drug. Common to most patients is the metabolism of the drug by CYPs, enzymes of the phase 1 of drug detoxification (Fig. 3). A reactive metabolite is formed during the hydroxylation reaction, which may either bind to the active center of the CYP or which may leave the active center and covalently modify other hepatic proteins. Up to this point, processes seem to be similar in all patients

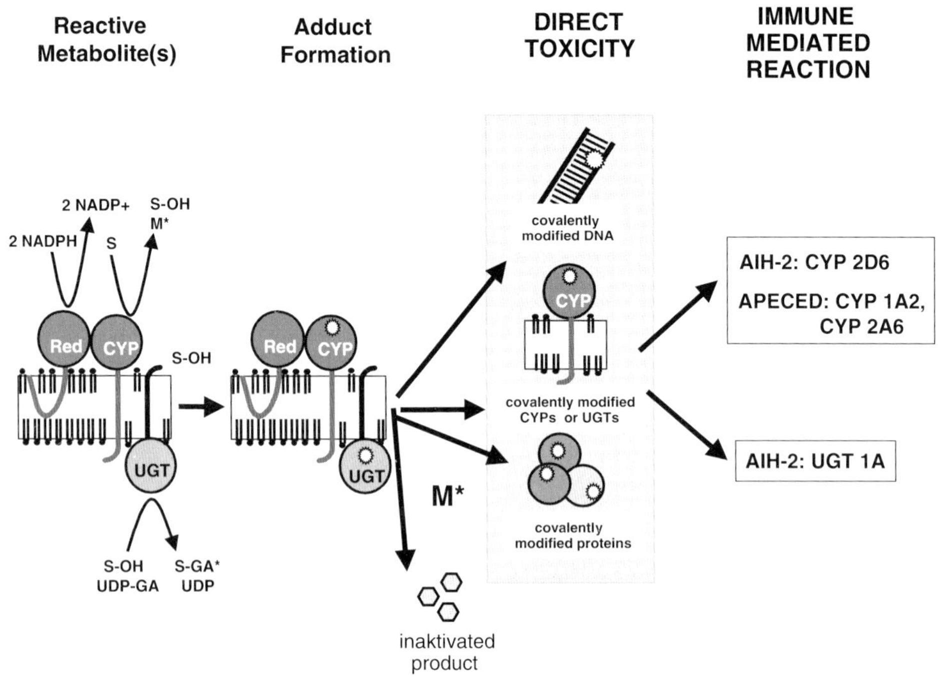

Fig. 3. The role of UDP-glucuronosyltransferases and cytochrome P450s (CYPs) in detoxification and adduct formation [67].

treated. However, in a few susceptible patients, drug adducts formed during these processes will be recognized by the immune system as non-self. If this immune reaction is not suppressed, it may lead to immune attacks directed against all cells, which harbor these modified proteins. This immune reaction may also be directed against native and modified hepatic proteins. Since the induction of an immune reaction is the critical event in drug-induced hepatitis, the severity and onset of disease are essentially independent of drug dosage. Time is necessary for the induction of the specific immune response; therefore, a significant latency period is observed, which may vary from a few weeks to several months. After withdrawal of drug modified proteins, the targets of the immune response and with them hepatitis decline. The disease recurs upon re-challenge with the drug, usually after a shorter latency period and hepatitis tends to be more severe upon re-exposure. Females tend to be more frequently affected by drug-induced hepatitis than men.

CONCLUSIONS

Currently, the etiology of AIH remains poorly understood. Clearly patients with AIH and their families share a genetic background, which favors the development of autoimmune diseases in general and several genes are believed to contribute to their genetic predisposition. With AIRE a model gene for the induction of autoimmune diseases has been identified, which will help to identify mechanisms active in the induction and maintenance of tolerance. However a disconcerting fact about genetic predisposition to AIH is the lack of concordance in identical twin pairs suggesting that other initiating events, such as the response to an environmental pathogen, are necessary for autoimmune disease manifestation. Triggers, which may favor the development of AIH, include infections with viruses or immune-mediated idiosyncratic reactions against drugs.

REFERENCES

[1] Manns MP, Strassburg CP. Autoimmune hepatitis: clinical challenges. Gastroenterology 2001; 120(6): 1502–1517.
[2] Manns MP, Krüger M. Genetics in liver diseases. Gastroenterology 1994; 106(106): 1676–1697.
[3] Gregorio GV, Portman B, Reid F, Donaldson PT, Doherty DG, McCartney M et al. Autoimmune hepatitis in childhood: a 20-year experience. Hepatology 1997; 25: 541–547.
[4] Alvarez F, Berg PA, Bianchi FB, Bianchi L, Burroughs AK, Cancado EL et al. International Autoimmune Hepatitis Group Report: review of criteria for diagnosis of autoimmune hepatitis. J Hepatology 1999; 31: 929–938.
[5] Strassburg CP, Obermayer-Straub P, Manns MP. Autoimmunity in liver diseases. Clin Rev Allergy Immunol 2000; 18(2): 127–139.
[6] Manns MP, Griffin KJ, Sullivan KF, Johnson EF. LKM-1 autoantibodies recognize a short linear sequence in P450IID6, a cytochrome P-450 monooxygenase. J Clin Invest 1991; 88: 1370–1378.
[7] Strassburg C, Obermayer-Straub P, Alex B, Durazzo M, Rizzetto M, Tukey RH et al. Autoantibodies against glucuronosyltransferases differ between viral hepatitis and autoimmune hepatitis. Gastroenterology 1996; 11: 1582–1592.
[8] Manns M, Gerken G, Kyriatsoulis A, Staritz M, Meyer zum Büschenfelde KH. Characterization of a new subgroup of autoimmune chronic active hepatitis by autoantibodies against a soluble liver antigen. Lancet 1987; I: 292–294.
[9] Wies I, Brunner S, Henninger J, Herkel J, Kanzler S, Meyer zum Buschenfelde KH et al. Identification of target antigen for SLA/LP autoantibodies in autoimmune hepatitis [see comments]. Lancet 2000; 355(9214): 1510–1515.
[10] Strettell MD, Thomson LJ, Donaldson PT, Bunce M, O'Neill CM, Williams RW. HLA-C genes and susceptibility to type 1 autoimmune hepatitis. Hepatology 1997; 26: 1023–1026.
[11] Strettel MDJ, Donaldson PT, Thomson LJ, Santrach PJ, Brenndan Moore S, Czaja AJ et al. Allelic basis for HLA-encoded susceptibility to type 1 autoimmune hepatitis. Gastroenterology 1997; 112: 2028–2035.
[12] Czaja AJ, Strettell M, Thomson LJ, Santrach P, Moore SB, Donaldson PT et al. Associations between alleles of the major histocompatibility complex and type 1 autoimmune hepatitis. Hepatology 1997; 25: 317–323.
[13] Donaldson P, Doherty D, Underhill J, Williams R. The molecular genetics of autoimmune liver disease. Hepatology 1994; 20: 225–229.
[14] Seki T, Ota M, Furuta S, Fukushima H, Kondo T, Hino K et al. HLA class II molecules and autoimmune hepatitis susceptibility in Japanese patients. Gastroenterology 1992; 103: 1041–1047.

[15] Marcos Y, Fainboim HA, Capucchio M, Findor J, Daruich J, Reyes B et al. Two-locus involvement in the association of human leukocyte antigen with the extrahepatic manifestations of autoimmune chronic active hepatitis. Hepatology 1994; 19(6): 1371–1374.

[16] Vazquez-Garcia MN, Alaez C, Olivo A, Debaz H, Perez-Luque E, Burguete A et al. MHC class II sequences of susceptibility and protection in Mexicans with autoimmune hepatitis. J Hepatol 1998; 28: 985–990.

[17] Fearon DT, Carroll MC. Regulation of B lymphocyte responses to foreign and self-antigens by the CD19/CD21 complex. Annu Rev Immunol 2000; 18: 393–422.

[18] Pickering MC, Walport MJ. Links between complement abnormalities and systemic lupus erythematosus. Rheumatology (Oxford) 2000; 39(2): 133–141.

[19] Scully LJ, Toze C, Sengar DPS, Goldstein R. Early-onset autoimmune hepatitis is associated with a C4A gene deletion. Gastroenterology 1993; 104: 1478–1484.

[20] Green EA, Flavell RA. Tumor necrosis factor-alpha and the progression of diabetes in non-obese diabetic mice. Immunol Rev 1999; 169: 11–22.

[21] Cope AP. Regulation of autoimmunity by proinflammatory cytokines. Curr Opin Immunol 1998; 10(6): 669–676.

[22] Brennan FM, Maini RN, Feldmann M. Role of pro-inflammatory cytokines in rheumatoid arthritis. Springer Semin Immunopathol 1998; 20(1-2): 133–147.

[23] Czaja AJ, Cookson S, Constantini PK, Clare M, Underhill JA, Donaldson PT. Cytokine polymorphisms associated with clinical features and treatment outcome in type 1 autoimmune hepatitis. Gastroenterology 1999; 117: 645–652.

[24] Cookson S, Constantini PK, Clare M, Underhill JA, Bernal W, Czaja AJ et al. Frequency and nature of cytokine gene polymorphisms in type 1 autoimmune hepatitis. Hepatology 1999; 30: 851–856.

[25] June CH, Bluestone JA, Nadler LM, Thompson CB. The B7 and CD28 receptor families. Immunol Today 1994; 15(7): 321–331.

[26] Mueller DL. T cells: A proliferation of costimulatory molecules. Curr Biol 2000; 10(6): R227–R230.

[27] Salomon B, Bluestone JA. Complexities of CD28/B7: CTLA-4 costimulatory pathways in autoimmunity and transplantation. Annu Rev Immunol 2001; 19: 225–252.

[28] Salomon B, Lenschow DJ, Rhee L, Ashourian N, Singh B, Sharpe A et al. B7/CD28 costimulation is essential for the homeostasis of the $CD4^+CD25^+$ immunoregulatory T cells that control autoimmune diabetes. Immunity 2000; 12(4): 431–440.

[29] Chambers CA, Allison JP. Costimulatory regulation of T cell function. Curr Opin Cell Biol 1999; 11(2): 203–210.

[30] Agarwal K, Czaja AJ, Jones DE, Donaldson PT. Cytotoxic T lymphocyte antigen-4 (CTLA-4) gene polymorphisms and susceptibility to type 1 autoimmune hepatitis. Hepatology 2000; 31(1): 49–53.

[31] Cantorna MT, Hayes CE, DeLuca HF. 1,25-Dihydroxyvitamin D3 reversibly blocks the progression of relapsing encephalomyelitis, a model of multiple sclerosis. Proc Natl Acad Sci USA 1996; 93(15): 7861–7864.

[32] Mathieu C, Waer M, Laureys J, Rutgeerts O, Bouillon R. Prevention of autoimmune diabetes in NOD mice by 1,25 dihydroxyvitamin D3. Diabetologia 1994; 37(6): 552–558.

[33] Vogel A, Strassburg CP, Manns MP. Genetic association of vitamin D receptor polymorphisms with primary biliary cirrhosis and autoimmune hepatitis. Hepatology 2002; (in press)

[34] Ahonen P, Myllärniemi S, Sipilä I, Perheentupa J. Clinical variation of autoimmune polyendocrinopathy-candidiasis-ectodermal dystrophy (APECED) in a series of 68 patients. New Engl J Med 1990; 322(26): 1829–1836.

[35] Betterle C, Greggio NA, Volpato M. Clinical review 93: Autoimmune polyglandular syndrome type 1. J Clin Endocrinol Metab 1998; 83(4): 1049–1055.
[36] Nagamine K, Peterson P, Scott HS, Kudoh J, Minoshima S, Heino M et al. Positional cloning of the APECED gene. Nat Genet 1997; 17: 393–398.
[37] Pitkänen J, Doucas V, Sternsdorf T, Nakajima T, Aratani S, Jensen K et al. The autoimmune regulator protein has transcriptional transactivating properties and interacts with the common coactivator CREB-binding protein. J Biol Chem 2000; 275(22): 16802–16809.
[38] Pitkänen J, Vahamurto P, Krohn K, Peterson P. Subcellular localization of the autoimmune regulator protein. characterization of nuclear targeting and transcriptional activation domain. J Biol Chem 2001; 276(22): 19597–19602.
[39] Heino M, Peterson P, Kudoh J, Nagamine K, Lagerstedt A, Ovod V et al. Autoimmune regulator is expressed in the cells regulating immune tolerance in thymus medulla. Biochem Biophys Res Commun 1999; 257: 821–825.
[40] Vogel A, Strassburg C, Obermayer-Straub P, Brabant G, Manns M. The Genetic Background of Autoimmune Polyendocrinopathy-candidiasis-ectodermal dystrophy and its Autoimmune disease components. J Mol Med 2002; (in press).
[41] Bjorses P, Halonen M, Palvimo JJ, Kolmer M, Aaltonen J, Ellonen P et al. Mutations in the AIRE gene: effects on subcellular location and transactivation function of the autoimmune polyendocrinopathy-candidiasis-ectodermal dystrophy protein. Am J Hum Genet 2000; 66(2): 378–392.
[42] Aaltonen J, Bjorses P. Cloning of the APECED gene provides new insight into human autoimmunity. Ann Med 1999; 31(2): 111–116.
[43] Heino M, Peterson P, Sillanpaa N, Guerin S, Wu L, Anderson G et al. RNA and protein expression of the murine autoimmune regulator gene (Aire) in normal, RelB-deficient and in NOD mouse. Eur J Immunol 2000; 30(7): 1884–1893.
[44] Wang CY, Davoodi-Semiromi A, Huang W, Connor E, Shi JD, She JX. Characterization of mutations in patients with autoimmune polyglandular syndrome type 1 (APS1). Hum Genet 1998; 103(6): 681–685.
[45] Vogel A, Liermann H, Harms A, Strassburg CP, Manns MP, Obermayer-Straub P. Autoimmune regulator AIRE: Evidence for genetic differences between autoimmune hepatitis and hepatitis as part of the autoimmune polyglandular syndrome type 1. Hepatology 2001; 33(5): 1047–1052.
[46] Vaidya B, Imrie H, Geatch DR, Perros P, Ball SG, Baylis PH et al. Association analysis of the cytotoxic T lymphocyte antigen-4 (CTLA-4) and autoimmune regulator-1 (AIRE-1) genes in sporadic autoimmune Addison's disease. J Clin Endocrinol Metab 2000; 85(2): 688–691.
[47] Nithiyananthan R, Heward JM, Allahabadia A, Barnett AH, Franklyn JA, Gough SC. A heterozygous deletion of the autoimmune regulator (AIRE1) gene, autoimmune thyroid disease, and type 1 diabetes: no evidence for association. J Clin Endocrinol Metab 2000; 85(3): 1320–1322.
[48] Meyer G, Donner H, Herwig J, Bohles H, Usadel KH, Badenhoop K. Screening for an AIRE-1 mutation in patients with Addison's disease, type 1 diabetes, Graves' disease and Hashimoto's thyroiditis as well as in APECED syndrome. Clin Endocrinol (Oxf) 2001; 54(3): 335–338.
[49] Benoist C, Mathis D. Autoimmunity provoked by infection: how good is the case for T cell epitope mimicry? Nat Immunol 2001; 2(9): 797–801.
[50] Behar SM, Porcelli SA. Mechanisms of autoimmune disease induction. The role of the immune response to microbial pathogens. Arthritis Rheum 1995; 38(4): 458–476.
[51] Gold DP. TCR V gene usage in autoimmunity. Curr Opin Immunol 1994; 6(6): 907–912.

[52] Mitchell T, Kappler J, Marrack P. Bystander virus infection prolongs activated T cell survival. J Immunol 1999; 162(8): 4527–4535.

[53] Robertson DA, Zhang SL, Guy EC, Wright R. Persistent measles virus genome in autoimmune chronic active hepatitis. Lancet 1987; 2(8549): 9–11.

[54] Vento S, Guella L, Mirandola F, Cainelli F, Di Perri G, Solbiati M et al. Epstein–Barr virus as a trigger for autoimmune hepatitis in susceptible individuals. Lancet 1995; 346(8975): 608–609.

[55] Vento S, Cainelli F, Renzini C, Concia E. Autoimmune hepatitis type 2 induced by HCV and persisting after viral clearance. Lancet 1997; 350(9087): 1298–1299.

[56] Vento S, Garofano T, Di Perri G, Dolci L, Concia E, Bassetti D. Identification of hepatitis A virus as a trigger for autoimmune chronic hepatitis type 1 in susceptible individuals. Lancet 1991; 337(8751): 1183–1187.

[57] Rahaman SM, Chira P, Koff RS. Idiopathic autoimmune chronic hepatitis triggered by hepatitis A. Am J Gastroenterol 1994; 89(1): 106–108.

[58] Cianciara J, Laskus T. Development of transient autoimmune hepatitis during interferon treatment of chronic hepatitis B. Dig Dis Sci 1995; 40(8): 1842–1844.

[59] Manns MP, Jentzsch M, Mergener K, Gerken G, Thiers V, Brechot C et al. Discordant manifestation of LKM-1 antibody positive autoimmune hepatitis in identical twins. Hepatology 1990; 12: 840.

[60] An autoimmune disease, APECED, caused by mutations in a novel gene featuring two PHD-type zinc-finger domains. The Finnish–German APECED Consortium. Autoimmune Polyendocrinopathy-Candidiasis-Ectodermal Dystrophy. Nat Genet 1997; 17(4): 399–403.

[61] Björses P, Halonen M, Palvimo JJ, Kolmer M, Aaltonen J, Ellonen P et al. Mutations in the AIRE gene: effects on subcellular location and transactivation function of the autoimmune polyendocrinopathy-candidiasis-ectodermal dystrophy protein. Am J Hum Genet 2000; 66: 378–392.

[62] Heino M, Scott HS, Chen Q, Peterson P, Maebppaa U, Papasavvas MP et al. Mutation analyses of North American APS-1 patients. Hum Mutat 1999; 13: 69–74.

[63] Pearce SHS, Cheetman T, Imrie H, Vaidya B, Barnes ND, Bilous RW et al. A common and recurrent 13-bp deletion in the autoimmune regulator gene in British kindreds with autoimmune polyendocrinopathy type 1. Am J Hum Genet 1998; 63: 1675–1684.

[64] Rosatelli MC, Meloni A, Meloni A, Devoto M, Cao A, Scott HS et al. A common mutation in Sardinian autoimmune polyendocrinopathy-candidiasis-ectodermal dystrophy patients. Hum Genet 1998; 103: 428–434.

[65] Scott HS, Heino M, Peterson P, Mittaz L, Laliotti MD, Betterle C et al. Common mutations in autoimmune polyendocrinopathy-candidiasis-ectodermal dystrophy patients of different origins. Mol Endocrinol 1998; 12: 1112–1119.

[66] Cihakova D, Trebusak K, Heino M, Fadeyev V, Tiulpakov A, Battelino T et al. Novel AIRE mutations and P450 cytochrome autoantibodies in Central and Eastern European patients with APECED. Hum Mutat 2001; 18(3): 225–232.

[67] Manns MP, Obermayer-Straub P. Cytochromes P450 and UDP-glucuronosyltransferases: model autoantigens to study drug-induced, virus-induced and autoimmune liver disease. Hepatology 1997; 26: 1054–1066.

Molecular Biology and Immunology in Hepatology
Edited by T. Tsuji, T. Higashi, M. Zeniya and K.-H. Meyer zum Büschenfelde

CHAPTER 16

Roles of Hepatitis C Virus Infection in Autoimmune Hepatitis

Hiroshi Miyakawa

Fourth Department of Internal Medicine, Teikyo University School of Medicine, Kanagawa, Japan

INTRODUCTION

Since the discovery of hepatitis C virus (HCV) [1], the most major causative agent of chronic hepatitis, issues regarding the pathogenesis and treatment of autoimmune hepatitis (AIH) have brought up. There is mounting evidence that HCV triggers and perhaps causes a multitude of autoimmune phenomena such as cryoglobulinemia [2], glomeluronephritis [3], Sjögren syndrome [4], and Hashimoto's disease [5]. Moreover, high prevalence of serological markers of autoimmunity in HCV infected patients have been reported [6,7]. Does HCV infection trigger the onset of AIH? In this review, new developments regarding these issues are described including findings obtained from our laboratory.

1. ANTI-GOR IN HCV INFECTION

The initial finding linking HCV infections with autoimmune disorders was the discovery of anti-GOR autoantibody in sera from patients with chronic hepatitis C (non-A, non-B) [8]. Anti-GOR is detected in 70% of sera from chronic hepatitis C patients. GOR is a nuclear antigen that appears to be expressed in the hepatic cell and has been implicated as a marker of HCV-induced autoimmunity. The autoantigen to anti-GOR have been identified to be the molecular motif: GRRGQKAKSNPNRPL. There exists a homological region in the HCV core protein which has been designated as CP10 [9]. Experimentally, GOR and anti-CP10 show cross-reactivity (see below).

2. POSSIBILITY OF HCV INFECTION AS THE TRIGGER OF AIH

There have been reports that certain types of hepatitis virus infections are able to trigger AIH. HAV and HBV are known to be such agents [10,11]. However, in HCV infections, an association with the onset of AIH has been rarely documented [12]. We have seen HCV-positive patients with AIH type I. These cases all had histories of blood transfusion. There have been other AIH patients with concurrent chronic HCV infections. Our experiences show that HCV RNA levels in these patients remain low in spite of receiving the usual dose of prednisolone for long periods. We have, however, seen a patient who developed HCV-induced post transfusion hepatitis following the appearance of anti-liver kidney microsome type 1 (anti-LKM-1) autoantibody. The patient's serum IgG levels gradually increased over a two-year period following the transfusion. Mackie et al. [13] have reported on the sequential appearance of IgM anti-LKM-1 followed by IgG anti-LKM-1 in a patient who developed HCV infection following orthotropic liver transplantation.

3. HCV-ASSOCIATED AUTOIMMUNITY: ANTI-LKM-1 IN HCV INFECTED PATIENTS

Anti-LKM-1, which is a hallmark of AIH type II [14], is also known to be present in a subset of chronic hepatitis C patients [15–18]. Earlier investigators divided such AIH type II patients into type IIa and IIb according to absence or presence of HCV infection [19]. Patients with AIH type IIa (without HCV infection) are usually young, serum aminoatransferase levels are high, and prednisolone is effective. However, it is now considered that the presence of anti-LKM-1 in chronic HCV infections is an epiphenomenon developing over the course of chronic HCV infection. We have emphasized that the so-called AIH type IIb should not be categorized as AIH, after analyzing the clinicopathological features of Japanese patients [20]. Predonisolone has been shown to be ineffective, and interferon (IFN) effective, for treatment of these patients. Such a case treated with IFN is shown in Fig. 1. Both HCV RNA and anti-LKM-1 disappeared following IFN therapy. Strassberg and Manns have designated this condition as HCV-associated autoimmunity [21].

4. ANTI-CYP2D6 AND HCV INFECTION

The major autoantigen to anti-LKM-1 has been identified as Cytochrome P450 IID6 (CYP2D6) [22–24]. CYP2D6 is one of the important phase I drug-metabolizing enzymes. This autoantibody is usually measured by immunofluorescence, ELISA, and immunoblotting. The prevalence of anti-LKM-1 (anti-CYP2D6) in chronic hepatitis C patients shows geographic heterogeneity. In Western countries, the following prevalences of anti-LKM-1 in HCV-infected patients have been reported: 0–3.0% in the USA, 2.1–3.7% in France, and 4.3–6.0% in Italy [25–27]. Anti-LKM-1 has been detected in 1–3% among chronic HCV-infected Japanese patients [20,28]. Our most recent analysis of chronic HCV-infected Japanese patients by ELISA using recombinant antigen is shown in Table 1.

There have been no reports on the appearance of anti-LKM-1 in non-HCV viral hepatitis patients. Thus, it may be considered that the relationship of anti-LKM-1 and HCV infections is a model for studying the interaction of autoantibody specificities and viral protein structures.

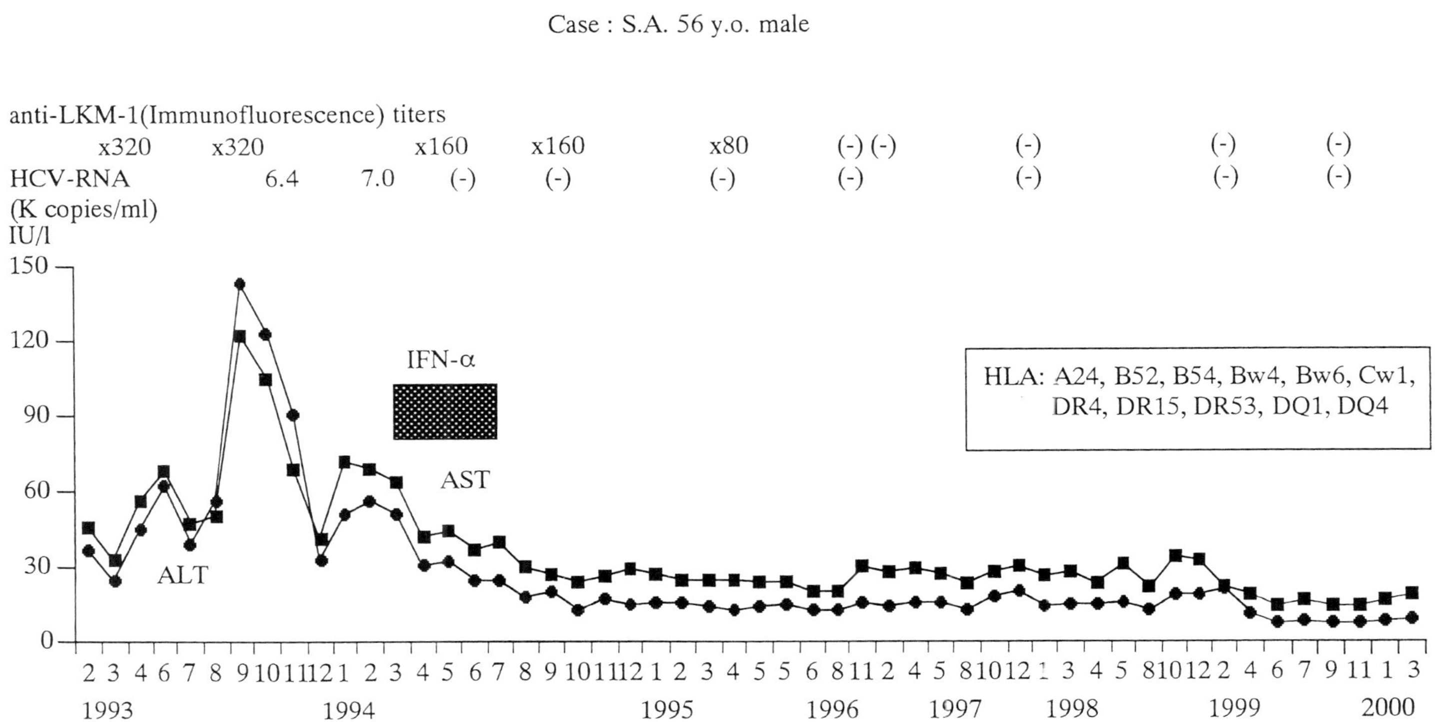

Fig. 1. Clinical course of an anti-LKM-1-positive chronic hepatitis C patient treated with IFN. Following IFN therapy, HCV RNA and then anti-LKM-1 disappeared in succession.

TABLE 1

Frequency of anti-LKM-1 (anti-CYP2D6) in adult patients with chronic HCV infection: a multicenter study conducted in Japan

	CH-C	LC-C
Teikyo University	3/100 (3.0%)	3/114 (2.6%)
Nagoya City University	3/203 (1.5%)	0/198 (0%)
Nagoya University	1/103 (1.0%)	
Niigata University	2/197 (3.0%)	0/74 (0%)
Kurume University	3/96 (3.0%)	3/97 (3.0%)
	12/699 (1.7%)	6/483 (1.2%)
Total	18/1182 (1.5%)	

CH-C = chronic hepatitis type C, LC-C = liver cirrhosis type C.

5. CROSS-REACTIVITY BASED ON MOLECULAR HOMOLOGY

One possible mechanism for such interactions is that cross-reactivity occurs based on molecular homology between the particular autoantigen and virus. Indeed, there are homological regions between the CYP2D6 molecule, which is the major autoantigen to anti-LKM-1, and HCV polyproteins [29]. We hypothesize that anti-LKM-1 appears as a result of cross-reactivity based on such molecular homologies. Several linear peptides spanning these homological regions were synthesized, and dose-dependence tests using an anti-GOR positive serum were performed by ELISA. However, as shown in Fig. 2, cross-reactivities could not be observed against the CYP2D6-derived peptides [30]. In contrast, reactivities were confirmed against the HCV-derived peptides. These results seem to indicate that the appearance of anti-GOR and anti-LKM-1 in HCV infections are due to separate mechanisms of antibody production. This interpretation is supported by the different frequencies of anti-GOR and anti-LKM-1 occurring in HCV infected patients.

6. *CYP2D6* GENETIC POLYMORPHISMS AND THE PRODUCTION OF ANTI-LKM-1

It is an established fact that *CYP2D6* genes exhibit genetic polymorphisms. At least, 21 polymorphisms have thus far been reported [31]. Many of these are associated with specific phenotypes. *CYP2D6*1* is associated with the extensive metabolizer phenotype, *CYP2D6*2*, **9*, and **10* with the intermediated metabolizer, *CYP2D6*3* with the poor metabolizer, and *CYP2D6*5* with the non-responder [32]. There exist ethnic variations in the frequencies of selected genotypes [33]. For example, 7% of Caucasians are of the non-responder genotype. Recently, we compared the frequencies of various *CYP2D6* genetic polymorphisms between anti-LKM-1-positive and -negative Japanese chronic hepatitis C patient. As shown in Table 2, there was a significant predominance of the *CYP2D6*1* genotype in anti-LKM-1-positive patients [34]. Although it is not clear why the extensive metabolizer-CYP2D6 genotype is associated with the presence of

TABLE 2

Analysis of *CYP2D6* allelic combination in patients with chronic hepatitis C

Allelic combination	(1) Anti-LKM-1-positive chronic hepatitis C ($n = 10$)		(2) Anti-LKM-1-negative chronic hepatitis C ($n = 36$)		(3) General Japanese population [a] ($n = 98$)		P [(1) vs (2)] (χ^2 test)
	No	Frequency (%)	No	Frequency (%)	No	Frequency (%)	
*1/*1	7	70	7	19	18	18	0.0021*
*1/*10	1	10	14	39	33	34	0.0847
*10/*10	0	–	5	14	17	17	0.2119
*1/*2	1	10	2	6	7	7	0.6146
*2/*5	1	10	0	–	2	2	0.5507
Others	0	–	8	23	21	22	

[a] Tateishi T et al. Clin Pharmacol Ther 1999; 65: 570–575.

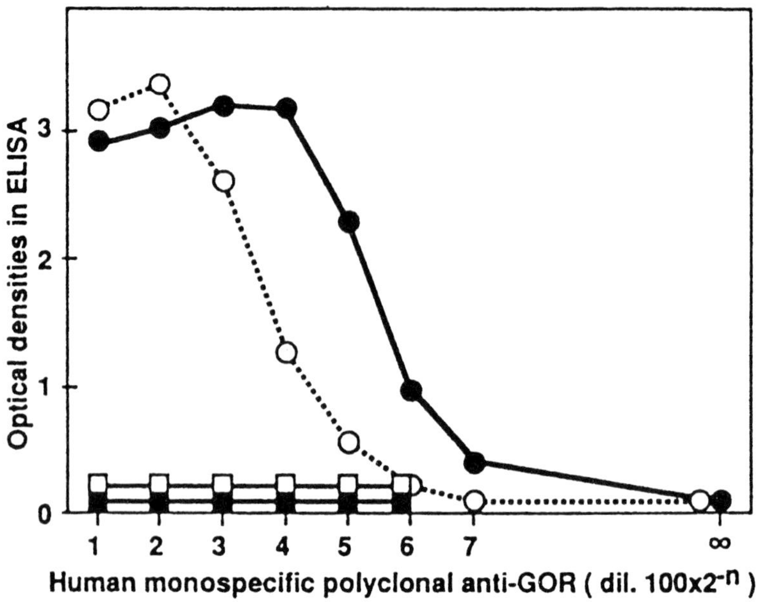

Fig. 2. Anti-GOR cross-reacts with HCV-derived synthetic peptides but not with CYP2D6-derived peptides. Titers of CP-10 were reduced by incubations with anti-GOR, but no changes were observed in reactivity of both CYP2D6-derived peptides (p450-uni and p450-gor) by incubations with anti-GOR. Closed circles, sp-GOR-2; open circles, HCV core (CP-10); open squares, p450-uni; closed squares, p450 gor. (Ref. [30]).

anti-LKM-1 in HCV infected patients, one may argue that the antigenicity of CYP2D6 is enhanced in extensive metabolizers either by overexpression or by alterations in B cell epitopes. However, the expression of *CYP2D6* genes are known to be down-regulated by IFN (or IFN inducers), and HCV-infected individuals who are already genetically predisposed to produce less *CYP2D6* mRNA should not be able to present the CYP2D6 antigen to the immune system efficiently. Further studies are required to clarify such inconsistencies.

7. IMMUNOREACTIVITY WITH CYP PROTEINS OTHER THAN CYP2D6 IN HCV INFECTION

CYP proteins other than CYP2D6 may also play a role in AIH or other autoimmune disorders. Regarding this issue, there is a well-established review by Manns et al. [35]. To investigate this possibility in the Japanese population, we tested for serum immunoreactivity against recombinant CYP1A2, 2C9, 2E1, and 3A4 proteins in patients with various chronic liver diseases including chronic hepatitis C [36]. CYP1A2 reacted with one out of 35 patients with AIH type I sera, CYP2E1 reacted with two out of 35 AIH type I sera, and with three out of 31 anti-LKM-1-negative chronic hepatitis C sera, and CYP3A4 reacted with one out of nine patients with AIH type II sera and with one out of 24 anti-LKM-1-positive chronic hepatitis C sera. CYP2C9 did not react with any of the sera tested. In contrast, none of the sera from 15 patients with chronic hepatitis B reacted with these CYP proteins. From these results, it is suggested that CYPs other than CYP2D6 can function as immunotargets in certain disease conditions.

8. TREATMENT FOR AIH PATIENTS WITH HCV INFECTION

There have been numerous reports regarding treatment of AIH patients infected with HCV. Earlier reports revealed that IFN enhanced host autoimmunity. However, these responses were found to occur only in patients having latent autoimmunity in the form of organ or non-organ specific autoantibodies. We have also experienced a case of acute aggravation of serum aminotransferases during IFN treatment, where the patient presented with several anti-thyroid autoantibodies. Reactivation of latent Hashimoto's disease was occurred. Therefore, a thorough understanding of the patient's autoantibody profile should be attained before commencing IFN treatment.

Another issue for these patients is the aggravation of serum HCV RNA levels during prednisolone treatment. Thorough studies utilizing the sensitive HCV RNA assays are indicated to clarify this phenomenon.

CLOSING REMARKS

There are few lines of evidence showing that HCV infections trigger the onset of AIH. However, various autoimmune phenomena are frequently observed in HCV infected patients. These are felt to be unique to HCV infections. The specific therapeutic strategy should be established on a case-by-case basis taking into consideration of clinical features and laboratory data including HCV loads.

REFERENCES

[1] Choo Q-L, Kuo G, Weiner AJ, Overby LR, Bradley DW, Houghton M. Isolation of a cDNA clone derived from blood-borne non-A, non-B viral hepatitis genome. Science 1989; 224: 359–362.

[2] Agnello V, Chung RT, Kaplan L. A role for hepatitis C virus infection in type II cryoglobulinemia. N Engl J Med 1992; 19: 1490.

[3] Johnson RJ, Gretch DR, Yamabe H et al. Membrano-proliferative glomerulonephritis associated with hepatitis C virus infection. N Engl J Med 1993; 18: 465–470.

[4] Haddad J, Deny P, Munz-Gotheil C et al. Lymphocytic sialadenitis of Sjögren's syndrome associated with chronic hepatitis C virus liver disease. Lancet 1992; 339: 989–990.

[5] Pateron D, Hardmann DJ, Duclos-Vallee JC, Jouanolle H, Beaugrand M. Latent autoimmune thyroid disease in patients with chronic HCV hepatitis. J Hepatol 1992; 16: 244–245.

[6] Abuaf N, Lunel F, Giral P et al. Non-organ specific autoantibodies associated with chronic C virus hepatitis. J Hepatol 1993; 18: 359–364.

[7] Pawlotsky JM, Ben Yahia M, Andre C et al. Immunological disorders in C virus chronic active hepatitis: a prospective case-control study. Hepatology 1994; 19: 841–848.

[8] Mishiro S, Hoshi Y, Takeda K et al. Non-A, non-B hepatitis specific antibodiers directed at host-derived epitope: implication for an autoimmune process. Lancet 1990; 336: 1400–1403.

[9] Mishiro S, Takeda K, Hoshi Y, Yoshikawa A, Gotanda T, Itoh Y. An autoantibody cross-reactive to hepatitis virus core and a host nuclear antigen. Autoimmunity 1991; 10: 269–273.
[10] Rahaman SM, Chira P, Koff RS. Idiopathic autoimmune chronic hepatitis triggered by hepatitis A. Am J Gastroenterol 1994; 89: 106–108.
[11] Laskus T, Slusarczyk J. Autoimmune chronic active hepatitis developing after acute type B hepatitis. Dig Dis Sci 1989; 34: 1294–1297.
[12] McFarlane BM, Bridger C, Tibbs CJ et al. Virus-induced autoimmunity in hepatitis C virus infections: a rare event. J Med Virol 1994; 42: 66–72.
[13] Mackie FD, Peakman M, Yun M et al. Primary and secondary liver/kidney microsomal autoantibody response following infection with hepatitis C virus. Gastroenterology 1994; 106: 1672–1675.
[14] Homberg JC, Abunaf N, Bernard O et al. Chronic active hepatitis associated with anti liver/kidney microsome type 1: a second type of "autoimmune hepatitis". Hepatology 1987; 7: 1333–1339.
[15] Lenzi M, Ballardini G, Fusconi M et al. Type 2 autoimmune hepatitis and hepatitis C virus infection. Lancet 1990; 335: 258–259.
[16] Garson JA, Lenzi M, Ring C et al. Hepatitis C viraemia in adults with type 2 autoimmune hepatitis. J Med Virol 1991; 34: 223–226.
[17] Miyakawa H, Kako M, Nagai K et al. HCV-RNA in type 2 autoimmune hepatitis. Am J Gastroenterol 1991; 86: 1688–1689.
[18] Todros L, Touscoz G, D'Urso N et al. Hepatitis C virus-related chronic liver disease with autoantibodies to liver/kidney microsomes (LKM). Clinical characterization from idiopathic LKM-positive disorders. J Hepatol 1991; 13: 128–131.
[19] Michel G, Ritter A, Gerken G, Meyer zum Büschenfelde KH, Decker R, Manns MP. Anti-GOR and hepatitis C virus in autoimmune liver diseases. Lancet 1992; 339: 267–269.
[20] Miyakawa H, Kitazawa E, Abe K et al. Chronic hepatitis C associated with anti-liver/kidney microsome-1 antibody is not a subgroup autoimmune hepatitis. J Gastroenterol 1997; 32: 769–776.
[21] Strassberg CP, Manns MP. Autoimmune hepatitis versus viral hepatitis C. Liver 1995; 15: 225–232.
[22] Manns MP, Johnson EF, Griffin KJ, Tan EM, Sullivan KF. Major antigen of liver kidney microsomal antibodies in idiopathic autoimmune hepatitis is cytochrome P450db1. J Clin Invest 1989; 83: 1066–1072.
[23] Zanger UM, Hauri HP, Loeper J, Homberg JC, Meyer UA. Antibodies against human cytochrome P-450db1 in autoimmune hepatitis type 2. Proc Natl Acad Sci USA 1988; 85: 8256–8260.
[24] Gueguen M, Boniface O, Bernard O, Clerc F, Cartwright T, Alvarez F. Identification of the main epitope on human cytochrome P450IID6 recognized by anti-liver kidney microsome antibody. J Autoimmun 1991; 4: 607–615.
[25] Todros L, Saracco G, Durazzo M et al. Efficacy and safety of interferon Alfa therapy with hepatitis C with autoantibodies to liver-kidney microsomes. Hepatology 1995; 22: 1374–1378.
[26] Reddy KR, Krawitt EL, Homberg JC et al. Absence of anti-LKM antibody in hepatitis C viral infection in the United States of America. J Viral Hepat 1995; 2: 175–179.
[27] Lenzi M, Johnson PH, McFarlane IG, Ballardine G et al. Antibodies to hepatitis C virus in autoimmune liver diseases: evidence for geographical heterogeneity. Lancet 1991; 338: 277–280.

[28] Nishioka M, Morshed SA, Kano K et al. Frequency and significance of antibodies to P450 2D6 protein in Japanese patients with chronic hepatitis C. J Hepatol 1997; 126: 992–1000.
[29] Michitaka K, Durazzo M, Tillmann HL et al. Analysis of hepatitis C virus genome in patients with autoimmune hepatitis type 2. Gastroenterology 1994; 106: 1603–1610.
[30] Miyakawa H, Kako M, Usuda S, Mishiro S. Reactivity of sera from Japanese patients with type 2 autoimmune hepatitis to peptides derived from host genes, Cytochrome HLD8.2, and GOR. In: Nishioka K et al. editors. Viral hepatitis and liver diseases. Springer-Verlag, 1994; pp. 229–231.
[31] Nabert DW. P450 genes: structure, evolution, and regulation. Ann Rev Biochem 1987; 56: 949–993.
[32] Nabert DW. Polymorphisms in drug-metabolizing enzymes; what is their clinical significance and why do they exist? Am J Hum Genet 1997; 60: 265–271.
[33] Nabert DW, Ingelmcn-Sundberg M, Dely AK. Genetic epidemiology of environmental toxicity and cancer susceptibility: human allelic polymorphisms in drug-metabolizing enzyme genes, their functional importance, and nomenclature issues. Drug Metabol Rev 1999; 31: 467–487.
[34] Hijikata M, Miyakawa H, Matsushita M, Kako M, Ohta Y, Mishiro S. *CYP2D6* polymorphism and the presence of anti-LKM-1 in patients with chronic hepatitis C. Biochem Biophys Res Commun 2000; 270: 922–926.
[35] Manns MP, Obermayer-Straub P. Cytochrome P450 and uridine triphosphate-glucuronosyltransferases: model autoantigens to study drug-induced, viral-induced, and autoimmune liver disease. Hepatology 1997; 26: 1054–1066.
[36] Miyakawa H, Kitazawa E, Kikuchi K et al. Immunoreactivity to various human Cytochrome P450 proteins of sera from patients with autoimmune hepatitis, chronic hepatitis B, and chronic hepatitis C. Autoimmunity 2001; 33: 23–32.

Edited by T. Tsuji, T. Higashi, M. Zeniya and K.-H. Meyer zum Büschenfelde

CHAPTER 17

Molecular Mechanisms of T cell Responses of Autoimmune Hepatitis

Mikio Zeniya, Hiroki Takahashi, Yoshio Aizawa and Gotaro Toda

Division of Gastroenterology and Hepatology, Department of Internal Medicine, Jikei University School of Medicine, Tokyo, Japan

BACKGROUND

Autoimmune hepatitis (AIH) has not been associated with a mode of transmission compatible with an infectious origin, such as that from hepatitis viruses, or with exposure to environmental agents thought to trigger an autoimmune response. Despite many efforts to elucidate the pathogenesis of AIH, the precise cellular and humoral immune-mechanisms responsible for this disease are unknown. However, recent understandings about the immune system based on research in molecular biology significantly advanced our understanding of the molecular basis of immunoregulation in AIH, especially the involvement of the T cell response.

In this chapter, we will review recent developments in our understanding of molecular-based T cell responses.

1. IMMUNOMOLECULAR MECHANISMS OF HEPATOCYTE DAMAGE

The autoimmune process involving a liver-specific antigen that was thought to be a key issue in the development of AIH is principally mediated through receptors: immunoglobulin (Ig) on the B lymphocyte surface and the T cell receptor (TCR) on the T lymphocyte. Important breakthroughs have recently been made in our understanding of the process of immune recognition involving the intracellular pathways of the immune signal at a molecular level. These two receptors are generated in a process that ensures maximum diversity to increase variety and to increase the probability of a reaction to all possible antigens, which includes autoantigens. The estimated diversity for Igs [1] and TCR [2] was reported to be in excess of 10 types. Consequently, this remarkable variety of receptors can recognize both host and foreign antigens, resulting in an autoreactivity that can lead to auto cell destruction. For example, it has been reported that T cells can react to self-proteins in the adult human immune system [3].

It has also been reported that B cell receptors can act differently in terms of their reactions with antigens and the manner in which they trigger cytotoxic responses. Immunoglobulin molecules react with soluble antigens by recognizing a tertiary structural complex, whereas TCR reacts with the relatively short peptide fragments of degraded proteins that are located in the cleft of MHC class I or II molecules on antigen-presenting cells (APC) [4]. The details of this antigen expression are shown in Figs. 1 and 2,

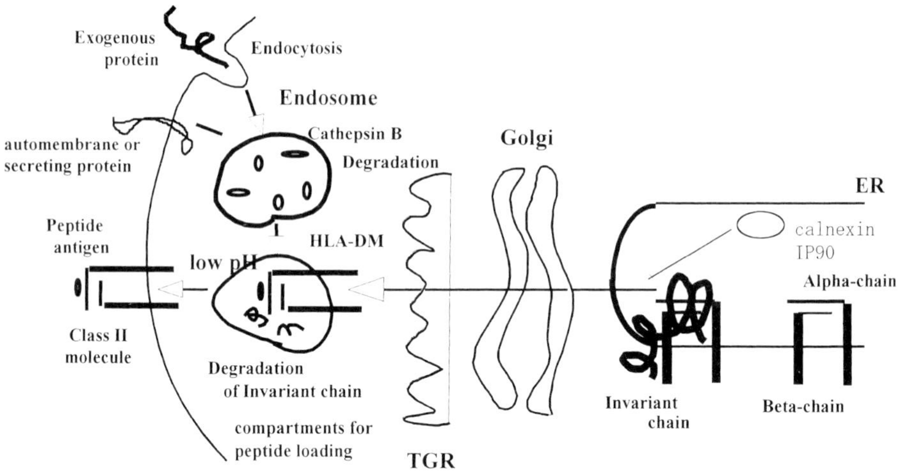

Fig. 1. Intracellular process of antigen presenting by HLA Class II molecules. Cathepsin and HLA-DM play a role in this process.

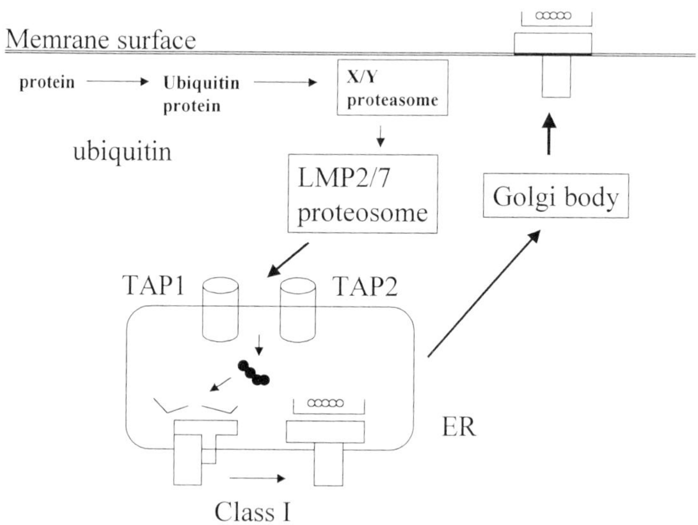

Fig. 2. Intracellular process of antigen presenting by HLA class I molecules. Note the TAP and LMP gene play a critical role in antigen processing.

which show the involvement of the intracellular factors TAP and LMP in processing of antigen presentation. These factors might be involved in liver autoreaction, although little is known about this process at present.

2. AUTOANTIGENIC PEPTIDE RECOGNITION IN AIH

Hepatocytes do not usually express HLA class II antigens, indicating that hepatocytes cannot play a role as APCs. Thus, there must be an APC that expresses a hepatocyte-specific antigen, and perhaps a critical antigen inducing autoreactivity specific to hepatocytes, which might be needed for the development of AIH. Similarly, molecular mimicry between hepatocyte-specific antigens and those of unknown origins, such as from an infectious agent, could induce an autoreaction in the hepatocyte through APCs. Lobo-Yeo et al. [5] reported that, based on an immune staining study using anti-HLA class II monoclonal antibody, hepatocytes from AIH patients do express class II HLA molecules. While it has only been observed in children with AIH, this aberrant expression of HLA class II molecules in hepatocytes might be involved in the pathogenesis of all cases of AIH.

3. HOW DOES AN AUTOANTIGEN TRIGGER AN AUTOIMMUNE REACTION?

3.1. Molecular mimicry

While hepatocytes may express self-antigens as autoantigens, the mechanism triggering the immune reaction has yet to be defined. Manns et al. [6] reported that the target peptide of liver–kidney microsome antibody-1 was cytochrome P450 2D6 (CYP2D6) and that its sequence showed partial homology to the HCV genome. This indicates that there is type 2 AIH that showed positive for both LKM-1 antibody and HCV antibody. Furthermore, these results suggest that an immune reaction to HCV may induce an autoimmune reaction to CYP2D6, a target of type 2 AIH. In hepatitis B infection, similar molecular mimicry might also be responsible for the positive results of autoantibodies, such as antinuclear antibody (ANA) and anti-smooth muscle antibody (ASMA). However, there was no definite proof that molecular mimicry can induce a sustained autoimmune reaction as an etiological factor in the development of AIH.

4. T CELL RESPONSE

Mononuclear cell infiltration in the portal area involving both lymphocytes and plasma cells is one of the histological features of AIH. Many reports have suggested that T cells are predominant among the infiltrating lymphocytes.

Clonal deletion of autoreactive T cells in the thymus is one of the key factors inducing tolerance to self-antigens. Among the autoreactive T cells, $CD4^+$ T cells might play a significant role in the development of autoimmunity. The lineage of regulatory $CD4^+$ T cells could be distinguished from effector cells by the expression of autoantigens that may exist on the hepatocyte membrane. Therefore, analysis of regulatory T cell function and search for a specific clone may be clinically valuable and may become a useful tool for immunotherapy in cases of AIH. Sakaguchi et al. [7] reported that one potential drawback of a unique lineage of regulatory T cells is critical for the susceptibility to a variety of environmental insults or genetic abnormality. They developed animal models of organ-specific autoimmune diseases by elimination of T cell subset [8]. Their data strongly suggested that different factors, such as drugs, radiation, infection etc., might lead to development of autoimmune disease involving AIH in a susceptible individual. It is well recognized that AIH has an immunogenetic component, i.e., HLA-DR3 or DR4, and the development of AIH is induced by an unknown trigger. This suggests that regulatory T cells play a crucial role in the development of AIH.

5. SPECIFIC T CELL CLONES IN AIH

Recently, TCR repertoires and CDR3 sequences have been investigated in several autoimmune diseases involving rheumatoid arthritis [9], multiple sclerosis [10], and experimental autoimmune encephalitis [11]. Through these analyses, an extensive search for corresponding autoantigenic determinants has been conducted and the existence of a disease-specific T cell [12] was confirmed.

6. TCR Vβ CHAIN REPERTOIRE IN AIH

Antigen-specific liver-infiltrating T cells were observed in the liver of AIH patients [13]. These specific T cell repertoires may recognize an autoantigen that expressed on a hepatocyte and may be concerned with the development of AIH. Hoshino et al. [14] reported the limited usage of TCR β chains and sequences of the complementary determining region (CDR) 3 of lymphocytes infiltrating in the liver of four Japanese female patients in 1995, by using a polymerase chain reaction (PCR) method with specific TCR primers. They sequenced the CDR3 region, and found that shared Vβ 3 expression was observed in the clones from all AIH patients. Moreover, they reported that Vβ 3-positive Jβ 1.2-positive T cells bearing an Asp–Arg–Pro motif were closely associated with HLA-DR4. Interestingly, one patient who was HLA-DR4-negative but HLA-DR2-positive also shared Vβ 3 expression. However this patient did not show Vβ 1.2.

Recently, Arenz et al. [15] reported similar results. They also analyzed the TCR Vβ repertoire of liver infiltrating T cells in 12 Caucasians with untreated AIH. Using lymphocytes isolated from biopsied liver tissue, they found that TCR Vβ 3 was also significantly overexpressed in the liver of patients with AIH compared with chronic hepatitis C patients. In their analysis, Vβ 13.1 molecules were also over-expressed compared with a healthy blood donor. Furthermore, they reported that TCR Vβ 3 T cells were found to be enriched in the liver tissue compared with autologous peripheral blood taken at the same time of liver biopsy. Taken together, in AIH the TCR Vβ 3-expressed T cells in liver tissue may play an important role in the pathogenesis of AIH.

However, the following factors should be studied. In the Japanese report, TCR Vβ 3 expression was closely associated with HLA-DR4, whereas in the Caucasian report, there was no association observed between HLA-DR4 and specific TCR Vβ expression. It is well known that both HLA-DR3 and -DR4 are significant genetic factors for AIH. It may be possible that both HLA-DR4 and -DR3 are strongly associated with TCR

Vβ 3 in AIH. However, Arenz et al also reported that over-expression of TCR Vβ 3 was observed in one patient with chronic hepatitis C.

Recently, it was reported that expressed autoimmune repertoires are not fixed but evolve over the course of the disease [16]. The reactivity of autoreactive T cells to secondary epitopes, which might be formerly cryptic, can regulate the response to the initially dominant epitopes. This delicate process is termed determinant spreading [17]. If determinant occurs in the course AIH, the different usage of the TCR Vβ repertoire might be explained.

TCR Vβ 3 over-expression has been reported in other liver diseases. Broome et al. [18] reported the preferential TCR Vβ 3 usage of hepatic T lymphocytes in primary sclerosing cholangitis which is thought to be an autoimmune liver disease having a different immunogenetic background. It has also been reported that TCR Vβ expression occurs in viral hepatitis [19]. From these observations, it is possible that the TCR Vβ 3-expressed T cell may be a liver-specific reactive lymphocyte, which plays a role in the development of liver diseases. However, overexpression of TCR Vβ 3 has not been reported in primary biliary cirrhosis [20] or autoimmune cholangitis [21].

7. TOLERANCE BREAKING

A defect in self-tolerance is also involved in the pathogenesis of autoimmune diseases. It has been reported that several immune cells play an important role in the maintenance of tolerance. The $CD4^+CD45RB^+$ cell (Tr cell) and γδT cell suppress autoreactive T cell activation through the secretion of interleukin (IL)-10 and TGF-β. The NKT cells, which express both TCR and NK cell receptor, has been reported as having a unique property [22]. The TCR of the NKT cell shows a quite limited invariant TCR, i.e. Vα24JαQ, and recognizes glycolipid, α-Gal-Ser expressed by CD1D [23]. The NKT cell secretes IL-4 or interferon (IFN)-γ and plays a role in self-tolerance maintenance. In several autoimmune diseases and animal models, it has been reported that the reduction of NKT cells was observed at the early stage of the disease [24], suggesting this reduction might be related to a break in self-tolerance. Furthermore, Goherty and colleagues [25] reported that liver-associated lymphocytes contain a high percentage (27%) of NKT cells compared with peripheral blood, and that CD1d is expressed on hepatocytes. These data strongly indicate that these factors might play a significant role in maintaining liver-related self-tolerance.

8. CYTOTOXIC EFFECTOR MECHANISMS

Fig. 3 shows the reported cytotoxic effector mechanisms [26]. The bulk of rapid target hepatocyte lysis is mediated by receptor- mediated mechanisms that depend mainly on cell–cell contact between CTL and its antigenic target. Perforin and granzymes are main casts for these mechanisms through CTL. Perforin exhibits many structural similarities to C9 and leads to membrane disruption and necrosis [27]. The granzymes A and B are known as the CTL granule and multiple neutral serine proteases. These granules enter the target cell through pores formed in the cell membrane by perforin. Granzyme B can also enter cells in the absence of perforin and is one of the proteases capable of specific

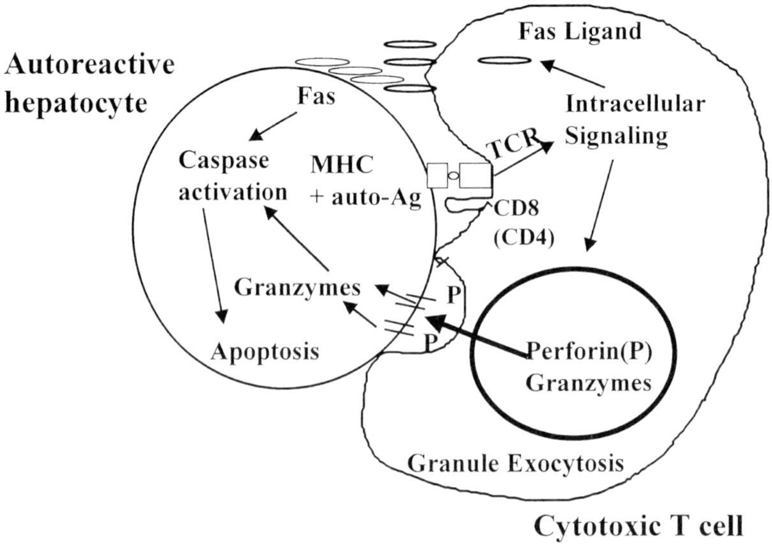

Fig. 3. T cell cytotoxicity-related molecules.

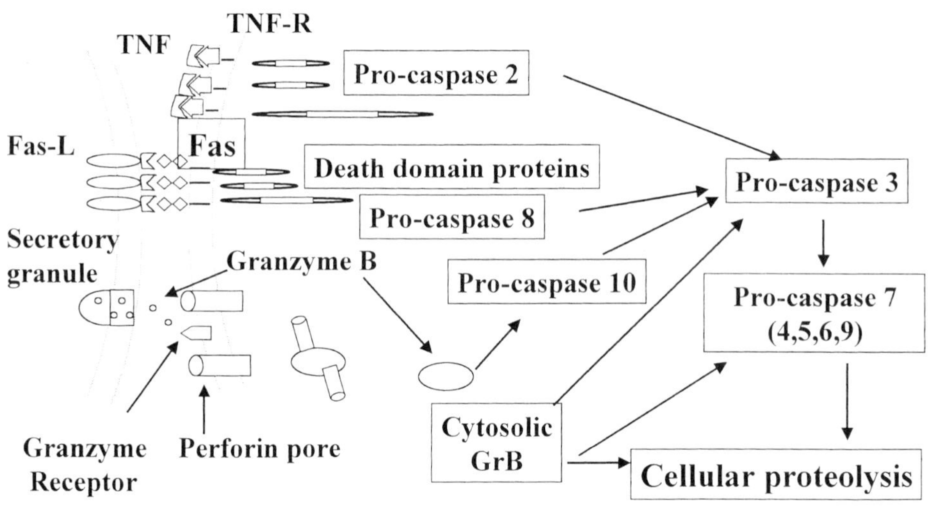

Fig. 4. Intracellular pathway of death signal. The signals reach caspase 3 and finally lead the cell to apoptosis.

cleavage and activation of the proenzyme forms of caspase 3 and other related caspases shown in Fig. 4. Granzyme A is a tryptase that does not cleave or activate the proenzyme form of caspase 3 but can cleave and activate caspase 1 of interleukin-1β-converting enzyme (ICE). Finally, the cleavage of the DNA-binding proteins, *caspases*, may explain the observed triggering of DNA fragmentation, resulting in cell death with *apoptosis*.

There is another distinct pathway that induces apoptosis in target cells that express a specific receptor designated as Fas receptor, which is one of several members of an extended family of death receptors that are structurally similar to tumor necrosis factor (TNF) receptor 1. Caspase 8 binds to Fas-associating protein with death domain (FADD) and then cleaves and activates caspase 3 and a cascade of proteases which leads to induction of apoptosis. Hepatocytes constitutively express Fas, and by inflammatory stimuli the expression of Fas in hepatocytes is further augmented [28].

At the same time, CTL can secrete several immune cytokines, such as TNF-α and IFN-γ, that can regulate the immune reaction involved in liver-specific autoreaction. TNF can activate a caspase cascade through type 1 TNF receptor (TNFR1) a manner similar to that triggered by Fas. The activation of TNFR1 can trigger a caspase death cascade and activate nuclear factor κB (NFκB) that induces the expression of genes encoding proteins that can block the apoptosis cascade. Furthermore, cytokines such as IFN-γ secreted by CTL might play an important role in moderating the immune reaction involving Kupffer cells and macrophages and can modify the clinical characteristics of AIH.

This system, including genetic differences in the immune response, may play an important role in the pathogenesis of AIH.

SUMMARY

Recent advances in molecular-based immunology have elucidated much about the basic autoimmune mechanism of AIH. However, the true mechanism of AIH remains unclear and the target epitope(s) has not been isolated. Furthermore, regulation of the T cell response has yet to be applied to clinical use. The lack of a proper animal model for AIH is one of the major challenges in improving our understanding of this process.

ACKNOWLEDGEMENTS

This work was supported by a Grant from the Japanese Ministry of Health and Welfare, and Research Grant (No. C2-11670536) from the Japanese Ministry of Health and Welfare and Mochida pharmaceutical company. We would like to express our sincere appreciation to Ms. Asako Takaki for her valuable assistance.

REFERENCES

[1] Grabar P. Autoantibodies and the physiological role of immunoglobulins. Immunol Today 1983; 4: 337–342.

[2] Blackman M, Keppler J, Marrack P. The role of T cell receptor in positive and negative selection of developing T cells. Science 1990; 248: 1335–1341.

[3] Kotani H, Mitsuya H, Jarret RF, Yonokisa GG, James SP, Strober W. An autoreactive T cell clone that can be activated to provide both helper and suppressor function. J Immunol 1986; 136: 1951–1959.

[4] German RN, Castellino F, Han R et al. Processing and presentation of endocytically acquired protein antigens by MHC class II and class I molecules. Immunol Rev 1996; 151: 5–30.

[5] Lobo-Yeo A, Mieli-Vergani G, Kenna G et al. Class I and class II major histocompatibility complex antigen expression on hepatocytes. A study in children with liver disease. Hepatology 1990; 12: 224–232.
[6] Manns MP, Griffin KJ, Sullivan KF, et al. LKM-1 autoantibodies recognize a short linear sequence in P450IID6, a cytochrome P-450 monooxygenase. J Clin Invest 1991; 88: 1370–1378.
[7] Sakaguchi S, Toda M, Asano M, Itoh M, Morse SS, Sakaguchi N. T cell mediated maintenance of natural self-tolerance: its breakdown as a possible cause of various autoimmune diseases. J Autoimmun 1996; 9: 211–920.
[8] Sakaguchi S, Fukuma K, Kuribayashi K, Masuda T. Organ-specific autoimmune diseases induced in mice by elimination of T cell subset. I. Evidence for the active participation of T cell subset as a possible cause of autoimmune disease. J Clin Med 1985; 161: 72–87.
[9] Uematsu Y, Wege H, Straus A, et al. The T-cell-receptor repertoire in the synovial fluid of a patient with rheumatoid arthritis is polyclonal. Proc Natl Acad Sci USA 1991; 88: 8534–8538.
[10] Kotzin BL, Karuturi S, Chou YK, et al. Preferential T-cell receptor-chain variable gene use in myelin basic protein-reactive T-cell clones from patients with multiple sclerosis. Proc Natl Acad Sci USA 1991; 88: 9161–9165.
[11] Urbam JL, Kumar V, Kondo C et al. Restricted use of T cell receptor V genes in murine autoimmune encephalomyelitis raises possibility of antibody therapy. Cell 1988; 54: 577–592.
[12] Hashim GA, Vanderbark J, Jones R et al. Antibodies specific for V β 8 receptor peptide suppress experimental autoimmune encephalomyelitis. J Immunol 1990; 144: 4621–4627.
[13] Lohr H, Treichel U, Poralla T et al. The human asialoglycoprotein receptor (hASGPR) is a target antigen for liver-infiltrating T cells in autoimmune chronic active hepatitis and primary biliary cirrhosis. Hepatology 1990; 12: 1314–1320.
[14] Hoshino Y, Enomoto N, Izumi N et al. Limited usage of T-cell receptor β chains and sequences of the complementarity determining region 3 of lymphocytes infiltrating in the liver of autoimmune hepatitis. Hepatology 1995; 22: 142–147.
[15] Arenz M, Meyer zum Bushenfelde K-H, Lohr HF. Limited T cell receptor V β-chain repertoire of liver-infiltrating T cells in autoimmune hepatitis. J Hepatol 1998; 28: 70–77.
[16] Lehmann PV, Forsthuber T, Alexander M et al. Spreading of T-cell autoimmunity to cryptic determinants of an autoantigen. Nature 1992; 358: 155–157.
[17] Lehmann PV, Sercarz EE, Forsthuber T et al. Determinant spreading and the dynamics of the autoimmune T cell repertoire. Immunol Today 1993; 14: 203–208.
[18] Broome U, Grunewald J, Scheynius A et al. Preferential V beta3 usage by hepatic T lymphocytes in patients with primary sclerosing cholangitis. J Hepatol 1997; 26: 527–534.
[19] Pham BN, Degos F, Mosnier JF et al. Restriction of V beta gene usage of liver-derived lymphocytes in chronic hepatitis B and C. Hum Immunol 1996; 49: 56–63.
[20] Mayo MJ, Combers B, Jenkins RN. T-cell receptor V beta gene utilization in primary biliary cirrhosis. Hepatology 1996; 24: 1148–1155.
[21] Shimizu Y, Higuchi K, Miyamoto M et al. Clonal accumulation of V beta 5.1-positive cells in the liver of a patient with autoimmune cholangiopathy. Liver 1997; 17: 7–12.
[22] Ithoh M, Takahashi T et al. Thymus and autoimmunity: production of $CD25^+$ $CD4^+$ naturally anergic and suppressive T cells as a key function of the thymus in maintaining immunogenetic self-tolerance. J Immunol 1999; 162: 5317–5326.
[23] Spada FM, Koezuka Y et al. CD1d-restricted recognition of synthetic glycolipid antigens by human natural killer T cells. J Exp Med 1998; 188: 1529–1534.

[24] Mieza MA, Ithoh T et al. Selective reduction of Va14$^+$NKT cells associated with disease development I autoimmune-prone mice. J Immunol 1996; 156: 4035–4040.
[25] Norris S, Goherty DG et al. Natural T cells in the human liver: Cytotoxic lymphocytes with dual T cell and natural killer cell phenotype and function are phenotypically heterogeneous and induce Va24JaQ and γδ T cell receptor bearing cells. Hum Immunol 1999; 60: 20–31.
[26] Froelich CJ, Dixit VM, Yang X. Lymphocyte granule-mediated apoptosis: matters of viral mimicry and deadly protease. Immunol Today 1998; 19: 30–36.
[27] Liu C-C, Young LHY, Young JD-E. Lymphocyte-mediated cytolysis and disease. New Engl J Med 1996; 335: 1651–1659.
[28] Tanaka M, Suda T, Yatomi T et al. Lethal effect of recombinant human fas ligand in mice pretreated with propionibacterium acnes. J Immunol 1997; 158: 2303–2309.

Molecular Biology and Immunology in Hepatology
Edited by T. Tsuji, T. Higashi, M. Zeniya and K.-H. Meyer zum Büschenfelde

CHAPTER 18

Primary Biliary Cirrhosis: Solving the Enigma

Kazuhide Yamamoto [1] and M. Eric Gershwin [2]

[1] *Department of Medicine and Medical Sciences, Okayama University Graduate School of Medicine and Dentistry, Okayama, Japan*
[2] *Division of Rheumatology, Allergy and Clinical Immunology, University of California at Davis, Davis, CA, USA*

INTRODUCTION

Primary biliary cirrhosis (PBC) is an autoimmune liver disease that predominantly affects women and involves obstruction of intrahepatic bile ducts. This interferes with bile secretion, causing fibrosis and eventually cirrhosis of the liver. Antimitochondrial antibodies (AMA) are present in 90–95% of patients with PBC and occur before clinical signs appear [1,2]. A puzzling feature of PBC, similar to certain other autoimmune diseases, is that the autoimmune attack is predominantly organ-specific, but the mitochondrial autoantigens are present in all nucleated cells and organs. A major advance towards defining the pathogenesis of PBC has been the precise identification of the mitochondrial proteins that are the targets of AMA [3,4].

Histopathologically, PBC is characterized by chronic progressive destruction of small intrahepatic bile ducts with portal inflammation, ultimately leading to cirrhosis [5]. The AMA targets are members of the family of 2-oxoacid dehydrogenase complexes (2-OADC), including the E2 subunit of the pyruvate dehydrogenase complex (PDC–E2), the E2 subunit of the branched chain 2-oxoacid dehydrogenase complex (BCOADC–E2), the E2 subunit of the 2-oxoglutarate dehydrogenase complex (OGDC–E2), and the dihydrolipoamide dehydrogenase binding protein (E3BP) [6]. The most common reactivity is against PDC–E2. Some patients have AMA that react with PDC–E2 alone, but most patients also show reactivity against OGDC–E2 or BCOADC–E2. These target antigens are located in the inner mitochondrial matrix and catalyze the oxidative decarboxylation of various keto-acid substrates [7]. The E2 enzymes have a common structure which consists of the N-terminal domain containing the lipoyl group(s), the peripheral subunit binding domain responsible, at least in part, for binding the E1 and E3 components together; and the C-terminal inner core that houses the active site responsible for the acyltransferase activity. Several studies using oligopeptides or recombinant proteins have shown that the predominant epitope of PDC–E2 is located within the lipoyl domain of PDC–E2 [6]. Although AMA are considered a hallmark feature of PBC, they are not the only disease-specific autoantibodies, and other autoantigens, usually nuclear located, are recognized by a minority of patients [8].

1. CLINICAL FEATURES OF DISEASE

Primary biliary cirrhosis presents insidiously with fatigue and pruritus; fatigue is found in up to 80% of patients [9]. However, fatigue is relatively non-specific and the cause is unknown, as is the case for fatigue in all other patients with chronic liver disease. The clinician needs to exclude other treatable causes of lethargy, such as depression or hypothyroidism. Severity of fatigue does not correlate with the severity of the disease, but is associated with depression and sleep disorder [10]. Pruritus is the second commonest symptom in PBC occurring in 50–60% of patients [9] and is characteristically worse on palms and soles and not associated with cutaneous changes. When pruritus occurs, it does not appear to be related to the disease stage and may remit as the disease progresses; in some patients, it can develop during the late stages of the disease. Although several hypotheses are proposed [11,12], the cause of pruritus is unknown.

Jaundice usually follows months or years later, but in 10% of patients, jaundice may be the presenting symptom. Darkening of the skin, hirsutism, anorexia, diarrhea, and weight loss may also be present. Less commonly, patients may present with a complication of portal hypertension, such as variceal bleeding or ascites — evidence of more advanced liver disease. Occasionally, patients may present with problems related to the complications of cholestasis, such as severe osteoporosis or symptoms resulting from fat-soluble vitamin deficiency. Some patients present with malabsorption, but this is usually more common in patients with advanced disease. PBC is associated with cutaneous changes of generalized hyperpigmentation and facial xanthelasmata. The latter changes result from raised total cholesterol concentration.

Physical findings are variable and depend on the extent of the disease. Hepatosplenomegaly, spider angiomas, palmer erythema, hyperpigmentation, hirsutism, and xanthoma may be present. An increasing susceptibility to urinary tract infection has been observed in women with PBC [13], but the cause of this associated problem is unknown. There also appears to be an increased prevalence of hepatocellular carcinoma among patients with PBC, but the magnitude of this is controversial [14,15].

In patients with PBC, elevation of serum alkaline phosphatase and γ-glutamyl transpeptidase levels are the most characteristic abnormalities of liver function tests. Hyperbilirubinemia is not frequently observed. However, serum bilirubin levels can rise to remarkably high levels as the disease progresses and serves as an excellent predictor of survival. Serum albumin levels and the prothrombin time are normal early in the course of the disease. A low serum albumin level and prolonged prothrombin time that is not corrected by vitamin K therapy are poor prognostic signs that indicate an advanced disease. Serum IgM levels is frequently increased, whereas IgG and IgA levels are usually within normal limits. The serologic hallmark of PBC is the high titer AMA and is positive in 95% of patients with PBC. The finding of a significant AMA titer (>1 : 40) is strongly suggestive of PBC, even in the absence of symptoms and the presence of normal levels of serum alkaline phosphatase [16]. Although demonstration of AMA by immunofluorescence has diagnostic specificity, newer techniques such as enzyme-linked immunosorbent assay and immunoblotting, are more sensitive and specific than immunofluorescence.

Ultrasound examination of the liver and biliary tree is mandatory in all patients with unexplained cholestasis. If the biliary system appears normal by ultrasound and the AMA test is positive, no further radiologic delineation of the bile duct is necessary. If the diagnosis of PBC is uncertain or a sudden rise in the serum bilirubin takes place, cholangiography may be necessary to exclude biliary obstruction.

The histological changes seen in the liver in PBC are well defined and are graded into four stages of severity as defined by Scheuer [17]. The biliary epithelial cells (BECs) lining the small intrahepatic bile ducts are the primary target for immunological damage, and thus the majority of early changes are seen in the portal and periportal regions. However, these histological changes develop at different rates in the different parts of the liver, an overlap among stages is frequently found. As only patients in stage IV have true histological cirrhosis, the term 'primary biliary cirrhosis' may be considered a misnomer.

2. EPIDEMIOLOGY

The disease predominantly occurs in middle-aged women of various ethnic and racial populations. Ninety percent of patients with PBC are female and the majority is diagnosed after the age of 40 years although the age at diagnosis varies from the low 20s to the high 80s. It has never been described in children, except one questionable case [18]. The basis for the gender and age predilections is unclear. The prevalence and the incidence vary widely, with high levels found among Northern European populations and a low level found in Japan. Estimates of disease prevalence range from 19 to 150 cases per million population and incidence between 4 and 30 cases per million per year [19]. The point prevalence of PBC has risen from 19 million in 1976 to 128 million in 1987 [20] and the reported incidence has also increased. Such apparent increases might only represent an improved diagnosis due to greater awareness and the increased use of autoantibody screening in primary care. However, it is impossible to exclude a genuine increase in the frequency of the disease. Geographical clusters of disease have been also reported, but no causative environmental agents have been identified [21].

3. BILE DUCT DESTRUCTION

The specificity of bile duct destruction, the presence of lymphoid infiltration in the portal tracts and the presence of MHC class II antigen on biliary epithelium in PBC have suggested that an intense autoimmune response is directed against biliary epithelial cells [2]. It has been hypothesized that the destruction of biliary cells in PBC is mediated by autoreactive liver-infiltrating T cells through either direct cytotoxicity or as a result of cytokine production. The evidence was initially derived from histochemical staining studies of tissue samples and later by analyzing T cell lines that proliferate in the presence of putative mitochondrial autoantigens [2]. Several years ago, we successfully obtained CD4$^+$ T cell lines from liver biopsies from patients with PBC [22]. Such T cell lines specifically produced IL-2 when stimulated with PDC–E2 or BCOADC–E2 whereas control proteins were not stimulatory. Recently, we explored T cell reactivity in more depth using peripheral blood mononuclear cells (PBMC), liver derived T cells and regional lymph node of patients with PBC and controls and derived T cell lines specific for PDC–E2 using a panel of 33 overlapping peptides spanning the entire PDC–E2 [23]. Phenotypically, these T cell clones were CD4$^+$, CD45RO$^+$, and T cell receptor α/β. The minimal epitopes of these cloned T cell lines all mapped to the amino acid sequence 163–176, GDLLAEIETDKATI within the inner lipoyl domain of PDC–E2 (the same as the B cell epitope). This would be consistent with more efficient uptake and processing of the autoantigen via the Ig receptor on autoimmune B cells, and protection of the epitopes from degradation during antigen processing [23]. Moreover, all T cell lines responded to the sequence 36–49, GDLIAEVETDKATV, which corresponds to the outer lipoyl domain of PDC–E2. These two reactive peptides share a common amino acid motif that includes E, D, and K at positions 170, 172, and 173, respectively (ExDK sequence motif), whereas other peptides which share amino acid sequence homology with PDC–E2 but do not have the ExDK motif did not induce T cell proliferation. One particular cloned T cell line also cross-reacted with an exogenous antigenic peptide, EQSLITVEGDKASM, homologous to part of the sequence of PDC–E2 from *Escherichia coli*, which has an ExDK motif. However, none of these PDC–E2-specific T cell clones cross-reacted with the HLA-DRα chain peptide 82–95, QGALANIAVDKANL, or the human glycogen phosphorylase peptide 354–367, despite both having some amino acid homology with PDC–E2 but lacking the requisite ExDK motif. Furthermore, we demonstrated, specifically in PBC, a high precursor frequency of PDC–E2 163–176 reactive T cells in the hilar lymph nodes and livers, 100–150 fold greater than for PBMC from the same patients [23]. T cell receptor analysis of PDC–E2-specific T cells within the liver revealed diverse usage of V and J [24].

4. AUTOANTIBODY PRODUCTION

The targets of AMA in PBC sera were initially found on mitochondria and have been proven to be members of the 2-oxoacid dehydrogenase complex (2-OADC) which catalyze the oxidative decarboxylation of various α-keto-acid substrates [4,25–27]. Components of this family include the E2 subunit of pyruvate dehydrogenase complex (PDC–E2), the E2 subunit of branched chain 2-OADC (BCOADC–E2), the E2 subunit of 2-oxoglutarate dehydrogenase complex (OGDC–E2) and the dihydrolipoamide dehydrogenase binding protein (E3BP) (Table 1). The most common reactivity of AMA is against PDC–E2 (Table 2). While some patients have AMA that react with PDC–E2 alone, most patients also show reactivity against OGDC–E2 or BCOADC–E2. Reactivity against OGDC–E2 or BCOADC–E2 alone is less common. Serologic cross-reactivity is only found between PDC–E2 and E3BP. There is no significant difference in the frequency and antigenic specificity of AMA between men and women, regardless of the predominance of the disease in women [28]. Interestingly, the immunodominant

TABLE 1

Molecular weights and functions of the 2-oxo-acid dehydrogenase complex

Enzymes	MW (kDa)	Function
Pyruvate dehydrogenase (PDC)		
E1α decarboxylase	41	Decarboxylates pyruvate with thiamine pyrophosphate (TTP) as a co-factor
E1α decarboxylase	36	Decarboxylates pyruvate with TTP as a co-factor
E2 acetyltransferase	74	Transfers acetyl group from E1 to coenzyme A (CoA)
E3 lipoamide dehydrogenase	55	Regenerates disulfide of E2 by oxidation of lipoic acid
E3 binding protein (protein X)	56	Anchors E3 to the E2 core of pyruvate dehydrogenase complex
2-Oxoglutarate dehydrogenase (OGDC)		
E1 oxoglutarate dehydrogenase	113	Decarboxylates α-ketoglutarate with TTP as a co-factor
E2 succinyl transferase	48	Transfers succinyl group from E2 to CoA
E3 lipoamide dehydrogenase	55	Regenerates disulfide of E2 by oxidation of lipoic acid
Branched-chain 2-oxo-acid dehydrogenase (BCOADC)		
E1α decarboxylase	46	Decarboxylates α-keto acids
E1β decarboxylase	38	Derived from leucine, isoleucine, and valine with TTP as a co-factor
E2 acyltransferase	52	Transfers acyl group from E1 to CoA
E3 lipoamide dehydrogenase	55	Regenerates disulfide of E2 by oxidation of lipoic acid

TABLE 2

PBC-associated autoantigens recognized by patient sera

Antigen	Prevalence (%)
Mitochondrial location	
PDC-E2	90–95
E3 binding protein	90–95
OGDC–E2	39–88
BCOADC–E2	53–55
PDC–E1α	41–66
PDC–E3	38
PDC–E1β	1–7
Nuclear location	
gp210	10–40
Nucleoporin p62	32
Sp100	20–30
Promyelocytic leukemia protein (PML)	20–30
Lamin B receptor	<1

epitopes of PDC–E2, OGDC–E2, BCOADC–E2, and E3BP are all lipoate-binding sites [29]. However, the findings of these highly specific autoantibodies and autoantigens have yet to be linked directly to the pathogenesis of PBC.

In addition to AMA, sera have been reported to contain other disease-specific autoantibodies, including antibodies against nuclear proteins (ANA). ANA have been identified in up to 52% of patients with PBC. These autoantigens include the nuclear pore protein, gp210, a 21-kDa transmembrane glycoprotein involved in the attachment of pore complex constituents to the nuclear membrane. Antibodies directed against gp210 are found in about 25% (range, 10–40%) of patients with AMA-positive PBC and up to 50% of those with AMA-negative PBC. The disease specificity for the detection of such autoantibodies by immunoblotting is over 99% [8]. In contrast to AMA, antibodies against gp210 have prognostic significance [30]. Other autoantigens include the nuclear pore protein p62, which is a nuclear pore glycoprotein specifically recognized by PBC sera and present in about 25% of patients with PBC [31]. The presence of anti-gp210 and p62 in PBC sera appears to be mutually independent. In about 20–30% of PBC patients, autoantibodies are directed against Sp100, a nucleoprotein of 100 kDa molecular weight and appear to exhibit a high specificity for PBC [32]. Antibodies against promyelocytic leukemia-associated protein (PML), a cell-encoded putative transcriptional transactivator, are associated with PBC and present concurrently with antibodies against Sp100 [33]. Finally, a minority of PBC sera also shows reactivity against the inner nuclear pore membrane protein lamin B receptor (LBR) [34]. LBR is an inner nuclear membrane protein that binds both nuclear lamins and double-stranded DNA; LBR may play a role in anchoring nuclear lamins and heterochromatin during interphase. Although <1% of PBC sera contains antibodies to LBR, there appears to be disease specificity for such autoreactivity. ANA detected in PBC frequently display unique immunofluorescence patterns, including nuclear dots (e.g. Sp100) or a nuclear ring-like pattern (e.g. gp210) while ANA in AIH are homogenous or speckled. In cases of patients with negative AMA, these PBC-associated ANA may be the only sero-immunological clues for establishing the diagnosis of PBC.

5. MOLECULAR MIMICRY

PDC–E2 is evolutionarily well conserved, especially at the lipoic acid binding sites and sera from patients with PBC react to both human and *E. coli* PDC–E2 [35]. However, using a functional assay that depends on epitope recognition, the level of cross-reactivity between mammalian and non-mammalian PDC enzymes do not support molecular mimicry, at least at the B cell level [36]. Still, molecular mimicry might still pertain at the T cell level [23]. Thus, in response to an infection, T cells would recognize the lipoyl domain of *E. coli* PDC–E2 or other enzymes containing an AVDKA sequence from the HLA-DRα chain, or an EDTDK sequence from human PDC–E2 presented by aberrantly expressed MHC class II molecules on bile duct cells. Finally, this reactivity would initiate the autoimmune cascade leading bile duct destruction in which AMA and/or T cells specific for mitochondrial antigens may play a pathogenic role. At this stage, the autoimmune process would take place in the absence of the exogenous antigens, such as *E. coli* PDC–E2, which initiated the original immune response. However, while some T cell clones crossreact with PDC–E2 from *E. coli*, the same T cells do not react with PDC–E2 purified from *Pseudomonas putida*, which not only has an ExDK sequence, but also has greater homology with human than *E. coli* PDC–E2. Epidemiologic data do not support an association of urinary tract infections and PBC [37].

6. IMMUNOGENETICS

A number of studies have investigated whether there is linkage between PBC and MHC markers by serological and PCR typing. Although a variety of associations have been reported, the data are not consistent and, thus far, no striking associations have been made [38]. MHC class II (HLA-DR) and ICAM-1, which are critical for the interaction and adhesion between lymphoid cells and target cells, have both been shown to be up-regulated on the BECs in PBC [39]. However, these molecules are commonly induced in a variety of liver diseases and are not specific for PBC, suggesting that this increased expression is secondary to the inflammatory response. This view is supported by the fact that MHC class-II expression is only detected during the intermediate stages of PBC and not during the early stages of the disease [40].

7. IMMUNOCHEMISTRY

Immunohistochemical studies using mAbs to the mitochondrial autoantigens have identified an accumulation of immunoreactive material in the apical region of BECs only in PBC [22]. The apically located material contains epitopes recognized by antibodies to PDC–E2, BCOADC–E2 and OGDC–E2 [41]. Furthermore, this accumulation is present early in PBC and precedes the appearance of B7 and MHC Class II [40].

The apically located material is also present in BEC in allografts of patients with recurrent PBC following liver transplantation [42]. Importantly, although BECs from PBC patients have mitochondria in the cytosol, there are no identifiable mitochondrial structures in the apical region; the apical region is also not stained by antibodies to other mitochondrial components, such as cytochrome oxidase [22]. The apically located material is not reactive with the full panel of antibody reagents to PDC–E2, or the other mitochondrial autoantigens, suggesting it differs in some respects to these proteins. Intensive studies have failed to identify an exogenous source for this material. Such an accumulation may be the result of enhanced synthesis, impaired degradation, and/or abnormal targeting of the PDC–E2 to the surface and apical regions of the BEC. However, there is no precedent for overexpression of a mitochondrial protein leading to deposition in a cytoplasmic location. Our consultant Dr. D. Danner has overexpressed each of the subunits of the BCOADC–E2 enzyme complex and never found any protein in the cytosol [43]. Furthermore, he has a BCOADC-kinase transgenic mouse; even with 100-fold overexpression, the only place the protein is found is in the mitochondria, with import being rapid and complete. Neither is there evidence that mistargetting due to alterations in trafficking signals would lead to this tissue-specific accumulation late in life, although such mutations have been reported as a cause of severe inherited disease of infancy [44]. An alternative analysis of AMA binding to purified BECs has suggested that the original target is PDC–E3BP [45], but these data have not been reproduced.

8. IS THERE A ROLE FOR IGA?

IgA is the principal immunoglobulin isotype on epithelial surfaces, including biliary epithelium. IgA is synthesized in plasma cells located in the lamina propria, and secreted IgA binds to a poly-Ig receptor which is present on the basolateral surfaces of biliary epithelial cells. Following internalization with the receptor, IgA is transported through the cytoplasm in a transport vesicle (transcytosis), and secreted into the bile ducts at the apical surface [46]. Relatively few cell types in the body are involved in the transcytosis of IgA, but of those that have been examined, both biliary epithelial cells and salivary duct epithelial cells are damaged in PBC [47]. These two cell types both show clear evidence of intense apical staining with specific anti-PDC–E2 antibodies that in the case of salivary gland epithelium is not found in tissue from patients with Sjögren's syndrome [48]. This suggests the hypothesis that the selective destruction of these cells in PBC may result from the pathogenic action of antimitochondrial IgA autoantibodies [46]. This process may be involved in the accumulation of apically located material and may also explain the specificity of tissue damage. BECs undergo apoptosis in PBC, although the mechanisms responsible for inducing such apoptosis need further study, particularly since cholestasis may also induce apoptosis [49].

9. MODELS OF DISEASE

There are no animal models of PBC. We have immunized a large number of species with PDC–E2 and although we produce an antibody response, the response most often is not directed at self and has a different specificity than human autoantibodies [50].

There is no liver pathology. There has been an abstract purporting that immunization of SJL mice with PDC–E2 leads to biliary pathology in a small number of mice but this work failed to include a control immunogen and has not been reproduced in our laboratory [51]. A number of other hypotheses about PBC etiology have been tested and discounted. (1) That PBC is a form of chronic graft versus host disease (GVHD). We were unable to find AMA in 89 patients with chronic GVHD [52]; (2) That PBC may be a cryptic infection that induces cross-reactive responses. To date, no one has succeeded in identifying bacteria by conventional culture techniques. By PCR, two groups, including ourselves, have attempted to detect bacterial genes in PBC livers using 16S rDNA and groEL [53]. Although a number of bacteria were found in PBC as well as control livers, we failed to define 'consensus' bacteria which were specifically detected only in PBC livers. (3) That retroviruses are present at high frequency in PBC patients. Recently, antibodies against retroviral elements were detected in the sera of patients with PBC [54]. However, this reactivity is clearly not disease-specific.

10. DO XENOBIOTICS CAUSE PBC?

In PBC, the major autoepitope recognized by both T and B cells is the inner lipoyl domain of the E2 component of pyruvate dehydrogenase (PDC–E2). To address the hypothesis that PBC is induced by xenobiotic exposure, we took advantage of ab initio quantum chemistry and synthesized the inner lipoyl domain of PDC–E2, replacing the lipoic acid moiety with synthetic structures designed to mimic a xenobiotically modified lipoyl hapten, and we quantitated the reactivity of these structures with sera from PBC patients. Interestingly, AMAs from all seropositive patients with PBC, but no controls, reacted against three of the 18 organic modified autoepitopes significantly better than to the native domain. By structural analysis, the features that correlated with autoantibody binding included synthetic domain peptides with a halide or methyl halide in the *meta*- or *para*-position containing no strong hydrogen bond accepting groups on the phenyl ring of the lysine substituents, and synthetic domain peptides with a relatively low rotation barrier about the linkage bond. Many chemicals, including pharmaceuticals and household detergents have the potential to form such halogenated derivatives as metabolites. These data reflect, the first time, that an organic compound has been shown to serve as a mimeotope for an autoantigen and further provide evidence for a potential mechanism by which environmental organic compounds may cause primary biliary cirrhosis.

Xenobiotics are foreign compounds that may either alter or complex to defined self proteins, inducing a change in the molecular structure of the native protein sufficient to induce an immune response. Such immune responses may then result in the recognition of not only the modified or altered protein, but also the unmodified native protein [55,56]. The chronic presence of the self protein serves to perpetuate the immune response initiated by the xenobiotic-induced adduct and leads to autoimmunity [57,58]. Many xenobiotics are metabolized in the liver, thereby increasing the potential for liver-specific alteration of proteins [59]. In fact, a liver-specific autoimmune disease can be observed in some patients exposed to chlorofluorohydrocarbon anesthetics [60,61]. Previous work has reported that immunization with halothane, whose trifluoroacetyl

(TFA) metabolite covalently links to lysine on cytochrome P450 2E1 [62], induces the formation of antibodies that cross-react with not only the haptenated (TFA) immunogen, but also to lipoated PDC–E2, the major autoantigen of PBC [63,64]. This finding has important implications in the pathogenic mechanisms associated with PBC, an autoimmune disease marked by the presence of AMAs [65,66]. The target of AMAs are the E2 components of the 2-oxo acid dehydrogenase pathway, particularly PDC–E2 [65], and the primary B cell epitope of PDC–E2 recognized by AMAs includes a lipoated lysine residue [67,68].

Our laboratory has had a long-standing interest in defining the etiological basis of PBC [65]. Thus, although we and others have identified the major autoantigens of PBC, it is not clear as to the event(s) that initiate(s) the recognition of these self-proteins as immunogenic. One of our working hypotheses has been that potential modifications of self proteins by agents such as xenobiotics may alter these self proteins enough to cause a breakdown of tolerance; that is immune responses that cross react with mature self molecules. In this way, the immune response would be perpetuated by the chronic low-level turnover of the self protein. The autoantigen PDC–E2 is essential for the function of mitochondria by using lipoic acid to rapidly transition between an oxidized and reduced state. Moreover, porcine PDC–E2 loses antigenicity when lipoic acid is removed [69] confirming our observation that lipoic acid is necessary for reactivity. Perhaps the preference for enzymes, containing substituents like lipoic acid, can be explained because the functional site of the enzymes are more accessible and therefore more susceptible to modification by exogenous agents (e.g. xenobiotics), thus providing neoantigens that can be recognized by the immune system [70].

The liver is an important organ for metabolism/degradation for xenobiotics and an altered immune response [71]. A large number of chemicals, including halogenated compounds, are detoxified through the liver and secreted in the bile. Hence, exposure to an agent that would uniquely modify the mitochondrial antigens within biliary epithelium, could lead to a breakdown of tolerance and induction of a self-reactive response that is target-specific. Moreover, there is evidence, based on in vivo studies in guinea pigs exposed to halothane, that Kupffer cells carry trifluoroacetylated protein adducts [72]; these protein adducts are not found in other organs, including hilar lymph nodes. This provides evidence that the generation of autoreactivity to the protein adducts is likely a local liver response. We should also note the possibility that xenobiotics have other immunotoxic potential, including a selective stimulation or inhibition of components of the immune system [57]. Such effects, of course, would be independent of any modification of autoantigens.

We postulate that people genetically predisposed to PBC have inherited such predisposition based on either the cytochrome P450 pathway or another metabolic process responsible for degrading halogenated compounds. A large number of common pharmaceuticals, such as diuretic agents, are halogenated structures. In fact, halogens are common substituents in pharmaceuticals that modulate binding, activity and metabolism. In addition, there are large numbers of detergents, commonly used at home and commercially, that are rich in halogenated derivatives. Estrogens have already been shown to modulate the expression of many liver metabolic pathways and may explain the preponderance of women with PBC. Finally, the presence of primarily small bile duct destruction may be reflective of the local mucosal immune response, which is more prominent on epithelial surfaces [47]. Indeed, PBC is often referred to as an epitheliitis with involvement not only of bile ducts, but also of salivary glands.

Defining the precise sequence and the molecular basis by which xenobiotics initiate the cascade of autoimmune responses is the next challenge for understanding the etiology and pathogenesis of PBC.

REFERENCES

[1] Metcalf J, James O. The geoepidemiology of primary biliary cirrhosis. Semin Liver Dis 1997; 17: 13–22.

[2] Gershwin ME, Ansari AA, Mackay IR, Nishio A, Rowley MJ, Coppel RL. Primary biliary cirrhosis: an orchestrated immune response against epithelial cells. Immunol Rev 2000; 174: 210–225.

[3] Fregeau DR, Prindiville T, Coppel RL, Kaplan M, Dickson ER, Gershwin ME. Inhibition of alpha-ketoglutarate dehydrogenase activity by a distinct population of autoantibodies recognizing dihydrolipoamide succinyltransferase in primary biliary cirrhosis. Hepatology 1990; 11: 975–981.

[4] Coppel RL, McNeilage LJ, Surh CD, Van de Water J, Spithill TW, Whittingham S et al. Primary structure of the human M2 mitochondrial autoantigen of primary biliary cirrhosis: dihydrolipoamide acetyltransferase. Proc Natl Acad Sci USA 1988; 85: 7317–7321.

[5] Nakanuma Y, Tsuneyama K, Gershwin ME, Yashoshima M. Pathology and immunopathology of primary biliary cirrhosis with emphasis on bile duct lesions: recent progress. Semin Liver Dis 1995; 15: 313–328.

[6] Van de Water J, Gershwin ME, Leung P, Ansari A, Coppel RL. The autoepitope of the 74-kD mitochondrial autoantigen of primary biliary cirrhosis corresponds to the functional site of dihydrolipoamide acetyltransferase. J Exp Med 1988; 167: 1791–1799.

[7] Harris R, Bowker-Kinley M, Wu P, Jeng J, Popov K. Dihydrolipoamide dehydrogenase complex: DNA-derived amino acid sequence, expression, and reconstitution of the pyruvate dehydrogenase complex. J Biol Chem 1997; 272: 6361–6369.

[8] Bandin O, Couvalin J, Poupon R, Dubel L, Homberg J, Johannet C. Specificity and sensitivity of gp210 autoantibodies detected using an enzyme-linked immunosorbent assay and a synthetic polypeptide in the diagnosis of primary biliary cirrhosis. Hepatology 1996; 23: 1020–1024.

[9] Witt-Sullivan H, Heathcote J, Cauch K, Blendis L, Ghent C, Katz A et al. The demography of primary biliary cirrhosis in Ontario, Canada. Hepatology 1990; 12: 98–105.

[10] Cauch-Dudek K, Abbey S, Stewart DE, Heathcote EJ. Fatigue in primary biliary cirrhosis. Gut 1998; 43: 705–710.

[11] Osborne EC, Wooten IE, DiSalva LC. Serum bile acid levels in liver disease. Lancet 1959; II: 1049–1053.

[12] Bergasa NV, Jones EA. The pruritus of cholestasis: potential pathogenic and therapeutic implications of opioids. Gastroenterology 1995; 108: 1582–1588.

[13] Burroughs AK, Rosenstein IJ, Epstein O, Hamilton-Miller JM, Brumfitt W, Sherlock S. Bacteriuria and primary biliary cirrhosis. Gut 1984; 25: 133–137.

[14] Nijhawan PK, Therneau TM, Dickson ER, Boynton J, Lindor KD. Incidence of cancer in primary biliary cirrhosis: the Mayo experience. Hepatology 1999; 29: 1396–1398.

[15] Floreani A, Baragiotta A, Baldo V, Menegon T, Farinati F, Naccarato R. Hepatic and extrahepatic malignancies in primary biliary cirrhosis. Hepatology 1999; 29: 1425–1428.

[16] Mitchison HC, Bassendine MF, Hendrick A, Bennett MK, Bird G, Watson AJ et al. Positive antimitochondrial antibody but normal alkaline phosphatase: is this primary biliary cirrhosis? Hepatology 1986; 6: 1279–1284.
[17] Scheuer P. Primary biliary cirrhosis. Proc R Soc Med 1967; 60: 1257–1260.
[18] Melegh B, Skuta G, Pajor L, Hegedus G, Sumegi B. Autoantibodies against subunits of pyruvate dehydrogenase and citrate synthase in a case of paediatric biliary cirrhosis. Gut 1998; 42: 753–756.
[19] Watson RG, Angus PW, Dewar M, Goss B, Sewell RB, Smallwood RA. Low prevalence of primary biliary cirrhosis in Victoria, Australia. Melbourne Liver Group. Gut 1995; 36: 927–930.
[20] Myszor M, James OF. The epidemiology of primary biliary cirrhosis in north-east England: an increasingly common disease? Q J Med 1990; 75: 377–385.
[21] Triger DR. Primary biliary cirrhosis: an epidemiological study. Br Med J 1980; 281: 772–775.
[22] Van de Water J, Ansari AA, Surh CD, Coppel R, Roche T, Bonkovsky H et al. Evidence for the targeting by 2-oxo-dehydrogenase enzymes in the T cell response of primary biliary cirrhosis. J Immunol 1991; 146: 89–94.
[23] Shimoda S, Van de Water J, Ansari A, Nakamura M, Ishibashi H, Coppel R et al. Identification and precursor frequency analysis of a common T cell epitope motif in mitochondrial autoantigens in primary biliary cirrhosis. J Clin Invest 1998; 102: 1831–1840.
[24] Van de Water J, Ansari A, Prindiville T, Coppel R, Ricalton N, Kotzin BL et al. Heterogeneity of autoreactive T cell clones specific for the E2 component of the pyruvate dehydrogenase complex in primary biliary cirrhosis. J Exp Med 1995; 181: 723–733.
[25] Yeaman SJ, Fussey SP, Danner DJ, James OF, Mutimer DJ, Bassendine MF. Primary biliary cirrhosis: identification of two major M2 mitochondrial autoantigens. Lancet 1988; 1: 1067–1070.
[26] Walker JG, Doniach D, Roitt IM, Sherlock S. Serological tests in the diagnosis of primary biliary cirrhosis. Lancet 1965; 1: 827–830.
[27] Gershwin ME, Mackay IR, Sturgess A, Coppel RL. Identification and specificity of a cDNA encoding the 70 kd mitochondrial antigen recognized in primary biliary cirrhosis. J Immunol 1987; 138: 3525–3531.
[28] Nalbandian G, Van de Water J, Gish R, Manns M, Coppel RL, Rudich SM et al. Is there a serological difference between men and women with primary biliary cirrhosis? Am J Gastroenterol 1999; 94: 2482–2486.
[29] Dubel L, Tanaka A, Leung PS, Van de Water J, Coppel R, Roche T et al. Autoepitope mapping and reactivity of autoantibodies to the dihydrolipoamide dehydrogenase-binding protein (E3BP) and the glycine cleavage proteins in primary biliary cirrhosis. Hepatology 1999; 29: 1013–1018.
[30] Itoh S, Ichida T, Yoshida T, Hayakawa A, Uchida M, Tashiro-Itoh T et al. Autoantibodies against a 210 kDa glycoprotein of the nuclear pore complex as a prognostic marker in patients with primary biliary cirrhosis. J Gastroenterol Hepatol 1998; 13: 257–265.
[31] Wesierska-Gadek J, Honenauer H, Hitchman E, Penner E. Autoantibodies against nucleoporin p62 constitute a novel marker of primary biliary cirrhosis. Gastroenterology 1996; 110: 840–847.
[32] Szostecki C, Krippner H, Penner E, Bautz FA. Autoimmune sera recognize a 100 kD nuclear protein antigen (sp-100). Clin Exp Immunol 1987; 68: 108–116.
[33] Sternsdorf T, Guldner HH, Szostecki C, Grotzinger T, Will H. Two nuclear dot-associated

proteins, PML and Sp100, are often co-autoimmunogenic in patients with primary biliary cirrhosis. Scand J Immunol 1995; 42: 257–268.
[34] Courvalin JC, Lassoued K, Worman HJ, Blobel G. Identification and characterization of autoantibodies against the nuclear envelope lamin B receptor from patients with primary biliary cirrhosis. J Exp Med 1990; 172: 961–967.
[35] Fussey SP, Ali ST, Guest JR, James OF, Bassendine MF, Yeaman SJ. Reactivity of primary biliary cirrhosis sera with Escherichia coli dihydrolipoamide acetyltransferase (E2p): characterization of the main immunogenic region. Proc Natl Acad Sci USA 1990; 87: 3987–3991.
[36] Teoh KL, Mackay IR, Rowley MJ, Fussey SP. Enzyme inhibitory autoantibodies to pyruvate dehydrogenase complex in primary biliary cirrhosis differ for mammalian, yeast and bacterial enzymes: implications for molecular mimicry. Hepatology 1994; 19: 1029–1033.
[37] Howel D, Fischbacher CM, Bhopal RS, Gray J, Metcalf JV, James OFW. An exploratory population-based case-control study of primary biliary cirrhosis. Hepatology 2000; 31: 1055–1060.
[38] Donaldson P, Doherty D, Underhill J, Williams R. The molecular genetics of autoimmune liver disease. [Review]. Hepatology 1994; 20: 225–239.
[39] Adams DH, Hubscher SG, Shaw J, Johnson GD, Babbs C, Rothlein R et al. Increased expression of intercellular adhesion molecule 1 on bile ducts in primary biliary cirrhosis and primary sclerosing cholangitis. Hepatology 1991; 14: 426–431.
[40] Tsuneyama K, Van de water J, Leung PSC, Cha S, Nakanuma Y, Kaplan M et al. Abnormal expression of the E2 component of the pyruvate dehydrogenase complex on the luminal surface of biliary epithelium occurs before major histocompatibility complex class II and BB1/B7 expression. Hepatology 1995; 21: 1031–1037.
[41] Migliaccio C, Nishio A, Van de Water J, Ansari AA, Leung PS, Nakanuma Y et al. Monoclonal antibodies to mitochondrial E2 components define autoepitopes in primary biliary cirrhosis. J Immunol 1998; 161: 5157–5163.
[42] Van de Water J, Gerson LB, Ferrell LD, Lake JR, Coppel RL, Batts KP et al. Immunohistochemical evidence of disease recurrence after liver transplantation for primary biliary cirrhosis. Hepatology 1996; 24: 1079–1084.
[43] McConnell BB, McKean MC, Danner DJ. Influence of subunit transcript and protein levels on formation of a mitochondrial multienzyme complex. J Cell Biochem 1996; 61: 118–126.
[44] Takakubo F, Cartwright P, Hoogenraad N, Thorburn D, Collins F, Lithgow T et al. An amino acid substitution in the pyruvate dehydrogenase E1 alpha gene, affecting mitochondrial import of the precursor protein. Am J Hum Genet 1995; 57: 772–780.
[45] Joplin R, Wallace L, Lindsay J, Palmer J, Yeaman S, Neuberger J. The human biliary epithelial cell plasma membrane antigen in primary biliary cirrhosis: pyruvate dehydrogenase X. Gastroenterology 1996; 113: 1727–1733.
[46] Reynoso-Paz S, Coppel RL, Mackay IR, Bass NM, Ansari AA, Gershwin ME. The immunobiology of bile and biliary epithelium. Hepatology 1999; 30: 351–357.
[47] Reynoso-Paz S, Leung PS, Van De Water J, Tanaka A, Munoz S, Bass N et al. Evidence for a locally driven mucosal response and the presence of mitochondrial antigens in saliva in primary biliary cirrhosis. Hepatology 2000; 31: 24–29.
[48] Tsuneyama K, Van de Water J, Nakanuma Y, Cha S, Ansari A, Coppel R et al. Human combinatorial autoantibodies and mouse monoclonal antibodies to PDC–E2 produce abnormal apical staining of salivary glands in patients with coexistent primary biliary cirrhosis and Sjögren's syndrome. Hepatology 1994; 20: 893–898.
[49] Koga H, Sakisaka S, Ohishi M, Sata M, Tanikawa K. Nuclear DNA fragmentation and expression of Bcl-2 in primary biliary cirrhosis. Hepatology 1997; 25: 1077–1084.

[50] Krams SM, Surh CD, Coppel RL, Ansari A, Ruebner B, Gershwin ME. Immunization of experimental animals with dihydrolipoamide acetyltransferase, as a purified recombinant polypeptide, generates mitochondrial antibodies but not primary biliary cirrhosis. Hepatology 1989; 9: 411–416.
[51] Jones DE, Palmer JM, Yeaman SJ, Kirby JA, Bassendine MF. Breakdown of tolerance to pyruvate dehydrogenase complex in experimental autoimmune cholangitis: a mouse model of primary biliary cirrhosis. Hepatology 1999; 30: 65–70.
[52] Quaranta S, Shulman H, Ahmed A, Shoenfeld Y, Peter J, McDonald GB et al. Autoantibodies in human chronic graft-versus-host disease after hematopoietic cell transplantation. Clin Immunol 1999; 91: 106–116.
[53] O'Donohue J, Fidler H, Garcia-Barcelo M, Nouri-Aria K, Williams R, McFadden J. Mycobacterial DNA not detected in liver sections from patients with primary biliary cirrhosis. J Hepatol 1998; 28: 433–438.
[54] Mason AL, Xu L, Guo L, Munoz S, Jaspan JB, Bryer-Ash M et al. Detection of retroviral antibodies in primary biliary cirrhosis and other idiopathic biliary disorders. Lancet 1998; 351: 1620–1624.
[55] Rose NR. Viral damage or 'molecular mimicry'-placing the blame in myocarditis. Nat Med 2000; 6: 631–632.
[56] Medzhitov R, Janeway C. How does the immune system distinguish self from nonself? Sem Immunol 2000; 12: 185–188.
[57] Powell J, Van de Water J, Gershwin ME. Evidence for the environmental agents in the initiation or progression of autoimmune conditions. Environ Health Perspect 1999; 107: 667–672.
[58] Rao T, Richardson B. Environmentally induced autoimmune diseases: potential mechanisms. Environ Health Perspect 1999; 107(Suppl. 5): 737–742.
[59] Kammer A, van der Burg S, Grabscheid B, Hunziker I, Kwappenberg K, Reichen J et al. Molecular mimicry of human cytochrome p450 by hepatitis C virus at the level of cytotoxic T cell recognition. J Exp Med 1999; 190: 169–176.
[60] Njoku D, Laster M, Gong D, Eger E, Reed G, Martin JL. Biotransformation of halothane, enflurane, isoflurane and desflurane to trifluroacetylated liver proteins: association between protein acylation and hepatic injury. Anesthesiol Anal 1997; 84: 173–178.
[61] Sinha A, Clatch R, Stuck G, Blumenthal S, Patel S. Isoflurane Hepatotoxicity: A case report and review of the literature. Am J Gastroenterol 1996; 91: 2406–2409.
[62] Bourdi M, Chen W, Peter RM, Martin JL, Buters JT, Nelson SD et al. Human cytochrome P450 2E1 is a major autoantigen associated with halothane hepatitis. Chem Res Toxicol 1996; 9: 1159–1166.
[63] Gut J, Christen U, Frey N, Koch V, Stoffler D. Molecular mimicry in halothane hepatitis: biochemical and structural characterization of lipoylated autoantigens. Toxicology 1995; 97: 199–224.
[64] Sasaki M, Ansari AA, Nakanuma Y, Coppel RL, Keeffe EB, Gershwin ME. The immunopathology of primary biliary cirrhosis: thoughts for the millennium. Arch Immunol Ther Exp 2000; 48: 1–10.
[65] Gershwin ME, Ansari AA, Mackay IR, Nakanuma Y, Nishio A, Rowley MJ et al. Primary biliary cirrhosis: an orchestrated immune response against epithelial cells. Immunol Rev 2000; 174: 210–225.
[66] Leung PS, Coppel RL, Ansari A, Munoz S, Gershwin ME. Antimitochondrial antibodies in primary biliary cirrhosis. Semin Liver Dis 1997; 17: 61–69.
[67] Coppel RL, Gershwin ME. Primary biliary cirrhosis: the molecule and the mimic. Immunol Rev 1995; 144: 17–49.

[68] Shimoda S, Van de Water J, Ansari A, Nakamura M, Ishibashi H, Coppel RL et al. Identification and precursor frequency analysis of a common T cell epitope motif in mitochondrial autoantigens in primary biliary cirrhosis. J Clin Invest 1998; 102: 1831–1840.

[69] Koike K, Ishibashi H, Koike M. Immunoreactivity of porcine heart dihydrolipoamide acetyl- and succinyl-transferases (PDC–E2, OGDC–E2) with primary biliary cirrhosis sera: characterization of the autoantigenic region and effects of enzymatic delipoylation and relipoylation. Hepatology 1998; 27: 1467–1474.

[70] Steinman L. Absence of 'Original Antigenic Sin' in autoimmunity provides an unforeseen platform for immune therapy. J Exp Med 1999; 189: 1021–1024.

[71] Bustmante J, Lodge J, Marcocci L, Tritshler H, Packer L, Rihn B. Alpha-lipoic acid in liver metabolism and disease. Free Radic Biol Med 1998; 24: 1023–1039.

[72] Furst SM, Luedke D, Gandolfi AJ. Kupffer cells from halothane-exposed guinea pigs carry trifluoroacetylated protein adducts. Toxicology 1997; 120: 119–132.

Edited by T. Tsuji, T. Higashi, M. Zeniya and K.-H. Meyer zum Büschenfelde

CHAPTER 19

Induction of T Cell Anergy by Peptide Analogues in Primary Biliary Cirrhosis

Hiromi Ishibashi, Shinji Shimoda, Hirohisa Shigematsu and Minoru Nakamura

Medicine and Biosystemic Science, Kyushu University Graduate School of Medical Sciences, Fukuoka, Japan

INTRODUCTION

Characteristic features of primary biliary cirrhosis (PBC) are; (1) the presence of autoantibody, antimitochondrial antibody (AMA) and/or antinuclear antibody, in patient's sera, (2) the specific destruction of small bile ducts in the liver, (3) marked infiltration of lymphocytes, predominantly T and B cells, around small bile ducts in the portal area [1], (4) frequent association of other autoimmune disease(s), and (5) familial clustering and a weak but significant association with HLA [2]. Thus, an autoimmune mechanism seems to be a cause of the bile duct damage [3]. However, the precise immune mechanism occurring at the molecular level remains to be elucidated.

The hallmark of this disease is the disease-specific appearance of AMA. Cloning and identification of major antigens recognized by AMA have been performed by Gershwin et al. since 1987, when they identified the major M2 antigens as the E2 component of pyruvate dehydrogenase complexes (PDC-E2). Other components of 2-oxo acid dehydrogenase complex have also been identified; OGDC-E2, BCOADC-E2, E3BP, E1α and E1β of PDC. Gershwin et al. and we have mapped the B cell epitope of PDC-E2 in the inner and outer lipoyl domains of PDC-E2 [4–6]. We have also generated the cloned B cell lines that produce the human monoclonal antibody to the PDC-E2 from a PBC patient, and analyzed the nucleotide sequences of complementarity determining region of the anti-human PDC-E2 immunoglobulin variable region. The results suggested that the B cells that produce the autoantibody with high specificity and high affinity to human PDC-E2 are stimulated and expanded by an antigen-driven, clonal selection process [7,8].

T cells play a central role in the immune response. T cell activation is initiated upon recognition of an antigen peptide bound to a major histocompatibility complex by the T cell receptor. With the aid of co-stimulatory signals, T cells exert effector functions by various biological activities of secreted lymphokines. T cell response can be altered by modulating the antigen peptide, and such peptide analogues can induce qualitative changes in the T cell response; T cell anergy, changes in proliferative responses of T cells or lymphokine production.

The aim of this study is to investigate the response of antigen-specific T cells to various analogue peptides to identify peptides that induce anergy or cause changes in the proliferative response of T cells. The strategy which we took to identify the analogue peptides that modulate the immune response is as follows: (1) identification of the T cell epitope in PDC, (2) generation of T cell clones reactive to the antigen peptide, (3) synthesis of peptides that are analogous to the epitope peptide: (a) one amino acid-substituted peptides or (b) mimicry peptides which have a homologous sequence to the epitope peptide, and finally, (4) an assay of the reactivity of the cloned T cell lines against synthetic analogue peptides.

The final goal of this study is the clinical application of antigen-specific immunotherapy for the treatment of PBC.

1. IDENTIFICATION OF T CELL EPITOPE

To identify the T cell epitope of the PDC-E2, we synthesized 33 peptides covering the entire molecule of human PDC-E2. The peptides were separated to seven groups, consisting of five peptides in each peptide mixture. Peripheral blood mononuclear cells (PBMC) obtained from PBC patients or healthy subjects were assayed for proliferation to these peptide mixtures. Since T cells responded to the peptide mixture groups 2 or 3, we tested the proliferation of T cells using each peptide in Group 3. Consequently, all T cells responded only to one peptide, PDC-E2 163–182, among 5 peptides in the Group 3 peptide mixture [9].

2. ANTIGEN SPECIFICITY AND HLA RESTRICTION OF THE T CELL RESPONSE

Antigen specificity of the PDC-E2 163–176-reactive T cells was studied. The T cells responded only to PDC in a dose-dependent manner, but not to other antigens such as ovalbumin or OGDC. The response was abolished by the addition of anti-CD3, anti-CD4 or anti-DR antibodies, suggesting that these T cells are CD3 and CD4 positive, and the reaction is restricted by DR antigens [9].

The HLA restriction of the PDC-E2 163–176-reactive T cell clone was studied using L cells transfected with the DRB1*0405, DRB1*0901 and DRB4*0101 genes, expressing DR4, DR9 and DR53 molecules on the cell surface, respectively. The T cell response was observed only when DR53 was used but not when DR4 or DR9 were used, suggesting that the T cells are restricted by DR53 [10].

3. MINIMAL EPITOPE MAPPING

To identify the minimal epitope of this peptide, we truncated the 163–182 peptide from both N- and C-terminals, and the truncated peptides were assayed for the proliferation of T cells. The minimal epitope was determined as 163–176 of PDC-E2. The T cell epitope thus identified is localized on the inner lipoyl domain of PDC-E2.

The region, 36–49, on the outer lipoyl domain was also determined as an epitope [9]. Interestingly, these T cell epitopes are mapped at almost the same region as the B cell epitopes [4–6].

Essential amino acids in this peptide for the proliferation of T cells were identified by substituting each amino acid of the peptide to alanine or serine. Glutaminic acid (E) at position 170, aspartic acid (D) at position 172 and lysine (K) at position 173 were found to be essential for the proliferation of all the cloned T cell lines, and an ExDK sequence appeared to be an important motif for the proliferation of T cells [9].

4. FREQUENCY OF T CELLS IN THE PERIPHERAL BLOOD AND THE LIVER

PDC-E2 163–176-reactive T cells are present among PBMC of PBC patients at 8-fold higher frequency than that in healthy subjects [10]. Furthermore, these T cells are present in the liver and regional lymph nodes of PBC patients at 100 to 150-fold higher frequency than that in the peripheral blood [11].

Thus, the characteristics of PDC-E2 163–176-specific T cells are summarized as follows; (1) PDC-E2 163–176 is the immunodominant epitope in mitochondrial antigens, (2) T cell epitopes are localized at almost the same regions as B cell epitopes on PDC-E2, (3) the T cells specific to this epitope are present in the peripheral blood of PBC patients at higher frequency than that of healthy subjects, (4) the T cells exist in the liver and regional lymph nodes at higher frequency than that in the peripheral blood, (5) all these T cells are $CD3^+CD4^+CD8^-CD45RA^-CD45RO^+TCR\alpha\beta^+$ cells, HLA DRB4*0101 (DR53)-restricted and cytokine production pattern being Th1-like. From these results, PDC-E2 163–176-specific T cells are considered to play an important role in the pathogenesis of PBC [3].

5. PROLIFERATIVE RESPONSE OF T CELLS AGAINST ANALOGUE PEPTIDES

We generated PDC-E2 163–176 specific T cells by repeated in vitro stimulation of peripheral T lymphocytes with human PDC-E2 163–176, and established four T cell clones from healthy subjects and six clones from PBMC of PBC patients. We synthesized peptides analogous to the epitope PDC-E2 163–176: (a) mimicry peptides that have an ExDK-sequence, (b) one amino acid-substituted peptides. Mimicry peptides were searched by the following criteria. Substituting an amino acid at positions 170, 172 and 173 with peptides of similar natures, peptides having the amino acid sequence <EDNQ> at position 170, <DENQ> at position 172 and <KRH> at position 173 were searched using the Swiss protein data base [13]. Thirty-seven homologous peptides having relatively higher homology with human PDC-E2 163–176 were selected from viruses, bacteria or human autoantigens. All peptides were synthesized using a solid-phase peptide synthesizer, based on an Fmoc strategy and were purified by reversed-phase HPLC.

We tested the proliferation of PDC-E2 163–176-specific T cells using 37 mimicry peptides having an ExDK sequence, some of which are derived from human autoantigens and others from bacteria. Response of PDC-E2 163–176-reactive T cells against mimicry peptides was unique to each T cell clone. Some T cell clones reacted to

Wild type	G	D	L	L	A	E	I	E	T	D	K	A	T	I
L165A	–	–	A	–	–	–	–	–	–	–	–	–	–	–
L165S	–	–	S	–	–	–	–	–	–	–	–	–	–	–
L166A	–	–	–	A	–	–	–	–	–	–	–	–	–	–
L166S	–	–	–	S	–	–	–	–	–	–	–	–	–	–
A167S	–	–	–	–	S	–	–	–	–	–	–	–	–	–
E168A	–	–	–	–	–	A	–	–	–	–	–	–	–	–
E168D	–	–	–	–	–	D	–	–	–	–	–	–	–	–
E168Q	–	–	–	–	–	Q	–	–	–	–	–	–	–	–
I169A	–	–	–	–	–	–	A	–	–	–	–	–	–	–
I169S	–	–	–	–	–	–	S	–	–	–	–	–	–	–
E170A	–	–	–	–	–	–	–	A	–	–	–	–	–	–
E170D	–	–	–	–	–	–	–	D	–	–	–	–	–	–
E170Q	–	–	–	–	–	–	–	Q	–	–	–	–	–	–
E170T	–	–	–	–	–	–	–	T	–	–	–	–	–	–
E170H	–	–	–	–	–	–	–	H	–	–	–	–	–	–
E170Y	–	–	–	–	–	–	–	Y	–	–	–	–	–	–
E170N	–	–	–	–	–	–	–	N	–	–	–	–	–	–
T171A	–	–	–	–	–	–	–	–	A	–	–	–	–	–
T171S	–	–	–	–	–	–	–	–	S	–	–	–	–	–
D172A	–	–	–	–	–	–	–	–	–	A	–	–	–	–
D172E	–	–	–	–	–	–	–	–	–	E	–	–	–	–
D172N	–	–	–	–	–	–	–	–	–	N	–	–	–	–
D172T	–	–	–	–	–	–	–	–	–	T	–	–	–	–
D172H	–	–	–	–	–	–	–	–	–	H	–	–	–	–
D172Y	–	–	–	–	–	–	–	–	–	Y	–	–	–	–
D172Q	–	–	–	–	–	–	–	–	–	Q	–	–	–	–
K173A	–	–	–	–	–	–	–	–	–	–	A	–	–	–
K173R	–	–	–	–	–	–	–	–	–	–	R	–	–	–
K173H	–	–	–	–	–	–	–	–	–	–	H	–	–	–

Fig. 1. One amino acid-substituted peptides of PDC-E2 163–176. One amino acid substituted peptides were synthesized using a solid-phase peptide synthesizer, based on an Fmoc strategy. All peptides were purified by reversed-phase HPLC. In total, 29 one amino acid-substituted analogue peptides were synthesized.

mimicry peptides derived from human E3BP or OGDC, and others to some mimicry peptides derived from bacteria [12].

In total, 29 one amino acid-substituted analogue peptides were synthesized (Fig. 1). Using these peptides, we assayed the proliferation of the cloned T cells against peptides. The dose–response curve to the set of analogue peptides was compared with that of the original peptide. The response was classified into 3 groups; group A consists of analogue peptides that were more potent than the wild type peptide, i.e., Q and A at position ^{168}E (Fig. 2A) [13]. Group B consists of peptides that decreased the response by one or two orders of magnitude, i.e., E at position ^{172}D and A at position ^{165}L (Fig. 2B). However, group C, as shown in Fig. 2C, consists of peptides that completely abrogated the proliferative response of the T cells; peptides with some substitutions, i.e., A, R and H at position ^{173}K [13].

6. ANERGY ASSAY

We performed an anergy assay to identify analogue peptides that induce anergy to the T cells. Briefly, T cells were preincubated for 24 hours with a test peptide in the

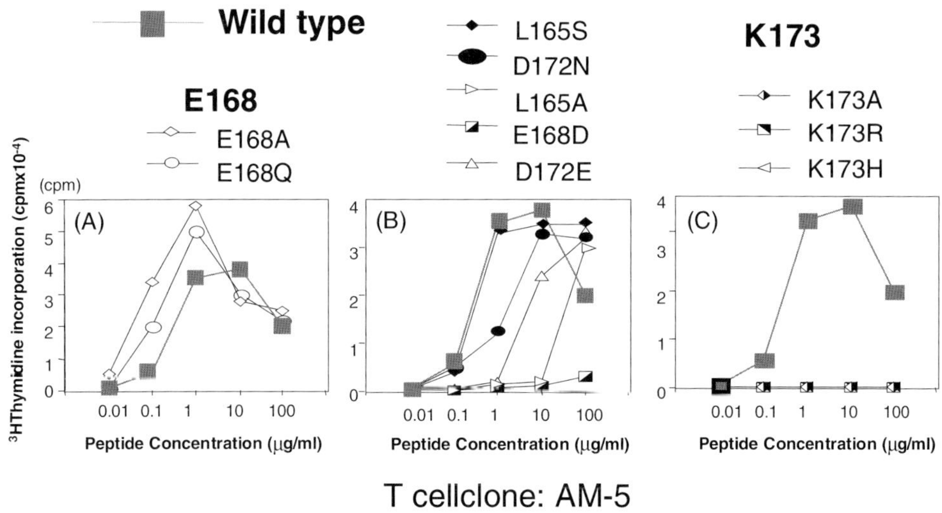

Fig. 2. Response of PDC-E2 163–176-reactive T cell clones to analogue peptides. The dose–response curve to the set of analogue peptides was compared with that of the original peptide. The response was classified into 3 groups. (A) Group consists of the analogue peptides that were more potent than the wild type peptide (i.e., Q and A at position ^{168}E). (B) Group consists of peptides that decreased the response by one or two orders of magnitude (i.e., E at position ^{172}D and A at position ^{165}L). However, (C) group peptides completely abrogated the proliferative response of the T cells; peptides with some substitutions (i.e., A, R and H at position ^{173}K). (Ref. [13])

presence of irradiated auto-PBMC as antigen-presenting cells. Then, the T cells were transferred to the well containing irradiated auto-PBMC pulsed with a wild-type peptide, then cultured for 72 hours. The T cell proliferation was assayed by thymidine uptake. If the test peptide has an antagonistic or partial agonistic activity, the proliferation of T cells by the wild type peptide would be altered. In T cell clone HT-6, one peptide with substitution of K (lysine) to H (histidine) at position 173 suppressed the T cell proliferation stimulated by the wild type 163–176 peptide. In clone IY-1, two peptides with substitution E (glutamic acid) to D (aspartic acid) or Q (glutamine) at position 165 suppressed the T cell proliferation stimulated by the wild 163–176 peptide (Fig. 3) [13]. This indicates that these analogue peptides have an ability to induce anergy to T cells.

SUMMARY

In summary, we localized immunodominant T cell epitopes on PDC-E2. The PDC-E2 163–176 peptide-reactive T cell is considered to be associated with pathogenesis of PBC. The pattern of the recognition of a peptide/HLA DR53 complex by PDC-E2 163–176 peptide-reactive T cells was diverse, but the ExDK motif is essential to recognition by T cells. Among T cells that recognize the ExDK motif, there exist T cells that respond to other autoantigens, such as human OGDC-E2 or E3BP peptide, indicating

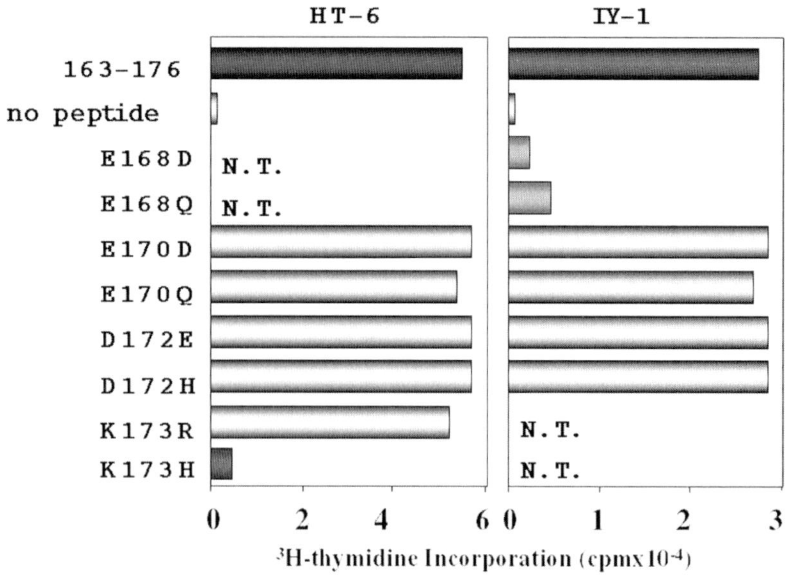

Fig. 3D. Induction of anergy by analogue peptides. In T cell clone HT-6, one peptide with substitution of K (lysine) to H (histidine) at position 173 suppressed the T cell proliferation stimulated by the original 163–176 peptide. On the other hand, in clone IY-1 two peptides with substitution of E (glutamic acid) to D (aspartic acid) or Q (glutamine) at position 165 suppressed the T cell proliferation stimulated by the original 163–176 peptide, indicating that these analogue peptides have an activity to induce anergy to T cells. (Ref. [13])

the molecular basis of cross-reactivity among proteins of 2-OADC. Several analogue peptides that induce anergy to PDC-E2 163–176-reactive T cells were identified.

At present, non-specific immunosuppressive drugs such as UDCA or corticosteroid are used for the treatment of PBC. However, specific immunotherapy based on the specific immune response of T cells is anticipated. To avoid various side effects, analogue peptides that can induce anergy in T cells, soluble analogue peptide/MHC complex, or anti-TCR antibody are under investigation as candidates of specific immunotherapy for PBC.

ACKNOWLEDGEMENTS

This work was supported in part by a Grant-in-Aid for Scientific Research from the Ministry of Education, Science, Sports, and Culture of Japan, a grant for research on Intractable Disease from the Ministry of Public Welfare of Japan, and a grant from a Clinical Research Foundation.

REFERENCES

[1] Nakamura M, Ishibashi H, Matsui M, Shimoda S, Hayashida K, Koike K et al. Peripheral B lymphocyte repertoire to mitochondrial antigen in primary biliary cirrhosis. Positive correlation between the disease activity and the frequency of circulating B lymphocytes specific for pyruvate dehydrogenase complex. Autoimmunity 1995; 21: 253–262.

[2] Mukai T, Kimura A, Ishibashi H, Sasazuki T, Sata M, Maruyama T et al. Association of HLA-DRB1*0803 and *1602 with the susceptibility to primary biliary cirrhosis. Int Hepatol Commun 1995; 3(4): 207–212.

[3] Ishibashi H, Shimoda S, Shigematsu H, Ichiki Y, Nakamura M, Hayashida K et al. Immune pathophysiology of primary biliary cirrhosis. In: Yamanaka M, Toda G, Tanaka T, editors. Progress in Hepatology Vol. 5 Liver and Immunology. Tokyo: Elsevier Science, 1999; pp. 105–115.

[4] Matsui M, Nakamura M, Ishibashi H, Koike K, Kudo J, Niho Y. Human monoclonal antibodies from a patient with primary biliary cirrhosis that recognize two distinct autoepitopes in the E2 component of the pyruvate dehydrogenase complex. Hepatology 1993; 18(5): 1069–1077.

[5] Koike K, Ishibashi H, Koike M. Immunoreactivity of porcine heart dihydrolipoamide acetyl- and succinyl-transferases (PDC-E2, OGDC-E2) with primary biliary cirrhosis sera: Characterization of the autoantigenic region and effects of enzymatic delipoylation and relipoylation. Hepatology 1998; 27(6): 1467–1474.

[6] Ishibashi H, Fukuhsima N, Matsui M, Ikematsu H, Shimoda S, Nakamura M et al. Identification of the epitope of anti-PDC-E2 antibodies and analysis of their immunoglobulin genes. Mechanism of the production of antimitochondrial antibody. In: Autoantibodies and Autoimmunity '99. Nagoya: MBL, 1999; pp. 25–32.

[7] Fukushima N, Nakamura M, Matsui M, Ikematsu H, Koike K, Ishibashi H et al. Establishment and structural analysis of human mAb to the E2 component of the 2-oxoglutarate dehydrogenase complex generated from a patient with primary biliary cirrhosis. Int Immunol 1995; 7(7): 1047–1055.

[8] Fukushima N, Ikematsu H, Nakamura M, Matsui M, Shimoda S, Hayashida K et al. Nucleotide variations amongst V_H genes of AMA-producing B cell clones in primary biliary cirrhosis. J Autoimmunity 2000; 14(3): 247–257.

[9] Shimoda S, Nakamura M, Ishibashi H, Hayashida K, Niho Y. HLA DRB4 0101-restricted immunodominant T cell autoepitope of pyruvate dehydrogenase complex in primary biliary cirrhosis: Evidence of molecular mimicry in human autoimmune diseases. J Exp Med 1995; 181(5): 1835–1845.

[10] Ichiki Y, Shimoda S, Hara H, Shigematsu H, Nakamura M, Hayashida K et al. Analysis of T-cell receptor β of the T-cell clones reactive to the human PDC-E2 163–176 peptide in the context of HLA-DR53 in patients with primary biliary cirrhosis. Hepatology 1997; 26(3): 728–733.

[11] Shimoda S, Van de Water J, Ansari A, Nakamura M, Ishibashi H, Coppel RL et al. Identification and precursor frequency analysis of a common T cell epitope motif in mitochondrial autoantigens in primary biliary cirrhosis. J Clin Invest 1998; 102(10): 1831–1840.

[12] Shimoda S, Nakamura M, Shigematsu H, Tanimoto H, Gushima T, Gershwin ME et al. Mimicry peptides of human PDC-E2 163–176 peptide, the immunodominant T-cell epitope of primary biliary cirrhosis. Hepatology 2000; 31(6): 1212–1216.

[13] Shigematsu H, Shimoda S, Nakamura M, Matsushita S, Nishimura Y, Sakamoto N et al. Fine specificity of T cells reactive to human PDC-E2 163–176 peptide, the immunodominant autoantigen in primary biliary cirrhosis: Implications for molecular mimicry and cross-recognition among mitochondrial autoantigens. Hepatology 2000; 32(5): 901–909.

Molecular Biology and Immunology in Hepatology
Edited by T. Tsuji, T. Higashi, M. Zeniya and K.-H. Meyer zum Büschenfelde

CHAPTER 20

Putative Mechanism of Overlap Syndrome: What is the Entity?

Morikazu Onji [1] and Kazuhide Yamamoto [2]

[1] *Third Department of Internal Medicine, Ehime University School of Medicine, Ehime, Japan*
[2] *First Department of Internal Medicine, Okayama University Medical School, Okayama, Japan*

INTRODUCTION

Autoimmune hepatitis (AIH), primary biliary cirrhosis (PBC) and primary sclerosing cholangitis (PSC) are autoimmune diseases of the liver. They share the presumed autoimmune pathogenesis, although clinical features, course of the disease, and response to therapy are quite distinct among these three conditions.

The factors underlying the breakdown of the immune regulatory mechanism responsible for protecting the liver from the occurrence of autoimmune diseases, may be different among these autoimmune liver diseases, but there have been several reports of patients presenting with clinical and biochemical, and/or histological features reminiscent of both AIH and PBC. Various names have been used for these patients such as overlap syndrome, mixed type chronic aggressive hepatitis (CAH) and PBC, and autoimmune cholangitis (AIC). With the advancement of serological and molecular biological diagnosis of chronic hepatitis due to hepatitis C virus, further experimental data on autoimmune liver diseases were piled up. However, the problems on the entity of overlap syndrome remain controversial. In the present review, we would like to provide a clinical, serological and histological description of the putative concept of overlap syndrome and the mixed type of autoimmune liver diseases.

1. OVERVIEW OF THE OVERLAP SYNDROME OF AUTOIMMUNE LIVER DISEASES

Some reports on borderline diseases of AIH and PBC have been described in the literature during the last 30 years. Popper et al. have reported that PBC–CAH overlap syndrome in 1970; the patients presented with scanty cholestasis, no distinct elevation of serum alkaline phosphatase (ALP) and cholesterol, positivity for anti-mitochondrial antibody (AMA) and anti-smooth muscle antibody (ASMA), and histological features of chronic non-suppurative destructive cholangitis (CNSDC) and chronic hepatitis [1]. These clinical features suggest that these patients were suffering mainly from the AIH type of autoimmune liver disease.

The CAH–PBC mixed type of autoimmune liver disease was described by Berg in 1976. These patients were positive for AMA in the sera, had histological features of both cholestasis and aggressive hepatitis in the liver and responded to glucocorticoid therapy [2,3]. Patients with this mixed form of CAH–PBC type of autoimmune liver diseases had clinical features characteristic of both AIH and PBC, and these patients were positive for type 2 and type 4 AMA, the target antigen for which was sulphite oxidase located in the external membrane of mitochondria [4]. For a while, type 4 AMA was considered to be a specific marker of a mixed form of AIH and PBC; however, the diagnostic specificity of this autoantibody was lost in the course of time. Though very rare, patients with a mixed form of AIH and PBC are still occurring in clinical practice. In these cases, AIH and PBC occur concurrently.

Cholangitis resulting from an autoimmune etiology such as immune-cholangitis, autoimmune cholangiopathy, and autoimmune cholangitis, was reported in 1987 [5]. This pathological condition is characterized by the clinical and histopathological features of chronic intrahepatic cholangitis with a negative test for AMA by immunofluorescence and a positive test for antinuclear antibody (ANA) of an uncharacterized type [6–9]. Initial reports indicated the therapeutic responsiveness of corticosteroid drugs in these patients. Opinions vary as to whether AIC is an independent disease entity, or a serological variant of PBC, or a cholangiopathic variant of AIH. Originally, AIC had three characteristic features: (1) intrahepatic cholestasis similar to PBC, (2) negativity for AMA, and (3) responsiveness to corticosteroid therapy. At present, all three points have become controversial. The most important confusion occurred around the issue of AMA negativity. Using the immunoblotting technique, a study has reported the presence of either one or multiple subclasses (IgG, IgA or IgM) of anti-M2 antibodies in sera from 23 patients with AIC [10]. Although AMA positivity evaluated by highly sensitive methods may indicate that cases with AIC may be nonexisting, it would be premature to conclude this because the significance of low titers of AMA is not still clear, both clinically and histopathologically. In fact, low titers of AMA may even be detected in some patients with typical AIH.

ANA positivity distinguish AIC from the classical PBC, although there is no specific type of ANA characteristics of AIC. Interestingly, some patients with PBC may be positive for ANA, especially the centromere type of ANA. Similar to PBC, patients with AIC also show CNSDC histologically. On the other hand, we have documented hepatitis-like features in patients with AIC both laparoscopically and histologically. Reddish markings were detected by laparoscopy, and focal and interface hepatitis were seen histologically in patients with AIC. It is to be noted that hepatitis-like lesions have also been reported from patients with PBC [11–13]. Hepatitis lesions in AIC are improved by corticosteroid therapy. Existence of hepatitis-like lesions in liver histology from patients with both AIC and PBC have raised new questions concerning the independent entity of these diseases. Good responsiveness to corticosteroid therapy in AIC may be a key point; however, recent studies indicate both good and poor responses to corticosteroid therapy in AIC patients [14]. Although steroid therapy improves the degree of hepatitis in patients with AIC, this therapy does not improve PBC-like biliary lesions; ursodeoxycholic acid is routinely administered in case of AIC.

Many reports about the overlap syndrome of AIH and PBC are now piling up. Czaja classified the overlap syndrome of AIH/PBC or AIH/PSC in concurrent features of autoimmune liver diseases, and the outlier syndrome as AIC [9]. Recent data in this regard have been summarized in Table 1.

2. PUTATIVE MECHANISM OF OVERLAP SYNDROME

PBC, AIH and PSC obviously represent a single entity of autoimmune liver disease, although they have some variant forms. AIC and overlap syndrome have not been established as one disease entity and may have diverse pathological processes. On the other hand, recent reports indicate that they are variant forms of PBC or AIH. How can one address these diversities about the overlapping features of autoimmune liver diseases? The following possibilities may be considered.

(1) Patients with overlap syndrome may suffer from two diseases at the same time.
(2) The diseases may represent the cholestatic form of AIH or the hepatitic form of PBC.
(3) Serological and histological variants of AIH or PBC. In this case, overlapping features of autoimmune liver diseases are manifested between AIH and PBC as part of a continuous spectrum of autoimmune liver diseases. Concurrent features of AIH and PBC are considered as the epiphenomena.
(4) Overlap syndrome may be an independent disease entity.

The mixed form of AIH and PBC is characterized by the presence of combined features of AIH and PBC, because they are serologically positive for both AMA and ANA and show biochemical and histological features of both chronic cholestasis and CAH. They are not an independent disease entity, but rather a simple combination of AIH and PBC. This conclusion is based on the fact that there is no specific clinical, biochemical or histological marker, except seropositivity for the M4 type of AMA. But the diagnostic specificity of the M4 type of AMA is doubtful. The frequency of the mixed form of AIH and PBC is also very low, indicating an accidental circumstantial association between AIH and PBC.

Also AIC is not considered as an independent disease entity. Recent reports have shown that 10–20% patients diagnosed as PBC may also be defined as AIH based on the conventional criteria or by using the AIH scoring system. Interestingly, the frequencies of mixed or overlapping cases of AIH and PBC constitute about 20–30% of the autoimmune liver diseases, although PBC and AIH are rare disease entities compared with other liver diseases [15,16].

The causes underlying the existence of hepatitis-like lesions in AIC and also in some cases with PBC are not known. It is elusive to consider that patients with AIC would have two types of cytotoxic T cells, one targeting the hepatocytes and the other destroying the bile duct epithelium. Lohse et al. provided evidences suggesting that the overlap syndrome of PBC and AIH is a hepatitic form of PBC, because these patients had HLA type characteristics of AIH (B8, DR3 or DR4), were positive for anti-M2

TABLE 1

Outline of autoimmune liver diseases

	AIH	AIH–PBC mixed form	AIC	PBC	Early PBC
Sex	female > male	female > male	female > male	female > male	female > male
Age of onset	middle-aged (peak; 50–59 years)	middle-aged (peak; 50–59 years)	middle-aged (peak; 50–59 years)	middle-aged (peak; 50–59 years)	middle-aged (peak; 50–59 years)
Biochemistry					
GOT–GPT	++–+++	++–+++	+–++	+	normal
ALP–γ GTP	+	++–+++	++–+++	++	normal
IgG	++	++–+++	+	+	normal
IgM	+	++–+++	++–+++	+++	normal
Hematology					
AMA [a]	0–15%	100%	0%	~90%	100
Anti-PDH–OGDH–BCODH antibody [b]	20%		50–100%	100%	
ANA	80–100%	100%	100%	20–70%	
SMA	60–90%	25–60%	~40%	5–10%	
Histology	Hepatitis	CNSDC Hepatitis	CNSDC Hepatitis	CNSDC	CNSDC
Therapy	Adrenocortical hormone Immunosuppressive UDCA	Adrenocortical hormone Immunosuppressive UDCA	Adrenocortical hormone UDCA	UDCA Bezafibrate	

[a] Immunofluorescence.
[b] Immunoblotting.

antibody and had CNSDC in the liver [17]. Although this report is logical, all patients with AIC may not have had AIH-specific HLA typing. At present, this syndrome may be considered as a variant form of AIH and PBC.

2.1. Our recent study on the overlap syndrome

We recently analyzed 111 Japanese patients with overlap syndrome who fulfilled both the diagnostic criteria for PBC and AIH proposed by the Intractable Hepatitis Research Committee of the Japanese Ministry of Health and Welfare. These cases were further classified into definite, PBC-dominant and AIH-dominant overlap depending on PBC and AIH criteria defined by Chazouilleres et al., with slight modifications [15]. PBC criteria included: (1) elevated ALP, at least 1.5 times of the upper limit of normal values, or γ-GTP, at least 3 times; (2) being positive for anti-mitochondrial antibody (AMA); and (3) histological findings such as CNSDC or bile ductopenia. AIH criteria included: (1) elevated ALT, at least 3 times; (2) elevated IgG, at least 1.5 times; and (3) histological findings of interface hepatitis. A definite overlap syndrome was defined when patients had at least two factors of both the PBC and AIH criteria. A PBC-dominant overlap syndrome was defined when patients had at least two PBC factors and one AIH factors. AIH-dominant overlap cases had at least two AIH factors and one PBC factor. Autoimmune cholangitis (AIC) was defined when patients fulfilled the PBC criteria but were negative for AMA and positive for anti-nuclear antibody (ANA).

Definite overlap cases showed elevated ALT levels, IgG and IgM, but neither ALP/ALT nor total cholesterol levels were increased. All cases were positive for both ANA and AMA. Histological examination showed interface hepatitis associated with bile duct lesions. PBC-dominant overlap cases showed elevated levels of ALP/ALT, total cholesterol and IgM, but neither ALT nor IgG levels were elevated. Most cases were positive for both AMA and ANA. Histological examination revealed PBC-like bile duct lesions. AIH-dominant overlap cases showed elevated ALT and IgG levels, but no increase in ALP, total cholesterol or IgM levels. Most cases were positive for ANA and some were positive for AMA. Histologically, the hepatitic feature was dominant with rare bile duct lesion. AIC cases showed biochemical and histological findings similar to PBC but some immunological findings were similar to AIH.

These results suggest that definite overlap cases show both PBC and AIH features in immunological and histological findings but resemble AIH in the biochemical findings. It is necessary to follow the definite overlap cases to find out whether they develop cholestatic liver disease or whether they respond to corticosteroid therapy. The PBC-dominant or AIH-dominant overlap syndrome resembles PBC or AIH but is associated with some immunological features of AIH or PBC, respectively. The feature of AIC resembles that of PBC except for some AIH-like immunological findings. There were few patients who had two distinct entities at the same time. These results suggest that the overlap syndrome manifested as a part of a continuous spectrum of autoimmune liver diseases and that the concurrent features of AIH and PBC are epiphenomena.

We recently introduced a PBC scoring system similar to that for AIH [18,19]. The scoring system includes biochemical, immunological and pathological factors similar to

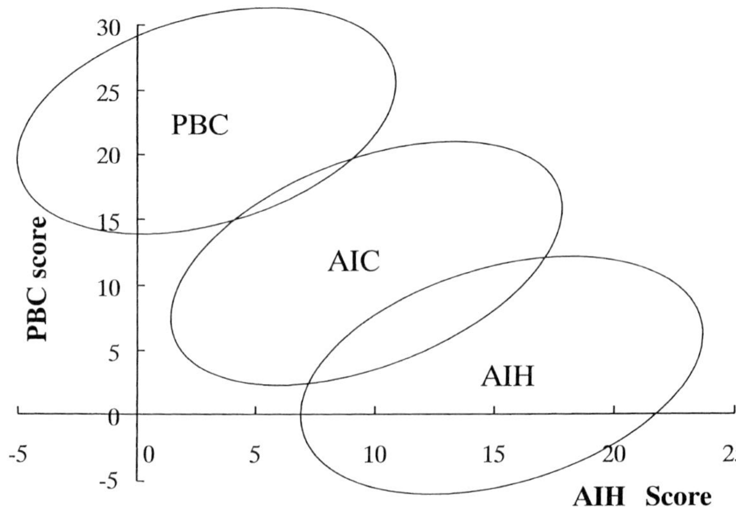

Fig. 1. PBC and AIH scores in PBC, AIC and AIH. PBC and AIH cases are plotted along the vertical axis and horizontal axis, respectively. AIC cases are plotted at the intermediate area.

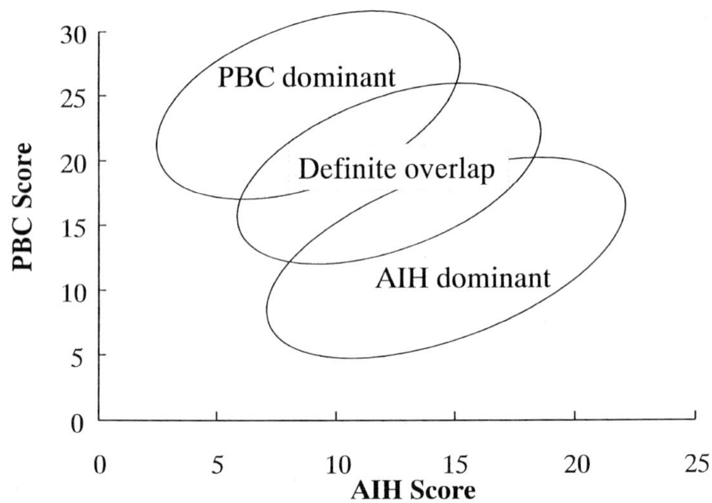

Fig. 2. PBC and AIH scores in overlapping cases of PBC and AIH. Both scores are high in the definite overlap cases. PBC-dominant and AIH-dominant overlap cases are located near PBC and AIH cases, respectively.

the AIH scoring system. Each case was scored using both the AIH and PBC scoring systems and plotted in a rectangular coordinate system (Figs. 1 and 2). Typical PBC and AIH cases are located along vertical or horizontal lines, respectively, while cases of overlap syndrome or autoimmune cholangitis plotted in the area where both scores are high. In particular, patients with a definite overlap syndrome showed high scores on both scoring systems. We suggest that the PBC scoring system is useful to analyze patients with the overlap syndrome or AIC.

3. PRESENT CONCEPT OF OVERLAP SYNDROME OF AUTOIMMUNE LIVER DISEASES

Because the exact etiology is unknown, it is very difficult to define and classify overlap syndrome of autoimmune liver diseases. However, we encounter many cases of overlap syndrome in the clinical practice. Naturally, there is an ethical need to use empirical therapy as treatment option for the overlap syndrome. The mixed form of AIH and PBC may be defined as a combination of both distinct AIH and PBC at the same time. The concept of AIC is a matter of international controversy. In Japan, most cases of AIC are regarded as PBC (AMA-negative by immunofluorescence). It is possible that some of these cases with AIC are different from PBC and the hepatitic form of PBC. Our study indicates that there are some cases of AIH with PBC-like clinical features. We would like to call them the AIH-dominant overlap syndrome.

According to the numerical scoring system of AIH proposed by the International Autoimmune Hepatitis Group, AIH may be diagnosed as definite, probable or other [19]. We propose that PBC and overlap syndrome may also be diagnosed as definite, probable or other. The 'other group' may include early and latent cases of autoimmune liver diseases. Mitchison described 'early PBC' as a disease entity with no apparent clinical features of PBC, a normal routine liver function test (ALP, alanine transaminase, bilirubin) and AMA positivity with histological features of PBC [20]. 'Latent AIH' was reported among patients with non-B, non-C chronic hepatitis in Japan [21] to indicate an early stage or very mild grade of autoimmune liver disease. From these observations we proposed a continuous spectrum of autoimmune liver diseases as presented in Fig. 3.

An overlapping syndrome of PSC and AIH has been repeatedly reported and this has been termed as autoimmune sclerosing cholangitis in children [21]. The prevalence of the so-called PSC-definite AIH overlap syndrome is about 1.8%–7.1% [22,23]. There is a report of a case of overlap syndrome of PSC and PBC. Although PSC and PBC are mutually exclusive, the normally distinctive features of PBC and PSC occasionally overlap. Fig. 4 shows the possibility of overlapping of different autoimmune liver diseases.

SUMMARY

It is certain that autoimmune liver diseases, especially AIH and PBC, overlap each other. Moreover, the prevalence of overlapping of AIH and PBC is higher as compared with the accidental simple combination of AIH and PBC (mixed form). At present, the overlap syndrome is considered to be a variant form of these diseases, but not an independent disease entity. The mechanism underlying the pathogenesis of the overlap syndrome is still completely unknown.

Further study is needed for piling-up of precise clinical data and also for analysis of genetic factors responsible for each autoimmune liver disease.

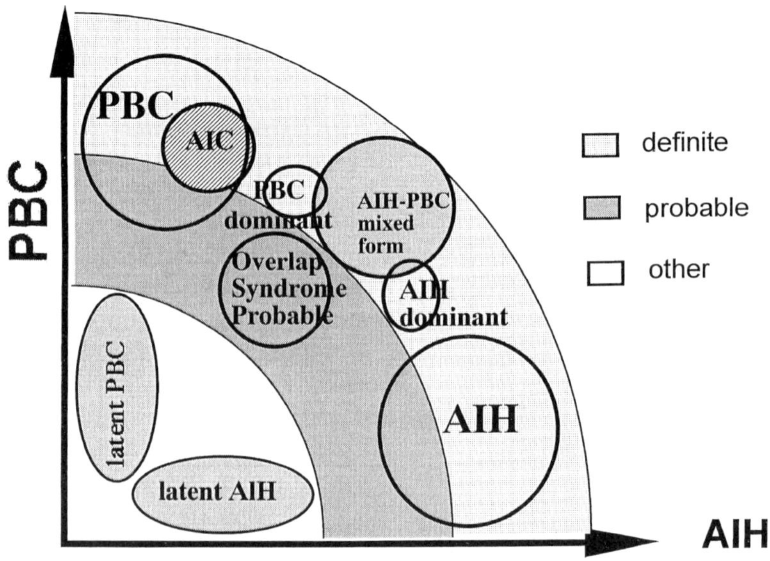

Fig. 3. Disease spectrum of autoimmune liver diseases. Horizontal (AIH) and vertical (PBC) lines show diagnostic reliability (definite, probable and other). AIC is mostly included into definite PBC. The AIH–PBC mixed form is thought to be a combined entity of definite PBC and AIH. Both dominant types of AIH and PBC exist in between AIH and PBC, and these entities will become a controversial issue from now on. There is a possibility that latent types of PBC and AIH exist.

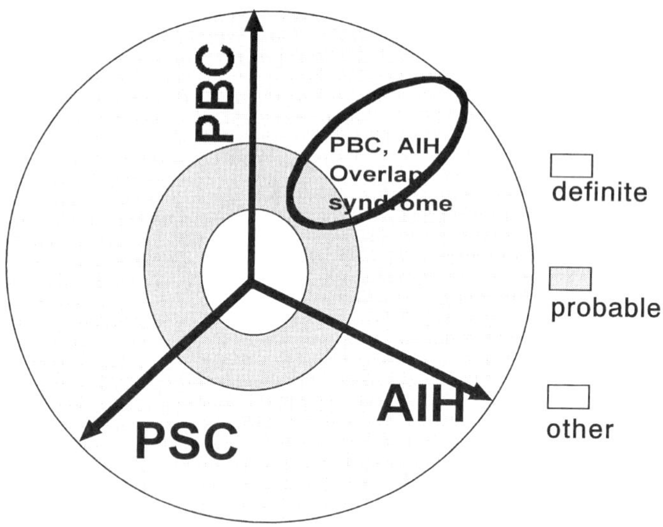

Fig. 4. Overlapping of three different autoimmune liver diseases. Definite cases of overlapping of PBC and AIH and of PSC and AIH have been reported; especially the PBC and AIH overlap syndrome is very popular. Although few cases of overlaps and of combinations of PSC and PBC have been reported, it may not be impossible.

REFERENCES

[1] Popper H, Shaffner F. Nonsuppurative destructive chronic cholangitis and chronic hepatitis. In: Popper H, Schaffner F, editors. Progress in liver disease, Vol. III. New York and London: Grune and Stratton, 1970; pp. 336–354.
[2] Berg PA, Binder T. Demonstration of mitochondrial antibodies in sera from patients with chronic liver disease reacting with two different types of complement-fixing antigens. In: Gentilini P et al., editors. Chronic hepatitis. Basel: Karger, 1976; pp. 79–85.
[3] Kloeppel G, Seifert G, Lindor H et al. Histopathological features in mixed type chronic aggressive hepatitis and primary biliary cirrhosis. Correlations of liver histology with mitochondrial antibodies of different specificity. Virchows Arch Pathol Anat Histol 1977; 373: 143–160.
[4] Berg PA, Wiedmann KH, Sayers T et al. Serological classification of chronic cholestatic liver disease by the use of two different types of antimitochondrial antibodies. Lancet II 1980; 1329–1332.
[5] Brunner G, Klinge O. A cholangitis with antimitochondrial antibodies (immuno-cholangitis) resembling chronic non-suppurative destructive cholangitis. Dtsch Med Wochenschr 1987; 112: 1454–1458.
[6] Ben-Ari Z, Dhillan AP, Sherlock S et al. Autoimmune cholangiopathy: part of the spectrum of autoimmune chronic active hepatitis. Hepatology 1993; 18: 10–15.
[7] Taylor SL, Dean PJ, Riely CA et al. Primary autoimmune cholangitis — an alternative to antimitochondrial antibody-negative primary biliary cirrhosis. Am J Surg Pathol 1994; 18: 91–99.
[8] Michieletti P, Wanless IR, Katz A et al. Antimitochondrial antibody negative primary biliary cirrhosis: a distinct syndrome of autoimmune cholangitis. Gut 1994; 35: 260–265.
[9] Czaja AJ. The variant forms of autoimmune hepatitis. Ann Intern Med 1996; 125: 588–598.
[10] Nakajima M, Shimizu H, Miyazaki A et al. Detection of IgA, IgM, and IgG subclasses of anti-M2 antibody by immunoblotting in autoimmune cholangitis: is autoimmune cholangitis an early stage of primary biliary cirrhosis? J Gastroenterol 1999; 34: 607–612.
[11] Masumoto T, Ninomiya T, Yamauchi Y et al. Laparoscopic findings in patients with autoimmune cholangiopathy. Gastroenterol Endosc 1997; 39: 1183–1188 (in Japanese).
[12] Masumoto T, Ninomiya T, Michitaka K et al. Three patients with autoimmune cholangiopathy treated with prednisolone. J Gastroenterol 1998; 33: 909–913.
[13] Nakanuma Y, Ohta G. Histometric and serial section observations of the bile ducts in primary biliary cirrhosis. Gastroenterology 1979; 76: 1326–1332.
[14] Czaja AJ, Carpenter HA, Santrach PJ et al. Autoimmune cholangitis within the spectrum of autoimmune liver diseases. Hepatology 2000; 31: 1231–1235.
[15] Chazouilleres O, Wendum D, Serfaty L, Montembault S, Rosmorduc O, Poupon R. Primary biliary cirrhosis-autoimmune hepatitis overlap syndrome: clinical features and response to therapy. Hepatology 1998; 28: 296–301.
[16] Czaja AJ. Frequency and nature of the variant syndromes of autoimmune liver diseases. Hepatology 1998; 28: 369–365.
[17] Lohse AW, Meyer zum Büschenfelde K-H, Franz B, Kanzler S, Gerken G, Dienes H-P. Characterization of the overlap syndrome of primary biliary cirrhosis (PBC) and autoimmune hepatitis: evidence for it being a hepatitic form of PBC in genetically susceptible individuals. Hepatology 1999; 29: 1078–1084.
[18] Yamamoto K, Okamoto R, Tsuji T et al. A scoring system for primary biliary cirrhosis (in preparation).

[19] Alvarez F, Berg PA, Bianchi FB et al. International autoimmune hepatitis group report: review of criteria for diagnosis of autoimmune hepatitis. J Hepatol 1999; 31: 929–938.

[20] Metcalf JV, Mitchison HC, Palmer JM et al. Natural history of early primary biliary cirrhosis. Lancet 1996; 348: 1399–402.

[21] Kaneko A, Kato M, Fujimoto K et al. Latent autoimmune hepatitis in non-B non-C chronic liver diseases. Acta Hepatol Jpn 1996; 37: 688–695 (in Japanese).

[22] Mieli-Vergani G. Autoimmune sclerosing cholangitis: a distinct clinical entity? J Hepatol 2000; 32(Suppl. 2): 7–8.

[23] Chazouilleres O. Diagnosis of primary sclerosing cholangitis–autoimmune hepatitis overlap syndrome: to score or not to score? J Hepatol 2000; 33: 661–663.

Fulminant Hepatic Failure

Molecular Biology and Immunology in Hepatology
Edited by T. Tsuji, T. Higashi, M. Zeniya and K.-H. Meyer zum Büschenfelde

CHAPTER 21

Etiology and Pathophysiology of Fulminant Hepatic Failure

Kenji Fujiwara and Satoshi Mochida

Third Department of Internal Medicine, Saitama Medical School, Saitama, Japan

INTRODUCTION

Acute liver failure is a clinical syndrome characterized by severe impairment of liver function, which develops in patients without preceding chronic liver diseases. Massive or sub-massive necrosis is a characteristic pathological feature in the liver. In Japan, this syndrome is defined as shown in Fig. 1. The patients with no hepatic encephalopathy or encephalopathy of coma grade I showing prothrombin time of less than 40% of the normal value are diagnosed as acute hepatitis severe type. When these patients present encephalopathy of grade II or more within 8 weeks of the disease onset, they are diagnosed as fulminant hepatitis, a partial synonym of fulminant hepatic failure. Fulminant hepatitis is classified into two subtypes, acute type and subacute type, in which the encephalopathy occurs within 10 days and later than 11 days, respectively. The patients in whom the encephalopathy develops between 8 and 24 weeks after the disease onset are regarded as late onset hepatic failure (LOHF).

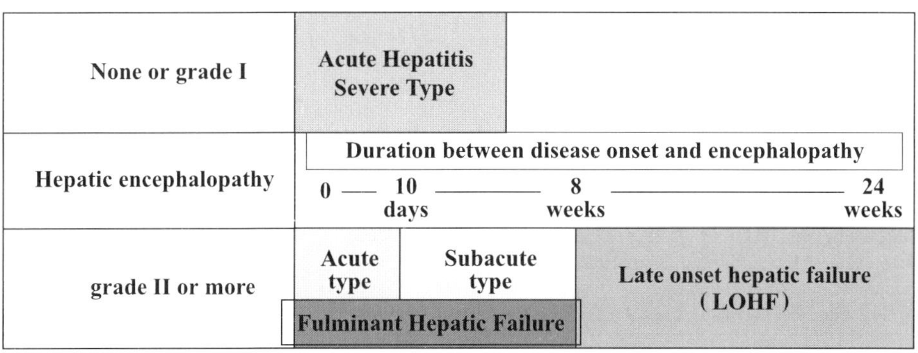

Fig. 1. Classification of acute liver failure in Japan.

In this article, demographic and clinical features and prognosis of fulminant hepatitis and LOHF in Japan are described. Also, therapies for these diseases are presented with proposed strategies based on the mechanisms of massive liver necrosis in rat models of acute liver failure.

1. CHARACTERISTICS OF FULMINANT HEPATITIS AND LOHF IN JAPAN

In Japan, the number of fulminant hepatitis patients is estimated as about 1000 per year. Demographic and clinical features of these patients are evaluated through the annual nation-wide survey by Saitama Medical School as a project of "Intractable Liver Diseases Study Group of Japan, the Ministry of Health and Welfare". According to this survey, 221 patients with fulminant hepatitis and 27 with LOHF were admitted to hospitals with hepatologists between January 1998 and December 1999 [1,2]. The fulminant hepatitis patients included 114 of acute type and 107 of subacute type.

1.1. Background of fulminant hepatitis and LOHF

As shown in Table 1, 20.9% of acute type and 23.9% of subacute type were hepatitis B virus (HBV) carriers in 1998. In these patients, complications other than liver diseases, such as diabetes, cancers and psychological diseases, were frequently seen; in

TABLE 1

Demographic and clinical features and prognosis of patients with fulminant hepatitis and LOHF in Japan

	Acute type	Subacute type	LOHF
Patients in 1998			
n	46	47	11
Male : Female	27 : 19	22 : 25	4 : 7
Ages (mean ± SD)	46.4 ± 17.0	50.0 ± 17.9	60.1 ± 13.8 **
HBV carrier (%)	20.9 (9/43)	23.9 (11/46)	9.1 (1/11)
Complications [a] (%)	28.9 (13/45)	41.3 (19/46)	63.6 (7/11) **
Daily medication (%)	20.9 (9/43)	37.0 (17/46)	63.6 (7/11) **
Survival rate (%): excluding transplanted patients	51.1 (23/45)	25.6 (11/43) **	0 (0/10) **
Number of transplanted patients	1	4	1
Survival rate (%): including transplanted patients	52.2 (24/46)	29.8 (14/47) **	9.1 (1/11) **
Patients in 1999			
n	68	60	16
Male : Female	35 : 32 (:1)	28 : 31 (:1)	4 : 12 *
Ages (mean ± SD)	42.8 ± 17.8	46.8 ± 14.4	53.3 ± 14.7 **
HBV carrier (%)	11.8 (8/68)	15.2 (9/59)	6.3 (1/16)
Complications [a] (%)	31.3 (21/67)	41.7 (25/60)	62.5 (10/16) **
Daily medication (%)	23.1 (15/65)	42.1 (24/57)	60.0 (9/15) **
Survival rate (%): excluding transplanted patients	62.7 (37/59)	29.5 (13/44) **	21.4 (3/14) **
Number of transplanted patients	9 (1)	16 (2)	2 (2)
Survival rate (%): including transplanted patients	66.2 (45/68)	45.0 (27/60) **	18.8 (3/16) **

[a] Diseases such as diabetes, malignancies and psychiatric disorders.
* $P < 0.1$ and ** $P < 0.05$ vs acute type.

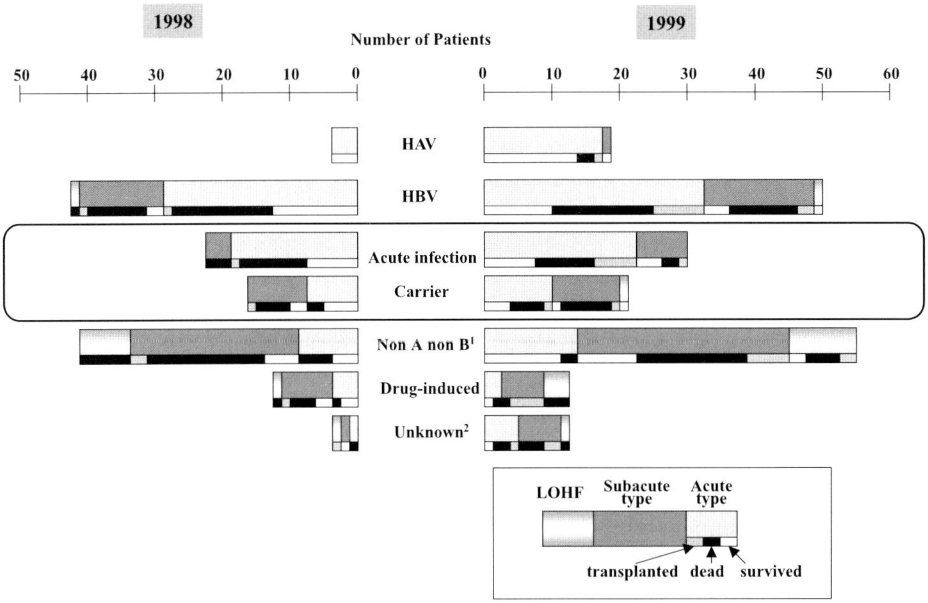

Fig. 2. Etiology and prognosis of fulminant hepatitis and LOHF in Japan (1998 and 1999). [1] Patients whose serum anti-HA IgM, HBs antigen and anti-HBc IgM were negative. [2] Patients whose serum anti-HA IgM, HBs antigen and anti-HBc IgM were not determined.

41.3% of subacute type patients and 63.6% of LOHF patients. It is noteworthy that most of these patients received daily medications. In contrast, the frequency of HBV carriers in fulminant hepatitis patients was less in 1999, since hepatitis A virus (HAV) infections prevailed during this year in Japan (Fig. 2). However, the patients with complications and daily medications were similarly frequent in subacute type and LOHF in 1999 (Table 1). There seems to be increasing frequency of HBV carriers and complications than before in patients with fulminant hepatitis and LOHF [3].

1.2. Etiology of fulminant hepatitis and LOHF

HAV and HBV infections and cryptogenic hepatitis are three major causes of fulminant hepatitis in Japan. The frequencies of these causes vary depending on the prevalence of HAV infection in each year. As shown in Fig. 2, HAV infection was the cause of fulminant hepatitis only in 4 patients (4.3%) in 1998, but in 18 patients (14.1%) in 1999. HBV infection was most frequent in patients with fulminant hepatitis; 42 and 48 patients (45.2% and 37.5%) in 1998 and 1999, respectively. These 90 patients included 51 of transient HBV infection, 31 of exacerbation of HBV carrier and 3 of undetermined. Most patients with transient HBV infection were in acute type, while HBV carriers were more frequent in subacute type than in acute type (Fig. 2).

There were 79 patients with no evidence of HAV and HBV infections; 34 (36.6%) in 1998 and 45 (35.2%) in 1999 (Fig. 2). Fifty-seven (72.2%) of these patients were in subacute type. It was reported that hepatitis C virus (HCV) infection seldom caused fulminant hepatic failure [4]. However, there were 5 patients in whom the etiology could be HCV infection based on viral markers and clinical course. Also, there was a patient with positive serum HBV-DNA, even though all serological markers reflecting HBV infection were negative. Silent HBV infection with X region mutation [5] might be involved in non-A and non-B fulminant hepatitis. It is noteworthy that serum anti-nuclear antigen was highly positive and serum IgG concentration was higher in patients with no evidence of HAV and HBV infections compared to patients with HAV and transient HBV infections. In 17 (21.5%) of these patients autoimmune hepatitis was suspected.

Although there were a lot of patients receiving daily medications due to complications, drug-induced fulminant hepatitis is not frequent in Japan; the etiology was drug allergy only in 18 patients (8.1%). The role of drugs in the development of massive and sub-massive liver necrosis should be investigated in future.

The etiology of LOHF was almost similar to that of fulminant hepatitis of subacute type (Fig. 2). Both HAV and HBV infections were not contributory in 18 patients (66.7%), and autoimmune hepatitis was suspected in 3 patients.

1.3. Acute hepatitis severe type and fulminant hepatic failure

Clinical features and prognosis of acute hepatitis severe type have been prospectively studied by Iwate Medical Collage as a project of "Intractable Liver Diseases Study Group of Japan" [6]. One hundred patients were enrolled in the study, and 29 of them developed hepatic encephalopathy of coma grade II or more, suggesting that acute hepatitis severe type progressed to fulminant hepatitis in about 30% of the patients. The extent of liver dysfunction was more severe in such patients than in those without the encephalopathy. It appears that massive liver necrosis causing hepatic encephalopathy has already been progressed even in acute hepatitis severe type patients.

2. THE MECHANISMS OF MASSIVE LIVER NECROSIS

The mechanisms of development of massive liver necrosis in fulminant hepatitis have been studied from three aspects: viral factors, immunological factors and local factors in the liver.

2.1. Viral factors

In Japan, δ-virus infection seldom contributes to fulminant hepatitis due to HBV infection. Super-infection or co-infection of HCV has been proposed in aggravation of HAV or HBV infection [7]. Also, the mutation of HBV-DNA, especially in pre-core and/or core regions, is assumed to be involved in fulminant hepatitis [8]. However, there is still no evidence that these viral factors cause massive liver necrosis.

Recently, we experienced a patient with fulminant hepatitis of subacute type, in whom TT virus (TTV) infection may be associated with liver injury [9]. This patient had HCV infection as well, and the genotype of TTV was 1b. Serum ALT levels changed in association with TTV-DNA levels. Nine TTV clones were isolated from the serum, and amino acid sequences of the hypervariable regions were completely identical in six clones, and sequence divergence was minimal even in the other three clones; there was 89% to 99% homology in the sequence of the major clones [9]. Considering that amino acid sequences of these regions showed quasispecies in patients with persistent TTV infection [10], such major clones might cause fulminant hepatitis in patients with HCV infection.

2.2. Immunological factors

In general, hepatitis virus itself is not cytotoxic to hepatocytes. Liver injury develops during eradication of virus-infected hepatocytes by cytotoxic T lymphocytes (CTL). CTL can recognize hepatocytes through adhesion molecules, and injure them by the perforin–granzyme B system [11]. Hepatocyte injury is further aggravated by CTL through the Fas/Fas ligand system and TNF-α [11]. Based on these observations, fulminant hepatitis can develop as a result of excessive immune reaction against virus-infected hepatocytes. Such mechanisms would be possible in the progression of fulminant hepatitis of subacute type and LOHF, but less possible in the development of fulminant hepatitis of acute type, because the number of CTL infiltrating into the liver is small.

2.3. Local factors in the liver

Microcirculatory disturbance due to sinusoidal fibrin deposition was first observed by King's College Hospital group in patients with fulminant hepatic failure [12]. They proposed early treatment of fulminant hepatic failure by heparin as an anticoagulant [13]. However, conflicting data were presented by other groups [14,15]. A controlled trial of heparin therapy performed in England showed no efficacy [15]. This theory has been paid attention in Japan based on experimental results by our group.

Massive liver necrosis was induced in rats by intraperitoneal injection of carbon tetrachloride (CCl4) or dimethylnitrosamine. When antithrombin III concentrate was infused in these rats, plasma antithrombin III activity was increased in a dose-related manner in both models [16]. However, an improvement of serum ALT activity was seen only in dimethylnitrosamine-treated rats. In these rats, coagulation activity in the circulation was significantly higher than in CCl4-treated rats. Electron microscopic examination revealed that fibrin deposition with endothelial cell damage in the hepatic sinusoids was present only in dimethylnitrosamine-treated rats [16]. Thus, sinusoidal fibrin deposition seemed to develop depending on the mechanisms of development of massive liver necrosis [16,17]. King's College Hospital group found sinusoidal fibrin deposition in patients with fulminant hepatic failure of viral origin [12], but conducted the control trial in patients with paracetamol-induced hepatic necrosis [15].

Massive liver necrosis develops in rats given heat-killed *Propionibacterium acnes* (*P. acnes*) or undergoing 70% partial hepatectomy after intravenous administration of endotoxin (Fig. 3) [18,19]. Both models present pathological features similar to fulminant hepatitis of acute type. When rats received heat-killed *P. acnes*, hepatic

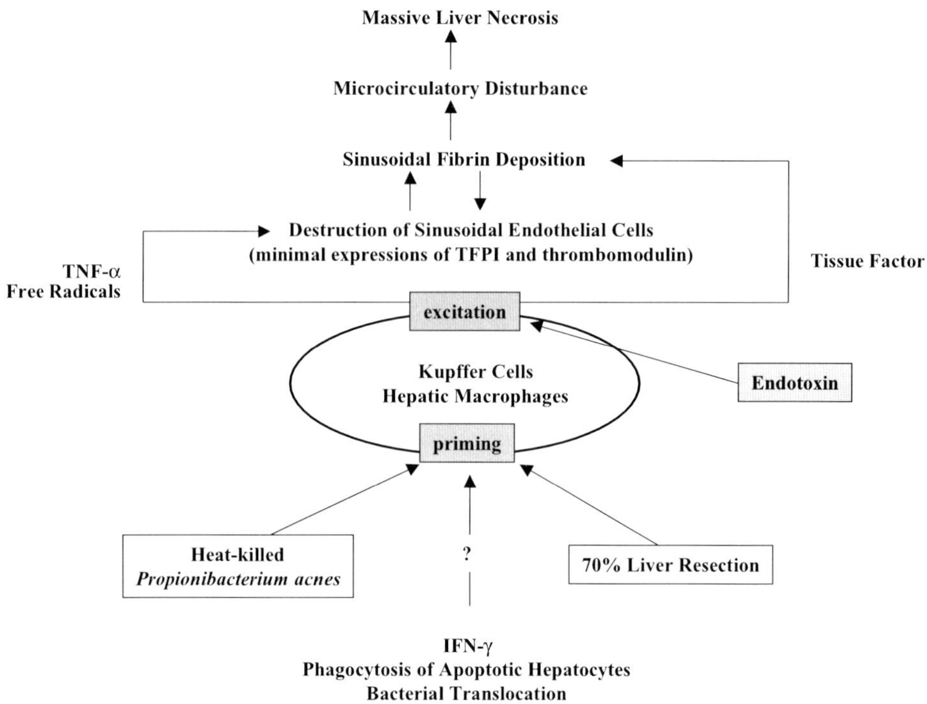

Fig. 3. The possible mechanisms of development of massive liver necrosis.

macrophages became activated through the cytokine network of IL-18, IL-2 and IFN-γ [20]. Chemokine network through osteopontin, an extracellular matrix that can also promote migration of macrophages, was associated with macrophage infiltration into the liver in this model [21,22]. These macrophages are activated to produce a large amount of TNF-α and superoxide anions [23,24] and cause destruction of endothelial cells leading to development of fibrin deposition in the hepatic sinusoids [24,25]. In contrast, Kupffer cells became activated through bacterial translocation from the gut to portal blood following 70% liver resection in rats [26,27]. These Kupffer cells produced abundant tissue factor, an initiator of blood coagulation cascade, and fibrin deposition develops after endotoxin administration as a result of deranged blood coagulation equilibrium in the hepatic sinusoids [28]. In both models, hepatocyte damage occurs through microcirculatory disturbance due to sinusoidal fibrin deposition [24,28].

Sinusoidal endothelial cells are unique in anticoagulation function, and this may contribute to the development of sinusoidal fibrin deposition. In general, blood coagulation cascade triggered by tissue factor is suppressed by tissue factor pathway inhibitor (TFPI) on endothelial cells. The cascade is further regulated by thrombomodulin on the cells through inactivation of thrombin and activation of protein C. However, both TFPI and thrombomodulin expressions in endothelial cells are minimal in the hepatic sinusoids compared to cells in other organs [29,30]. Thus, microcirculatory disturbance due to fibrin deposition can easily develop in the hepatic sinusoids following activation of Kupffer cells and hepatic macrophages [30]. Also, the derangement of blood coagulation equilibrium is caused by endothelial cell injury in the hepatic sinusoids [24].

3. THERAPEUTIC STRATEGIES FOR PREVENTION OF MASSIVE LIVER NECROSIS

Peripheral platelets are frequently decreased in number in patients with acute hepatitis severe type due to HAV or HBV transient infection. In these patients, hepatocyte injury can be produced by microcirculatory disturbance due to sinusoidal deposition, and thereby anticoagulant therapy using antithrombin III concentrate is preferable [31]. In contrast, when peripheral platelets are unchanged, as was seen in HBV-carrier patients taking a course of hepatitis exacerbation, anti-viral therapy such as lamivudine administration would be recommended.

Considering the unique function of sinusoidal endothelial cells, anticoagulant therapy using TFPI or thrombomodulin can be a candidate for prevention of sinusoidal fibrin deposition. When recombinant TFPI was intravenously administered in rats, it rapidly disappeared from the circulation and was detected in the hepatic sinusoids [30]. Heparin administration caused its reappearance in the circulation with disappearance from the sinusoids, suggesting that TFPI was trapped by heparinoid in the hepatic sinusoids. Electron microscopic examination revealed that TFPI was present on the surface of sinusoidal endothelial cells and microvilli of hepatocytes exposing in the Disse space [30]. Intravenous administration of recombinant TFPI significantly attenuated liver injury induced by endotoxin in partially hepatectomized rats [28]. Recombinant TFPI may be an anticoagulant targeting the hepatic sinusoids, even when endothelial cells are lost [30,32].

Another candidate for anticoagulant therapy is an oral administration of polymyxin B sulfate [26,27]. Massive liver necrosis develops in rats following orthotopic liver transplantation through microcirculatory disturbance due to sinusoidal fibrin deposition [33]. In these rats, tissue factor activity was markedly increased in Kupffer cells [33], but attenuated in rats pretreated with polymizin B sulfate before the operation with the improvement of liver injury [26].

4. TREATMENT AND PROGNOSIS OF FULMINANT HEPATITIS AND LOHF IN JAPAN

According to the survey by "Intractable Liver Diseases Study Group of Japan" [1,2], most patients with fulminant hepatitis and LOHF received artificial liver support with combination of plasma exchange and blood dialysis and filtration. Anticoagulant therapy was done in about 60%. Lamivudine for HBV infection has become prevalent. Seven (38.8%) and 10 (47.6%) of 18 and 21 HBV carriers received lamivudine in 1998 and 1999, respectively. Various complications occurred in patients with fulminant hepatitis and LOHF, and the therapies for these complications were also given. Bacterial and fungal infections occurred in 42.3% and 43.8%, DIC in 42.1% and 38.5%, brain edema in 40.1% and 14.3%, renal failure in 31.0% and 25.0% and gastrointestinal bleeding in 20.7% and 25.0% of patients with fulminant hepatitis and LOHF, respectively [2].

It appeared that such therapeutic procedures have improved the prognosis of patients with fulminant hepatitis and LOHF. Survival rates in patients who did not undergo liver transplantation were 62.7% and 29.5% for fulminant hepatitis of acute and subacute types, respectively, and 21.4% for LOHF in 1999 [1]. These rates were higher than the rates reported previously [2,3]. Fifteen of 17 patients (88.2%) with HAV infection survived without liver transplantation. In contrast, the rates in patients with transient and persistent HBV infections were 50.0% and 30.0%, respectively. The rate in patients with no HAV and HBV infections was 45.6%.

Living-donor related liver transplantation became prevelant in Japan as a therapeutic procedure for fulminant hepatitis and LOHF. Liver transplantation was performed only in 6 patients (5.8%) in 1998 [2], but in 27 patients (18.8%) in 1999; 9, 16 and 2 patients with fulminant hepatitis of acute and subacute types and LOHF, respectively [1]. The survival rates in patients with fulminant hepatitis of acute and subacute types and LOHF including those undergoing liver transplantation were 66.2%, 45.0% and 18.8%, respectively in 1999 [1].

In Japan, the patient selection for liver transplantation in fulminant hepatitis is based on the criteria made in 1996 by Acute Liver Failure Study Group of Japan [34]. The predictive accuracy of this guideline was 82% in the retrospective study of 196 patients in 42 hospitals 4 years ago [34]. However, the accuracy of the guideline, assessed from the prognosis of patients undergoing no liver transplantation in 1999, was 73.7% and 73.5% for fulminant hepatitis of acute and subacute types, respectively [1]. In the subacute type, 9 (29.0%) survived among 31 patients who were evaluated as fatal and thereby indicative for liver transplantation. The guideline should be regularly revised by taking recent therapeutic modalities into consideration.

REFERENCES

[1] Fujiwara K, Mochida S, Matsui A. Fulminant hepatitis and late onset hepatic failure in Japan (1998). Intractable Liver Diseases Study Group of Japan, The Ministry of Health and Welfare. Annual Report at 1999, 2000, pp. 59–62.

[2] Fujiwara K, Mochida S, Matsui A. Fulminant hepatitis and late onset hepatic failure in Japan (1999). Intractable Liver Diseases Study Group of Japan, The Ministry of Health and Welfare. Annual Report at 2000, 2001, pp 24–31.

[3] Sato S, Suzuki K, Takigawa Y. Fulminant hepatitis and late onset hepatic failure in Japan (1998). Intractable Liver Diseases Study Group of Japan, The Ministry of Health and Welfare. Annual Report at 1998, 1999, pp. 62–66.

[4] Fukai K, Yokosuka O, Fujiwara K, Tagawa M, Imazeki F, Saisho H, Omata M. Etiologic considerations of fulminant non-A, non-B viral hepatitis in Japan: Analyses by nucleic acid amplification method. J Infect Dis 1998; 178: 325–333.

[5] Uchida T, Saitoh T, Shinzawa H. Mutations of the X region of hepatitis B virus and their clinical implications. Pathol Int 1997; 47: 183–193.

[6] Suzuki K. Prospective study for prognosis of fulminant hepatic failure and acute hepatitis severe type in Japan. Intractable Liver Diseases Study Group of Japan, The Ministry of Health and Welfare. Annual Report at 1999, 2000, pp. 66–67.

histological damage. At the same time, inflammatory cells like neutrophils are recruited by means of the activation of endothelial cells, fibroblasts, and the like. At this point, severe hepatic histological damage occurs due to the further recruitment of highly activated inflammatory cells such as macrophages.

Experimental results from studies using HBV transgenic mice have shed light on the mechanisms of hepatic histological damage [7]. Extensive hepatic cellular necrosis can be induced by administration of HBVAg-specific CTLs to the HBV transgenic mouse resulting in death. This process can be separated into three stages [7]. In the first stage, HBVAg-specific CTLs act on HBVAg-positive cells and at about one hour after injection of the CTLs, a response is induced in the form of apoptosis. In the second stage, 4–12 hours later, a response is initiated when infiltration by inflammatory cells such as antigen-nonspecific lymphocytes, neutrophils, and macrophages occurs in the area around hepatic cells that have undergone apoptosis, inducing a response in the form of focal necrosis. In the final stage, 24 72 hours post-injection, a response occurs that is thought to be a delayed hypersensitivity response. In this final stage the high level of activation of macrophages infiltrating in the liver is caused by IFN-γ produced by CTLs that encountered target cells, and the extensive necrosis of hepatic cells produces a pathology closely resembling fulminant hepatic failure [7].

2. CYTOKINE DYNAMICS IN VIRAL HEPATITIS

As mentioned previously, CTLs and NK cells play a pivotal role in the elimination of hepatic cells with hepatitis viral infection; however, helper T cells govern the activation of those cells. Helper T cells recognize viral antigens presented by antigen presenting cells (APCs), such as dendritic cells, and are activated, promoting the secretion of IL-2 and Th1-types of cytokines (pro-inflammatory) like IFN-γ [8], activation and expansion of CTLs and NK cells and the production of Th2-types of cytokines (anti-inflammatory) as well, e.g. IL-4, 5, 6, and 10. They also promote differentiation and expansion of APCs that act on B cells. In addition, the APCs themselves produce and secrete IL-12 due to stimulation by activated helper T cells, acting to promote production of Th1 cytokines and to activate CTLs and NK cells, thus helping eliminate the hepatitis virus [9]. On the other hand, IL-10 secreted by Th2 cells acts on APCs, suppressing the activation of Th1 cells by suppressing IL-12 production. Consequently, the cellular immune response is suppressed, which is thought to finally bring an end to hepatitis [10]. Additionally, the pathology of viral hepatitis involves the activation of lymphocytes as well as of liver macrophages, as was noted previously, and inflammatory cytokines that are produced by these cells, such as TNF-α, are also thought to be extensively involved.

3. CYTOKINE DYNAMICS IN FULMINANT HEPATIC FAILURE

To this point hepatic cytotoxicity and histological damage in viral hepatitis as well as cytokine dynamics have been discussed. The following section addresses findings obtained with animal models in relation to cytokine dynamics in fulminant hepatic failure and results obtained from actual cases of fulminant hepatic failure in humans.

3.1. Animal models

An important point that must be addressed when investigating cytokine dynamics in fulminant hepatic failure using animal models is whether the extensive hepatic cellular necrosis in a model is mediated by activated T-cells or activated macrophages. As was described earlier, activated T-cells and activated macrophages do not act independently in the pathology of fulminant hepatic failure. Therefore, these mechanisms are believed to be related as part of the complicated pathology by means of the cytokine network. Accordingly, animal models of acute hepatopathy are separated into activated T cell-mediated and activated macrophage-mediated types, and attention has been focused on the pro-inflammatory and anti-inflammatory cytokines.

3.1.1. Activated T cell-mediated model

A model in which mice are administered concanavalin A (ConA) has recently been reported as an activated T cell-mediated model [11]. In the model, T cell activation is accomplished by administration of ConA and selective hepatic cellular necrosis is subsequently induced. Infiltrating inflammatory cells in the periportal and perivenous areas were found to be $CD4^+$ T cells and polymorphonuclear leucocytes [12]. ConA administration induces the production of TNF-α, IL-1, 2, 6, granulocyte macrophage colony-stimulating factor (GMCSF) and IFN-γ. In further experiments using monoclonal antibodies, TNF-α [12–14] and IFN-γ [15,16], in particular, were noted as extremely inflammatory cytokines involved in the induction of hepatopathy.

In addition, Louis et al. [17] paid particular attention to IL-10, which is an anti-inflammatory cytokine. In the ConA model, IL-10 was produced in the initial stages after ConA administration. This endogenous IL-10 causes an increase in the secretion of inflammatory cytokines like TNF-α, IFN-γ, and IL-12 and can be inhibited by monoclonal antibodies. In contrast, administration of exogenous IL-10 decreases the secretion of these inflammatory cytokines. The activated T cell-mediated model then, gives information about inflammatory cytokines like TNF-α, IFN-γ, and IL-12 and highlights the involvement of the anti-inflammatory action of IL-10.

3.1.2. Activated macrophage-mediated model

The galactosamine/lipopolysaccharide (LPS) model [18] or the Corynebacterium/LPS model [19] are familiar as activated macrophage-mediated models. In the former model, the mouse is sensitized with galactosamine and is administered LPS; TNF-α increases significantly [20]. In addition, the hepatic histological damage and fatality rate decrease upon treatment with anti-TNF-α monoclonal antibodies [21]. In a TNF-α receptor-deficient mouse, hepatic histological damage is not induced [22]. Given the results from this model, TNF-α is thought to play an important role in this hepatopathy.

With regard to the latter of the two models, a study by Yamada et al. [23] showed that liver macrophage sensitization by Corynebacterium resulted in increased TNF-α and active oxygen production capacity. The hepatopathy in this model could be alleviated by administration of an anti-TNF-α monoclonal antibody or superoxide dismutase (SOD) causing the authors to hypothesize that TNF-α produced and secreted by liver macrophages, and active oxygen production capacity are important in this activated macrophage-mediated model. In addition, Kayano et al. [24] used a *Propionibacterium acnes* (*P. acnes*)/LPS model where sensitization was accomplished with *P. acnes*, and the liver macrophage TNF-α production capacity obtained was found to be significantly enhanced. The production and secretion of TNF-α by liver macrophages has been clearly demonstrated to be vital with regard to the induction of hepatopathy in this acute hepatopathy model.

3.2. Cases of fulminant hepatic failure

There are a number of reports regarding the analysis of the cytokine dynamics in serum or hepatic tissue obtained from actual cases of fulminant hepatic failure. Muto et al. [25] found an increase in the TNF-α and IL-1 production capacity of mononuclear leukocytes in peripheral blood from cases of fulminant hepatic failure in comparison to healthy subjects or cases of acute hepatitis. In addition, Tokushige et al. [26] measured TNF-α and soluble TNF receptors I and II, soluble Fas antigens and Fas ligands, in the serum of patients with fulminant hepatic failure. While no significant difference was noted between patients with fulminant hepatic failure and acute hepatitis in levels of soluble Fas antigens and Fas ligands, the levels of serum TNF-α and soluble TNF receptors I and II were higher with the acute type of fulminant hepatic failure. In particular, TNF receptor-1 was reported to be significantly higher for patients with the acute type of fulminant hepatic failure in comparison to patients with the subacute type of fulminant hepatic failure, patients with the severe type of acute hepatitis, patients with acute hepatitis, and healthy subjects. In cases of mortality due to the acute type of fulminant hepatic failure, the concentration of TNF receptor-1 in serum is often found to be 10 ng/ml or higher, while surviving patients are often found to have concentrations lower than 10 ng/ml. These results suggest that TNF-α may be involved in extensive hepatic cellular necrosis for actual cases of fulminant hepatic failure as well.

Further, with regard to the involvement of TNF-α in the pathology of fulminant hepatic failure, Streetz et al. [27] found that the levels of serum TNF-α and soluble TNF receptors I and II were significantly higher in cases of fulminant hepatic failure. The extent of that increase has been reported to be correlated with patient prognosis. The authors' hypotheses about TNF-α expression of infiltrating mononuclear lymphocytes in the hepatic tissues of these patients and the enhanced expression of TNF receptors in hepatic cells were confirmed with immunohistochemical staining. In particular, they found an increase in the number of infiltrating mononuclear lymphocytes and apoptosis in hepatic cells in areas with increased TNF-α expression. It is clear from these studies that the TNF/TNF-receptor system plays a vital role in the pathology of fulminant hepatic failure. Furthermore, Nagaki et al. [28] measured the serum TNF-α, IL-1β, IL-6, IL-10, IL-12, and soluble TNF receptors p55 and p75 levels in cases of fulminant hepatic failure, the severe form of acute hepatitis, and acute hepatitis. In cases of fulminant hepatic failure, the levels of TNF-α, IL-10, and soluble TNF receptor p55 were reported to be significantly higher in comparison to other groups.

Finally, Kimura et al. [29] focused on IFN-γ, which induces production of $CD8^+$ CTLs. In patients with fulminant hepatic failure, the level of IFN-γ that induces production of $CD8^+$ CTLs is significantly higher than in patients with acute hepatitis and normal subjects. This suggests that IFN-γ may be involved in the pathology of fulminant hepatic failure, possibly through the induction $CD8^+$ CTLs.

4. FUTURE PERSPECTIVES

This paper has restricted its focus to cytokine dynamics with regard to the pathology of fulminant hepatic failure. Analysis of findings obtained from animal models of fulminant hepatic failure and actual cases of fulminant hepatic failure, showed that IFN-γ and TNF-α are key pro-inflammatory cytokines. In addition, IL-10 is an important pro-inflammatory cytokine that appears to be deeply involved in the pathology of fulminant hepatic failure. The important point to note is that the pro-inflammatory cytokines, the anti-inflammatory cytokines, or both types of cytokines together, act as part of an extremely complicated system called the cytokine network. Nonetheless, they can perform suppression by means of an extremely consistent cascade. In the future, the elucidation of detailed mechanisms, to include new cytokines that may be discovered to be involved in this cytokine network, is an area of intense interest.

In addition, the most important differences between normal viral hepatitis, or what is called 'acute hepatitis,' and 'fulminant hepatic failure' are that acute hepatitis is essentially a self-limited form of hepatitis that is transient and self healing, while fulminant hepatic failure is a non self-limited form. The latter initiates a pathology called systemic inflammatory response syndrome (SIRS) [30], or hypercytokinemia, as a result of extensive hepatic cellular necrosis. In the end, liver failure and multiple organ failure are induced and this leads to death.

Accordingly, it is possible to predict the existence of essential differences between fulminant hepatic failure and acute hepatitis, though these differences remain unclear at this point. The most important point then, is the elucidation of the essential differences between fulminant hepatic failure and acute hepatitis in terms of the cytokine network or from an immunological standpoint.

REFERENCES

[1] Penna A, Chisari F, Bertoletti A et al. Cytotoxic T lymphocytes recognize an HLA-A2-restricted epitope within the hepatitis B virus nucleocapsid antigen. J Exp Med 1991; 174: 1565–1570.

[2] Tsai SL, Chen PJ, Yang PM et al. Characterization of T cell clones specific to a determinant of hepatitis B virus core and e antigens in chronic type-B hepatitis: Implication for a T cell mechanism of HBV immunopathogenesis. J Biomed Sci 1994; 1: 105–118.

[3] Chisari FV, Ferrari C. Hepatitis B virus immunopathogenesis. Annu Rev Immunol 1995; 13: 29.

[4] Tschopp J, Nabholz M. Perforin-mediated target cell lysis by cytotoxic T lymphocytes. Annu Rev Immunol 1990; 8: 279–302.

[5] Kagi D, Vignaux F, Ledermann B et al. Fas and perforin pathways as major mechanisms of T cell-mediated cytotoxicity. Science 1994; 265: 528–530.

[6] Vassalli P. The pathophysiology of tumor necrosis factors. Annu Rev Immunol 1992; 10: 411–452.

[7] Ando K, Moriyama T, Guidotti LG et al. Mechanism of class 1 restricted immunopathology. A transgenic mouse model of fulminant hepatitis. J Exp Med 1993; 178: 1541–1554.
[8] Mosmann TR, Sad S. The expanding universe of T-cell subsets: Th1, Th2 and more. Immunol Today 1996; 17: 138–146.
[9] Lamont AG, Adorini L. IL-12, a key cytokine in immune regulation. Immunol Today 1996; 17: 214–217.
[10] Meyyaard L, Hovenkamp E, Otto SA et al. IL12-induced IL-10 production by human T cells as a negative feedback for IL12-induced immune responses. J Immunol 1996; 156: 2776–2782.
[11] Tiegs G, Hentschel J, Wendel A. A T cell-dependent experimental liver injury in mice inducible by concanavalin A. J Clin Invest 1992; 90: 196–203.
[12] Mizuhara H, O'Neil E, Seki N, Ogawa T, Kusunoki C, Otsuka K, Satoh S et al. T cell activation-associated hepatic injury: mediation by tumor necrosis factors and protection by interleukin-6. J Exp Med 1994; 179: 1529–1537.
[13] Gantner F, Leist M, Lohse AW, Germann PG, Tiegs G. Concanavalin A-induced T cell-mediated hepatic injury in mice: the role of tumor necrosis factor. Hepatology 1995; 21: 190–198.
[14] Trautwein C, Rakemann T, Brenner DA, Streetz K, Licato L, Manns MP, Tiegs G. Concanavalin A-induced liver cell damage: activation of intracellular pathways triggered by tumor necrosis factor in mice. Gastroenterology 1998; 114: 1035–1045.
[15] Mizuhara H, Uno M, Seki N, Yamashita M, Yamaoka M, Ogawa T, Kaneda K et al. Critical involvement of interferon gamma in the pathogenesis of T cell activation-associated hepatitis and regulatory mechanisms of hepatitis. Hepatology 1996; 23: 1608–1615.
[16] Kusters S, Gantner F, Kunstle G, Tiegs G. Interferon gamma plays a critical role in T cell-dependent liver injury in mice initiated by concanavalin A. Gastroenterology 1996; 111: 462–471.
[17] Louis H, Moine OL, Peny MO, Quertinmont E, Fokan D, Goldman M, Deviere J. Production and role of interleukin-10 in concanavalin A-induced hepatitis in mice. Hepatology 1997; 25: 1382–1389.
[18] Galanos C, Freudenberg MA, Reutter W. Galactosamine-induced sensitization to the lethal effects of endotoxin. Proc Natl Acad Sci USA 1979; 76: 5939–5943.
[19] Nagakawa J, Hishinuma I, Hirota K, Miyamoto K, Yamanaka T, Tsukidate K, Katayama K et al. Involvement of tumor necrosis factor-α in the pathogenesis of activated macrophage-mediated hepatitis in mice. Gastroenterology 1990; 99: 758–765.
[20] Santucci L, Fiorucci S, Chiorean M, Brunori PM, Matteo FMD, Sidoni A, Migliorati G, Morelli A. Interleukin 10 reduces lethality and hepatic injury induced by lipopolysaccharide in galactosamine-sensitized mice. Gastroenterology 1996; 111: 736–744.
[21] Tiegs G, Wolter M, Wendel A. Tumor necrosis factor is a terminal mediator in D-galactosamine-endotoxin-induced hepatitis in mice. Biochem Pharmacol 1989; 38: 627–631.
[22] Pfeffer K, Matsuyama T, Kundig TM, Wakeham A, Kishiara K, Shahinian A, Wiegmann K, Ohashi PS, Kronke M, Mak TW. Mice deficient for the 55kd tumor necrosis factor receptor are resistant to endotoxic shock, yet succumb to L. monocytogenes infection. Cell 1993; 73: 457–467.
[23] Yamada S, Ogata I, Hirata K et al. Intravascular coagulation in the development of massive hepatic necrosis induced by Corynebacterium parvum and endotoxin in rats. Scand J Gastroenterol 1989; 24: 293.
[24] Kayano K, Sakaida I, Kubota M, Yasunaga M, Okita K. Functional differences between activated and normal rat liver macrophages: LPS uptake capacity by flow cytometric analysis in contrast with TNF-α release. LIVER 1995; 15: 253–259.

[25] Muto Y, Nouri-Aria K, Meager A, Alexander GJM, Eddleston ALWF, Williams R. Enhanced tumor necrosis factor and interleukin-1 in fulminant hepatic failure. Lancet II 1988; 72–74.

[26] Tokushige K, Yamaguchi N, Ikeda I, Hashimoto E, Yamauchi K, Hayashi N. Significance of soluble TNF receptor-I in acute type fulminant hepatitis. Am J Gastroenterol 2000; 95: 2040–2046.

[27] Streetz K, Leifeld L, Grundmann D, Ramakers J, Eckert K, Spengler U, Brenner D, Manns M, Trautwein C. Tumor necrosis factor α in the pathogenesis of human and murine fulminant hepatic failure. Gastroenterology 2000; 119: 446–460.

[28] Nagaki M, Iwai H, Naiki T, Ohnishi H, Muto Y, Moriwaki H. High levels of serum interleukin-10 and tumor necrosis factor-α are associated with fatality in fulminant hepatitis. J Infect Dis 2000; 182: 1103–1108.

[29] Kimura K, Ando K, Tomita E, Ohnishi H, Ishikawa T, Kakumu S, Muto Y, Moriwaki H. Elevated intracellular IFN-γ levels in circulating $CD8^+$ lymphocytes in patients with fulminant hepatitis. J Hepatol 1999; 31: 579–583.

[30] Rolando N, Wade J, Davalos M et al. The systemic inflammatory response syndrome in acute liver failure. Hepatology 2000; 32: 734–739.

Molecular Biology and Immunology in Hepatology
Edited by T. Tsuji, T. Higashi, M. Zeniya and K.-H. Meyer zum Büschenfelde

CHAPTER 23

Treatment and Prognosis of Fulminant Hepatic Failure

Makoto Yoshiba

Division of Gastroenterology, Department of Medicine, Showa University Fujigaoka Hospital, Yokohama, Japan

INTRODUCTION

The term 'fulminant hepatic failure (FHF)' is commonly used in Western countries to indicate acute severe liver diseases. This term implies acute liver diseases complicated by coma within 8 weeks after onset of the first symptoms [1]. The term fulminant hepatitis (FH) is more often used in Japan. Most authors in Japan use these two terms interchangeably because they seem to find no substantial differences between them.

However, there is a fundamental difference between FHF and FH. FHF is a group of symptoms or a syndrome brought about by massive liver cell necrosis or degeneration from any of many causes (Table 1). Most of the liver diseases lead to FHF except for those which never cause severe liver dysfunction such as hypernutritional fatty liver. Alcohol is usually excluded from the cause of FHF because it induces liver failure after long-term abuse. Only in Sherlock's textbook is it listed as a cause of FHF [2].

FH has pathogenetically much in common with acute self-limiting hepatitis and chronic hepatitis (CH). The difference between FH and acute self-limiting hepatitis is only that hepatic necrosis is more extensive in FH. Chronic hepatitis B sometimes suddenly leads to liver failure, either spontaneously or following immunosuppressive treatment [3].

The recognition of differences in the pathogenesis between FHF and FH is of primary importance in the development of a reliable medical treatment.

1. DIFFERENCE BETWEEN FHF AND FH

FHF is caused by a variety of factors. Liver cell damage in FHF is divided into two categories. One is caused by direct hepatotoxicity. For example, ischemic liver failure is induced by direct anoxic damage to hepatocytes [4]. A paracetamol overdose causes hepatocellular damage by depleting intracellular glutathione [5].

The other is caused by host reactions. The majority of the cases are mediated by destructive host immune reactions. The diagnosis of 'hepatitis' is made when pathologists witness lymphocyte infiltration along with liver cell necrosis. Cytotoxic

TABLE 1

Etiology of fulminant hepatic failure [a]

(1) Fulminant hepatitis
Hepatic viruses:
Acute hepatitis A
Reactivation of hepatitis B virus
Acute aggravation of hepatitis B by the superinfection of hepatitis D virus
Fulminant hepatitis in hepatitis B virus carriers
Acute non-A, non-B hepatitis and acute hepatitis C
Acute hepatitis E
Other viruses:
Herpes simplex 1, 2
Herpes zoster
Cytomegalovirus
Epstein–Barr
Adenovirus
Giant-cell hepatitis (by paramyxovirus)
Drug-induced
Autoimmune
(2) Others (non-fulminant hepatitis)
Toxic liver injury:
Acetaminophen overdose
Amanita, mushroom intoxication
Ischemic liver injury:
Hepatic vein obstruction (Budd–Chiari syndrome)
Hyperpyrexia
Infiltration by malignant cells
Wilson's disease
Small-droplet fatty liver (acute fatty liver of pregnancy, Reye's syndrome)
Liver transplantation
Partial hepatectomy

[a] From the Oxford Textbook of Clinical Hepatology [13] (modified).

T lymphocytes which are mainly responsible for hepatocyte necrosis in viral hepatitis are involved in the lymphocyte infiltration. Thus, 'hepatitis' represents damage of hepatocytes by host immune reactions.

For an accurate diagnosis of FH every patient should undergo a liver biopsy, and the FH-characteristic lymphocyte infiltration should be confirmed. However, liver biopsy is hazardous in FHF where blood clotting is impaired. Therefore, FHF is diagnosed without a liver biopsy on the assumption that it is caused by one of the following three diseases in which lymphocyte infiltration is confirmed in acute self-limiting hepatitis or chronic hepatitis: viral, drug-induced or autoimmune hepatitis.

Viral hepatitis is diagnosed by viral markers for type A, type B, type C, type D, type E and type G. The diagnosis of type A is made by IgM antibody to HA (anti-HA). Type B is diagnosed by IgM anti-HB core antigen (anti-HBc) because HB surface antigen (HBsAg) is already negative at the onset of coma in half of the patients with type B FH. Rarely, IgM anti-HBc is negative, and the diagnosis of non-B is made by negative

HBV DNA by polymerase chain reaction. Type C is diagnosed by a positive test for HCV RNA. The viral load is usually high in type C FH [6]. The diagnosis of type D is made by the positive result for IgM antibody to the HDV virus or HDV RNA. Type E is diagnosed by the positive result for HEV RNA. Both type D and type E FH are rare in Japan. Type G is diagnosed by positive GBV-C or HGV RNA.

The problem is that there is a substantial number of patients with negative results for all the virus markers, usually called 'non-A' to 'non-G' hepatitis, although the presence of type F is doubted. The cause of the 'non-A' to 'non-G' has not been identified; however, it should be diagnosed as viral in Asian countries where viral hepatitis prevails.

The diagnosis of drug-induced hepatitis is based on the patient's history of recent drug intake, eosinophilia, rash, and a positive result with the lymphocyte stimulation test. Caution should be exercised in that there are two sorts of drug-induced hepatic injuries: toxic liver injury and drug-induced hepatitis. Toxic liver injury affects every individual in a dose-dependent fashion, and typical of this sort is a paracetamol overdose. Drug-induced hepatitis affects certain individuals caused by idiosyncratic allergic reactions, and is unpredictable. A typical example of this is halothane hepatitis. FHF caused by the latter should be in the same category as FH.

Autoimmune hepatitis is diagnosed by a positive antinuclear antibody (ANA) and elevated IgG level (>2000 mg/dl).

2. SYMPTOMATIC TREATMENT OF FHF

Many attempts have been made to treat FHF by artificial liver support (ALS). Until the King's College group reported a beneficial effect of charcoal hemoperfusion in 1974 [7], exchange transfusion (ET) was a standard method of liver support. A small-scale controlled trial, however, found no beneficial effect of ET [8]. Opolon and coworkers in France reported a favorable effect of polyacrylonitrile (PAN) membrane hemodiafiltration (HDF) on hepatic coma in patients with FHF [9]. Many low-molecular substances such as ammonia, mercaptan, amino acid amines, short chain fatty acids, and GABA have been incriminated for hepatic coma [10]. However, the contribution of these low-molecular substances other than ammonia to hepatic coma is doubted because renal dialysis which eliminates low-molecular materials shows little effectiveness in the treatment of hepatic coma [11].

Charcoal hemoperfusion and PAN membrane HDF are characterized by the elimination of plasma molecules with a molecular weight of 1500–5000 Da. Based on the improvement of coma by these treatments, it is postulated that there must be some as yet unidentified middle-molecular substances responsible for hepatic coma [12]. The effect of the charcoal hemoperfusion treatment was later refused by a control study [13], and is no longer used except for the removal of toxic drugs. A similar trial was done in our country. The method was original in that the patient's plasma was separated from the whole blood, and the plasma was perfused through a column containing uncoated charcoal. The survival rate was disappointingly low, and disseminated intravascular coagulation was induced probably through the activation of clotting factor XII on the surface of the charcoal [14].

Currently, plasma exchange (PE) is prevailing in Japan as ALS treatment, owing to the established supply system by the Japanese Red Cross and a relatively low risk of human immunodeficiency virus infection. We have demonstrated that although PE is effective in the replenishment of plasma components, including coagulation factors, it has a limited effectiveness in the removal of accumulated toxic substances that are excessively accumulated [15].

To overcome this limitation we developed a HDF method using 'high-performance membranes' with larger pores than the PAN membrane used by Opolon. The purpose of this HDF is to safely and efficiently remove the middle-molecular substances assumed as responsible for coma. Cellulose acetate membranes (Nihon Shoji, Co., Tokyo) and polysulfon membranes (Kawasumi Co., Tokyo) are the most suitable for carrying out HDF.

The effect of the combined PE and HDF treatment is remarkable. Of the initial 68 patients with FHF treated with this ALS, 66 (97%) regained full consciousness from initial coma. Brain edema, a frequent complication of FHF, was observed in only four patients with grade IV coma. Hepatorenal syndrome, also a frequent accompaniment of FHF, was found in only two cases. The favorable effect of this new ALS is confirmed by other institutions, and has been adopted by 79.4% of the major hospitals in Japan according to the annual surveillance study in 1999 supported by the Ministry of Health and Welfare, although the method is modified to an easier but less effective continuous HDF (CHDF) in some institutions.

3. ARTIFICIAL LIVER

Efforts have been made to develop various types of artificial liver. Most of them use cultured porcine hepatocytes. Some are combined by absorbents such as charcoal (hybrid artificial liver) [16]. They seem to have some capability for the detoxification of toxic substances and the decompression of intracranial pressure. However, they are of a limited effectiveness in the replenishment of depleted human plasma components. Artificial livers now available block the permeation of porcine proteins using membranes. Taking into consideration the fact that the liver detoxication capacity can be easily and efficiently compensated using only buffers (water) by our HDF, artificial liver that is more efficient in the production of human plasma components should be developed. However, a number of problems should be overcome concerning biohazards such as unidentified animal virus infections and biocompatibility such as immune reactions to animal proteins.

4. TREATMENT OF UNDERLYING LIVER DISEASES

Little attention has been paid to the underlying liver disease in the treatment of FHF. Major causes of FHF in Western countries are type B FH due to acute infection of HBV, type A, a paracetamol overdose and other drug-induced liver injuries, Reye's syndrome and unknown causes [17]. It is well known that causal viruses are rapidly eradicated in type A FH and type B FH due to acute HBV infection [18]. The toxicity of paracetamol disappears rapidly with its rapid metabolization. Thus, treatment of underlying liver diseases is not necessary in Western countries.

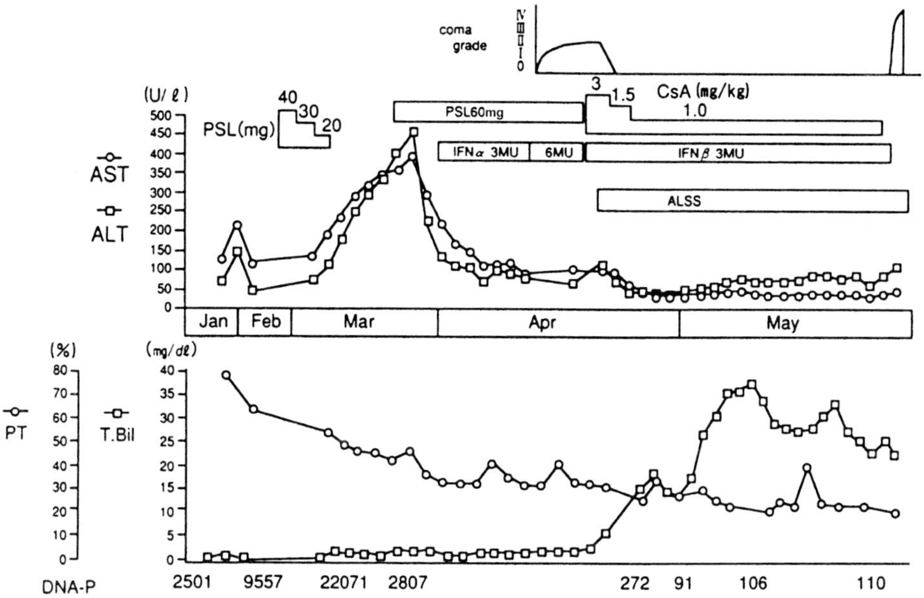

Fig. 1. Clinical course of a patient with chronic hepatitis B who developed fulminant hepatic failure after corticosteroid withdrawal therapy. CsA = cyclosporin A; AST (—○—) = aspartate aminotransferase; ALT (—□—) = alanine aminotransferase; PT (—○—) = prothrombin time; T.Bil (—□—) = total bilirubin; DNA-P = DNA polymerase; PSL = prednisolone; UN = interferon; ALSS = artificial liver support system.

Furthermore, in the decision for liver transplantation, which is regarded as the only reliable treatment for FHF in Western countries, consideration of underlying liver diseases is not necessary because liver transplantation is an ultimate 'symptomatic' treatment of FHF.

In Asian countries where HBV infection is endemic, HBV carriers often develop FHF. In a follow-up study before the onset of symptoms it is found that HBV highly replicates itself before the elevation of transaminases [19]. HBV DNA polymerase reaches peak values on average 20 days before the onset of coma (Table 2). Replication of HBV is usually persistent after the onset of coma, and liver destruction is also persistent or even progressive.

Fig. 1 shows a typical example of such a case. A patient with chronic hepatitis B underwent a corticosteroid withdrawal therapy as a priming therapy for interferon. HBV highly propagated as is shown by the highly elevated DNA-P activity. Transaminases were increased following the elevation of DNA-P activity, and a liver failure occurred. (This case should not be included in FHF even according to the Japanese criteria which include aggravation of asymptomatic HBV carriers because the patient had chronic hepatitis.) HBV continuously replicated itself for a long period in spite of IFN administration, and transaminases fluctuated continuously. The patient died of progressive liver failure.

TABLE 2

Clinical characteristics and viral markers in 24 patients with fulminant hepatitis B who had a primary or a persistent hepatitis B virus infection.

Disease and patient no.	Age (yr), sex	Outcome	HBsAg	HBeAg/anti-HBe	IgM anti-HBc	HBV DNA (PCR)	HBV DNA polymerase (cpm/ml)	
							at onset of coma	peak
Primary HBV infection								
1	21, F	survived	−	−/+	+	+	−[a]	NA
2	38, F	survived	+	−/+	+	+	−	NA
3	43, M	survived	+	−/+	+	+	−	NA
4	54, M	survived	−	−/+	−	+	−	NA
5	70, M	survived	+	+/−	+	+	−	NA
6	53, M	died	−	−/+	+	+	−	NA
7	67, M	died	+	−/+	+	+	−	NA
8	47, M	survived	−	−/+	+	+	−	NA
9	82, M	died	+	−/+	+	+	−	NA
10	45, F	survived	+	−/+	+	+	−	NA
11	51, M	survived	−	−/+	+	+	−	NA
Persistent HBV infection								
1	31, M[b]	died	+	+/−	−	+	272	22071
2	35, M	survived	+	+/−	−	+	357	NA
3	52, F	died	+	+/−	−	+	−	NA
4	54, F	survived	+	+/−	+	+	1564	5504
5	39, M	died	+	−/+	−	+	−	NA
6	31, M	survived	+	+/−	−	+	−	5479
7	40, M[c]	survived	+	−/+	−	+	−	18444
8	41, M	died	+	−/+	−	+	−	NA
9	46, M[c]	died	+	−/+	−	+	−	2746
10	55, F[c]	survived	+	−/+	−	+	−	8983
11	70, F	died	+	+/−	−	+	3040	5840
12	66, M[c]	died	+	−/+	−	+	1797	15400
13	46, M[c]	died	+	−/+	−	+	811	4290

HBsAg = hepatitis B surface antigen; HBeAg = hepatitis B e antigen; anti-HBe = antibody to hepatitis B e antigen; IgM anti-HBc, IgM antibody to hepatitis B core antigen; HBV = hepatitis B virus; PCR = polymerase chain reaction; NA = not available.

[a] Count per minute less than 30 was considered negative.

[b] After steroid withdrawal.

[c] After chemotherapy. Data from Inoue et al. [18].

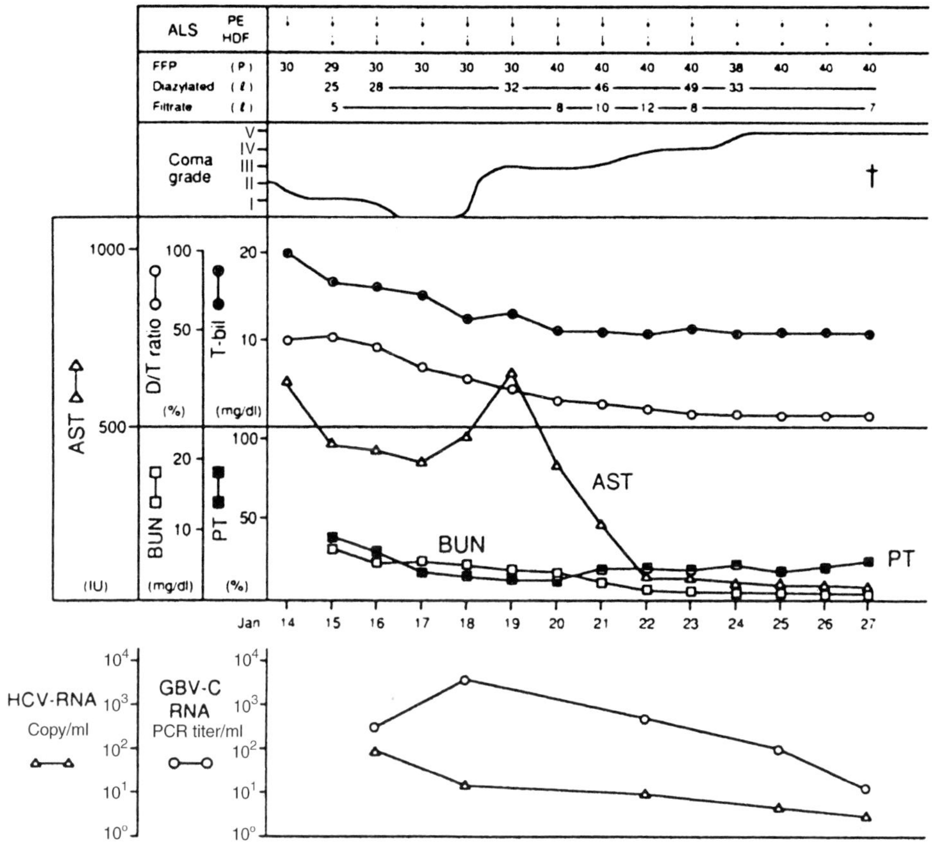

Fig. 2. Time line of clinical characteristics and chemistry in a patient with hepatitis C and hepatitis G shows persistent RNA replication for both viruses despite the development of fulminant hepatitis. ALSS = artificial liver support system; PE = plasma exchange; HDF = hemodiafiltration; FFP = fresh frozen plasma; PCR = polymerase chain reaction; T. bil (—•—) = total bilirubin; PT (—■—) = prothrombin time; HCV virus C RNA = D/T (—○—), direct bilirubin/total bilirubin; PT = prothrombin time; AST (—△—), aspartate transaminase; —□— = BUN.

Type C FH and type G FH also lead to persistent infection, Fig. 2 showing a typical example of this. In this case HCV RNA and GBV-C RNA remained high during the clinical course until the patient died of liver failure.

In cases of persistent replication of the causal virus the use of antivirals is warranted. IFN is a nonspecific antiviral, and it is currently used for type B, type C and type D chronic hepatitis. We reported that IFN is effective for type A AH which is prolonged due to persistent HAV replication [20]. Recently, lamivudine (3TC) and famciclovir (FCV) have been reported to be effective in suppressing replication of HBV [21,22]. We have already treated HBV carriers who had developed FHF with a combination of IFN, 3TC and FCV therapy. Compared with IFN monotherapy, the serum HBV DNA level is more reliably decreased (unpublished observation).

Immunosuppressive treatment is another important treatment of FH because host immune responses are assumed to be enhanced in viral FH. This is illustrated by the high titers of antibodies to hepatitis B surface and core antigen (anti-HBs and anti-HBc, respectively) [23,24]. Type B FH often develops after the cessation of immunosuppressive treatments [25]. Even type C FH is observed after a rapid decrease in cyclosporin A doses in patients receiving bone marrow transplantation [26]. However, a control trial showed no beneficial effect of a low-dose corticosteroid therapy [27]. Currently, corticosteroid is disputed because of an increased risk of infection. Immunosuppressive treatment alone without ascertaining the virological state may not be successful.

Aiming at a safer and more specific suppression of cytotoxic T lymphocytes, we have administered CsA instead of corticosteroid. Of 14 patients with FH in HBV carriers, type C and type non-A to non-C, all of whom were indicated for liver transplantation according to the criteria by the King's College group, 8 survived [28].

We recently started with 1000 mg of methyl prednisolone for 3 days which was gradually diminished. Cyclosporin A was started on the 4th day with a dose of 0.5 mg/kg and was gradually increased to 1.0 mg/kg to maintain the serum CsA concentration between 200 and 500 ng/ml. During the treatment, the transaminase level is closely monitored, and the doses of immunosuppressive agents are adjusted to reduce transaminases as rapidly as possible without inducing a flare-up. During the immunosuppressive treatment patients are kept isolated in a special room of the emergency ward, and every possible measure should be taken to protect patients from viral, bacterial and fungal infections.

Table 3 summarizes the results of this treatment. The patients were not selected, and every referred patient was accepted as far as our capacity permitted.

5. LIVER TRANSPLANTATION

Failure to develop a reliable liver support system facilitated the introduction of orthotropic liver transplantations into the treatment of FHF in 1980 by the Pittsburgh group [29]. The treatment has been rapidly adopted worldwide because the average survival rate is nearly 70%. As in Japan brain death has been only recently legally accepted, orthotropic liver transplantations have not been performed for the treatment for FHF. Instead, the living-related donor liver transplant (LRDLT) has prevailed in which children with FHF receive a part of their parent's liver [30]. Recently, LRDLT has been extended to FHF in adults. A strikingly high 5-year survival rate of 80% is reported by Shinshu University.

However, because FHF needs emergency surgery, there is usually not much time to obtain compatible livers. Consequently many patients die while waiting for a compatible liver [31]. Some patients suffer from primary graft rejection and need a second transplant surgery, and some die of liver failure. All patients who undergo liver transplantation must take immunosuppressive agents for the rest of their lives, and sometimes suffer adverse effects such as opportunistic infections. It is noteworthy, as Chapman states, that there are no controlled trials to ascertain whether liver transplantation is more effective than medical treatments [32]. However, such a controlled trial is not possible, because no patient would willingly accept assignment to the control group.

TABLE 3

Prognosis of 31 patients with fulminant hepatic failure treated in Showa University Fujigaoka Hospital over a 3.5 year period (overall survival rate was 74%)

Type	Age (yr), sex	Cause [a]	Prognosis
Acute [b]	37, M	A	survived
	45, M	A	survived
	46, M	A	survived
	34, M	A	survived
	34, M	A	survived
	49, M	A	survived
	83, M	B (acute) [c]	died
	47, M	B (acute)	survived
	38, F	B (acute)	survived
	60, F	B (acute)	survived
	50, F	B (acute)	died
	28, F	B (acute)	died
	57, F	B (acute)	survived
	25, F	B (acute)	survived
	21, F	B (acute)	died
	38, F	drug	survived
	49, F	drug	survived
Subacute [d]	40, M	B (chronic) [e]	survived
	31, M	B (chronic)	survived
	37, M	B (chronic)	survived
	65, M	B (chronic)	died
	33, M	B (chronic)	survived
	21, M	B (chronic)	survived
	52, F	B (chronic)	died
	23, M	B (chronic)	survived
	41, M	B (chronic)	died
	61, F	GBV-C	died
	23, F	GBV-C	survived
	21, F	non-A to non-G	survived
	30, F	non-A to non-G	survived
	66, M	non-A to non-G	survived

[a] A = caused by hepatitis A virus; B = caused by hepatitis B virus; GBV-C = caused by GB virus-C.
[b] Coma occurred within 10 days of the onset of the first symptoms; survival rate in this subgroup is 76%.
[c] Fulminant hepatic failure caused by acute HB infection.
[d] Coma occurred between 11 days and 2 months after the onset of the first symptoms; survival rate in this subgroup was 71%.
[e] Fulminant hepatic failure developing in chronic hepatitis B virus infection.

6. PROGNOSIS

Before the introduction of liver transplantation, prognosis of FHF was regarded as poor. A survival rate of FHF by medical treatment is currently at most 30% worldwide [33], and that justifies liver transplantations for FHF.

However, as shown in Table 2, recent results of our treatment which is based on the most intensive ALS and the most effective treatment of underlying liver diseases show a survival rate of more than 70%. Strikingly enough, an annual surveillance study on FHF tells us that the survival rate of the acute type of FHF (coma occurring within 10 days of first symptoms), which mainly includes type A FH and type B FH due to acute HBV infection and paracetamol overdose, is 66.7%. This high survival rate is not exceptional or episodic because a survival rate in a 1998 surveillance exceeded 50%. Introduction of our ALS comprising PE + HDF in nearly 80% of the institutions which answered the questionnaire is regarded as the main reason for the high survival rate.

Because this type of FHF can recover spontaneously, if the patient can be kept alive for a sufficient period, the survival rate will rise with technical progress. However, there are about 20% cases with a 'hyperacute' form of FHF in type B FH due to acute HBV infection in which liver destruction is so rapid that the liver has already been extensively destroyed by the time the the first symptoms appear. Although a liver transplantation is absolutely necessary for such cases, it is difficult to guarantee that the patient will stay alive until the liver transplantation, even with ALS.

In the 1999 surveillance a survival rate for the subacute form of FHF (coma occurring between 11 days and 24 weeks) which consists mainly of acute aggravation of HBV, type C, type G, type non-A to non-G, drug-induced hepatitis and autoimmune hepatitis was 45.0%. This high survival rate is also impressive because the survival rate was at most 20% for many years. The gradual spread of medical treatment of underlying liver diseases may affect the result.

A problem in the treatment of this form is a delay in the appearance of coma. In our experience the occurrence of coma is delayed when liver destruction proceeds slowly. Consequently, the liver has been already destroyed beyond the limit of regeneration when coma appears. In order to obtain a higher survival rate accurate prediction of FHF during the stage of acute severe hepatitis (PT < 40–50%) and an early start of treatment of hepatitis as described above is mandatory. Such attempts have already been started in our hospital.

REFERENCES

[1] Trey C, Davidson CS. The management of fulminant hepatic failure. In: Popper H, Schaffner F, editors. Progress in liver disease, Vol. 3. New York: Grune and Stratton, 1970; pp. 282–298.

[2] Sherlock S, Dooley J, editors. The haematology of liver disease. In: Sherlock S, Dooley J, editors. Diseases of the liver and biliary system, 10th ed. London: Blackwell Science, 1997; pp. 43–62.

[3] Thung SN, Gerber MA, Klion F, Gilbert H. Massive hepatic necrosis after chemotherapy withdrawal in a hepatitis B virus carrier. Arch Intern Med 1985; 145: 1313–1314.

[4] Fried MW. The liver in systemic illness. In: Zakim D, Boyer TD, editors. Hepatology – a textbook of liver disease, 3rd ed. Philadelphia, PA: WB Saunders, 1996; pp. 1706–1725.

[5] Rumack BH, Peterson RC, Koch GG, Amara IA. Acetaminophen overdose: 662 cases with evaluation of oral acetylcystein treatment. Arch Intern Med 1981; 141: 380–385.

[6] Farci P, Alter HJ, Shimoda A, Govindarajan S, Cheung L, Melpolder JC et al. Hepatitis C virus-associated fulminant hepatic failure. N Engl J Med 1996; 335: 631–634.

[7] Gazzard BG, Weston MJ, Murray-Lyon IM, Frax H, Record CD, Portmann B et al. Charcoal haemoperfusion in the treatment of fulminant hepatic coma. Lancet 1974; 1: 1301–1307.

[8] Redeker AG, Yamahiro HS. Controlled trial of exchange transfusion therapy in fulminant hepatitis. Lancet 1973; 1: 3–6.
[9] Denis J, Opolon P, Nusinovici V, Granger A, Darnis F. Treatment of encephalopathy during fulminant failure by hemodialysis with high permeability membrane. Gut 1978; 19: 787–793.
[10] Zeive L. The mechanism of hepatic coma. Hepatology 1981; 1: 360–365.
[11] Lepore M, Martel A. Plasmapheresis in hepatic coma. Lancet 1967; 2: 771–772.
[12] Opolon P. Significance of middle molecules in the pathogenesis of hepatic encephalopathy. In: Kleinberger G, Ferenci P, Riederer P, Thuler H, editors. Advances in hepatic encephalopathy and urea cycle diseases. Basel: Karger, 1984; pp. 310–314.
[13] O'Grady JG, Gimson AES, O'Brien CJ, Pucknell A, Hughes RD, Williams R. Controlled trials of charcoal hemoperfusion and prognostic factors in fulminant hepatic failure. Gastroenterology 1988; 94: 1186–1192.
[14] Yoshiba M, Sanjo T, Yamazaki Z, Inoue N, Sakai T, Okada Y et al. Aggravation of coagulation abnormality by charcoal plasma perfusion in dogs with experimental acute liver failure. Acta Hepatol Jpn 1983; 24: 426–431.
[15] Yoshiba M, Inoue N, Sanjo T, Yamazaki Z, Okada Y, Oda et al. Plasmapheresis in acute liver failure. In: Nose Y, Malchelsky PS, Smith JW, Krakauer RS, editors. Plasmapheresis therapeutic applications and new techniques. New York, NY: Raven Press, 1983; pp. 399–406.
[16] Rozca J, Demetriou AA. Artificial liver evolution and future perspectives. ASAID J 1995; 41: 831–837.
[17] Bernau J, Benhamou J-P. Fulminant and subfulminant liver failure. In: Bircher J, Benhamou J-P, McIntyre N, Rizzetto M, Rodes J, editors. Oxford textbook of clinical hepatology, 2nd ed. Oxford: Oxford Medical Publications, 1999; pp. 1341–1376.
[18] Brechot C, Bernuau J, Thiers V. Multiplication of hepatitis B virus in fulminant hepatitis B. Br Med J 1984; 288: 270–271.
[19] Inoue K, Yoshiba M, Sekiyama K, Okamoto H, Mayumi M. Clinical and molecular differences between fulminant hepatic failures following acute and chronic infection with hepatitis B virus. J Med Virol 1998; 55: 35–41.
[20] Yoshiba M, Inoue K, Sekiyama K. Interferon for hepatitis A. Lancet 1994; 343: 288–289.
[21] Dienstag JL, Schiff ER, Wright TL, Perrillo RP, Hann H-WL, Goodman Z et al. Lamivudine as initial treatment for chronic hepatitis B in the United States. N Engl J Med 1999; 341: 1256–1263.
[22] De Man RA, Marcellin P, Habel F, Desmond P, Wright T, Rose T et al. A randomized, placebo-controlled study to evaluate the efficacy of 12-month famciclovir treatment in patients with chronic hepatitis B e antigen-Positive hepatitis B. Hepatology 2000; 32: 413–417.
[23] Woolf I, Elsheikh N, Cullens H. Enhanced HBsAb production in pathogenesis of fulminant viral hepatitis type B. Br Med J 1976; II: 669–671.
[24] Trepo CG, Robert D, Motin J. Hepatitis B antigen (HBsAg) and/or antibodies (anti-HBs and anti-HBc) in fulminant hepatitis: pathogenic and prognostic significance. Gut 1976; 17: 10–13.
[25] Yoshiba M, Sekiyama K, Iwabuchi S, Takatori M, Tanaka F, Uchikoshi T et al. Recurrent fulminant hepatic failure in an HB carrier after intensive chemotherapy. Dig Dis Sci 1993; 38: 1751–1755.
[26] Yoshiba M, Sekiyama K, Inoue K, Okamoto H, Mayumi M. Contribution of hepatitis C virus to non-A, non-B fulminant hepatitis in Japan. Hepatology 1994; 19: 829–835.
[27] Rakela J, Mosley JW, Edwards VM, Govindarajan S, Alpert E. A double-blinded, randomized trial of hydrocortisone in acute hepatic failure. Dig Dis Sci 1991; 36: 1223–1228.

[28] Yoshiba M, Sekiyama K, Inoue K, Fujita R. Interferon and cyclosporin A in the treatment of fulminant viral hepatitis. J Gastroenterol 1995; 30: 67–73.
[29] Iwatsuki S, Stieber AC, Marsh JW. Liver transplantation for fulminant hepatic failure. Transplant Proc 1989; 21: 2431–2434.
[30] Shimahara Y, Awane M, Yamoka Y, Tanaka A, Morimoto T, Mori K et al. Analyses of the risk and operative stress for donors in living-related partial liver transplantation. Transplantation 1992; 54: 983–988.
[31] McCaughan GW. Selection of patients for liver transplantation. J Gastroenterol Hepatol 1993; 8: 185–194.
[32] Chapman RW, Forman D, Peto R, Smallwood R. Liver transplantation for acute hepatic failure? Lancet 1990; 335: 32–35.
[33] Bernuau J, Benhamou J-P. Fulminant and subfulminant liver failure. In: McIntyre N, Benhamou J-P, Bircher J, Rizzetto M, Rodes J, editors. Oxford textbook of clinical hepatology. Oxford: Oxford Medical Publications, 1991; pp. 921–944.

Living Related Liver Transplantation

Molecular Biology and Immunology in Hepatology
Edited by T. Tsuji, T. Higashi, M. Zeniya and K.-H. Meyer zum Büschenfelde

CHAPTER 24

Current Strategy of Living Related Liver Transplantation: Overview

Koichi Tanaka and Satoshi Kaihara

Department of Transplantation and Immunology, Graduate School of Medicine, Kyoto University, Kyoto, Japan

INTRODUCTION

Currently, liver transplantation has been the successful and fully accepted treatment for end-stage liver disease; however, organ donor shortage continues to be the most critical problem. Over the past 10 years, the number of patients listed for liver transplantation has increased more than 15-fold [1]. Consequently, about 20,000 patients are on the waiting list and the median waiting time is 500 days [1]. To solve this critical shortage of graft organs, living related liver transplantation (LRLT) has been receiving much attention as one of the options to expand the donor reserves.

LRLT was first performed in two patients by Raia et al. in 1988 [2]. Both recipients died shortly after the operation; however, they lived long enough to demonstrate the technical feasibility. The first successful LRLT came from Strong et al. in 1989 [3]. Since then, LRLT has expanded rapidly around the world, especially in countries in which cadaveric organ transplantation is not available or rarely performed. LRLT has several advantages compared to cadaveric liver transplantation (CLT). First, it increases the number of available organs directly. Second, most recipients receive their transplant electively and thus would induce lower morbidity and mortality. Finally, the preservation time can be minimized in LRLT with synchronous performance of donor and recipient operations.

Our institute started the living related liver transplant program in 1990 and entered the eleventh year in 2000. This LRLT program is the longest-running in Japan and the largest in the world as well. The number of transplants has been increasing every year and reached 600 cases on March in 2000. In the subsequent sections, we discuss the current strategy of LRLT including the problems and their solutions, and the future directions.

1. DONOR SELECTION

1.1. Informed consent

Full informed consent is imperative for living donation. It will be achieved in two steps. The initial consent will focus on the evaluation needed for a donor candidate and the donor's operation as well as an outline of transplantation. If the donor candidate agrees with it, the evaluations will be performed. After the donor is considered medically and psychologically suitable as a donor, the second consent will be retrieved. It will focus on the donor's operation including potential risk factors and surgical complications based on the results of the evaluations. The published data and personal experiences should be reviewed as well.

1.2. Evaluation

As a first step, social and psychological-, historical-, and physical evaluations are thoroughly assessed. In addition, blood type, complete blood count, blood chemistry, and hepatitis serology are evaluated. Next, the donor is subjected to Doppler ultrasound (Doppler US) and computed tomography (CT) or magnetic resonance imaging (MRI) to assess the anatomical variation in the vasculatures, the volume of the graft segment, and the possible latent disease in the donor [4–6]. The precise blood test will be performed again. The CT is also important to evaluate the grade of fatty infiltration in the graft liver.

Any invasive methods should be avoided as much as possible, considering the potential risk accompanied with the procedures. Angiogram is effective to rule out any anomalies of the hepatic artery that may render LRLT technically unfeasible; however, adopting a microsurgical technique has eliminated the necessity of the preoperative evaluation of the donor's hepatic artery [5,6]. Endoscopic retrograde cholangiography (ERC) can be avoided by applying the intra-operative cholangiography to assess the biliary anatomy [7]. Only one indication is in parents of children with Alagille's syndrome. Liver biopsy is imperative to assess the viability of the graft liver in CLT; however, the indication is limited in case of LRLT because the routine evaluations of the donor will be enough to assess the graft condition.

1.3. Contraindications

Several studies indicate a limitation in donor suitability. Renz et al. reported that only 10% of the first evaluated 75 potential living donors were acceptable for donation [4]. Emond et al. reported that 62 out of 134 potential donors were excluded: because of ABO incompatibility in 16 (12%), medical findings in 27 (20%), and social reasons in 19 (14%) donors [8]. In contrast, 120 out of 135 candidates were accepted as suitable donors in our early experience [9]. The wide variations between the institutions would be due to the different social and religious background in each country.

1.4. Risk for the donor

LRLT involves potential risks for the donor and there is still some discussion whether the excellent results and the situation on the waiting list can excuse the possible risks to a healthy person. To our knowledge there have been at least 6 deaths out of over 1200 living liver donors for an incidence of 0.5% [10].

The most critical complication in the donor is lung embolization. We experienced it in one donor who was fortunately fully recovered with conservative therapy. One case of donor death was also reported due to lung embolism occurred two days after the operation [11]. If the donor has risk factors such as massive overweight, smoking, or oral contraceptive steroids, special attention should be paid on the hazard of the lung embolization. In our institute, the high-risk donors are evaluated for the existence of deep vein thrombosis pre-operatively with radioisotope angiography. A special mechanical device has been routinely used as well to prevent the thrombus formation until the donor starts moving.

Intra-operative massive bleeding is not common. In our initial experience, the mean blood loss during the donor operation was 550 g for a left lobectomy and 370 g for a left lateral segmentectomy [12]. We used to prepare autologous blood just in case of massive bleeding; however, it is currently unnecessary. Other major complications in the literature include splenic injury requiring splenectomy, vascular complications, bile duct stenosis, bile leakage, intra-abdominal abscess, and psychiatric disorder [13–15]. The incidence of re-operation has been reported to be between 0 to 6% and the indications were gastro-intestinal tract obstruction, bile leakage, and incisional hernia [7,16,17].

2. RESULTS OF LRLT

2.1. Patient survival

The overall results of LRLT are reported to be between 71 and 100%, which are quite similar to those of CTL. Gross et al. compared the long term results of LRLT to CLT and found no differences in patient survival [7]. The one-year survival for LRLT was 87% and that for CLT was 81%. They concluded that the use of living related graft has reduced the waiting time and has improved patient survival.

In our series, 1-, 3-, and 5-year survival rates of 618 recipients by November 2000 was 78, 77, and 76% (data not published). Pediatric cases showed 83% of patient survival. A survival rate of 158 children transplanted for biliary atresia was 85% and it was over 90% in the last two years [18]. On the other hand, the survival rate of children who underwent LRLT for fulminant hepatic failure was 57%, especially 38% for those under 2 years old, and we need to analyze the reason for this undesirable result (data not published). The 1-year survival rate of adult LRLT was 70% survival, which was worse than pediatric cases and thus would be due to the graft size matching (data not published). It has been improving after applying right lobe graft to adult recipients and the 1-year survival rate of 117 cases of right lobe LRLT for adult patients was 75% versus 67% for adults who underwent left lobe LRLT.

ABO compatibility has a great impact on the survival of the recipients after liver transplantation. In our initial results, 1-year survival rate of 13 ABO incompatible cases was 77%, which was favorably comparable to that of CLT [19,20]. However, most of the initial recipients were younger children and, with the increase in the number of older children and adult recipients, the result has come down to 64.9% (data not published). Primary graft non-function is rare in LRLT and we have not encountered it at all. The overall incidence has been reported as 0.8%, which is much smaller than that of CLT [8,16,18,21]. The lower incidence can be attributed to several factors; better graft quality because of preoperative donor evaluation, stable hemodynamics before and during the donation, and a shorter preservation time.

2.2. *Surgical complications*

2.2.1. *Vascular complications*

Hepatic artery thrombosis (HAT) is a critical complication especially in the early post-transplant period. The incidence has been reported as low as 1.7% and this good result was achieved by adopting microsurgical techniques for arterial anastomosis [6]. The onset of HAT could be prevented with close monitoring and management of the coagulation after LRLT [22].

Complication of portal venous system is significantly higher in LRLT than CLT, especially in recipients younger than 1 year old. The incidence of hepatic vein related complications is low except the recipients who underwent LRLT for Budd-Chiari syndrome.

2.2.2. *Biliary complications*

The incidence of biliary complications is higher in LRLT than CLT. Cronin et al. reported that 35 out of 91 cases (38%) had biliary complications [23]. The left hepatic duct, used for LRLT, is much smaller in diameter than the common bile duct, which is used for CLT. In some cases of LRLT, the graft has multiple hepatic ducts to be reconstructed. The smaller bile duct in the graft may make the anastomosis more difficult and may cause a stricture or leakage at the anastomotic site. The elevation of the intraductal pressure may easily induce bile leakage from the cutting surface, resulting in biloma formation. ABO incompatibility may also be a risk factor for non-anastomotic biliary strictures after LRLT [24]. The incidence of biliary complication after LRLT did not affect the survival of those patients, which was significantly higher than in the CLT group [23].

2.3. *Rejection*

LRLT was expected to show a lower rate of rejection than CLT because the majority of the donors are relatives of the recipients. Actually, genetic advantages have been demonstrated in living related kidney transplantation. However, the incidence and severity of acute cellular rejection (ACR) in LRLT is not different from that of CLT. The occurrence of ACR in LRLT has been reported at between 25% and 50%, depending on the immunosuppressive regimens. In our initial series, 29% of recipients after LRLT treated with tacrolimus had at least one episode of ACR [25]. Regarding chronic rejection, LRLT has been reported to have some advantages compared to CLT. In our initial series, only 3 out of 120 patients developed chronic rejection [26]. Alonso et al. also reported the low incidence of chronic rejection in LRLT recipients than that in CLT recipients (8 vs 20%) [27]. Hyperacute rejection has not been reported in LRLT.

3. GRAFT SIZE MATCHING

3.1. Small-for-size graft

LRLT has been successfully performed on pediatric patients using left lateral or left segment, because further resection might compromise the peri-operative safety of the donor. On the other hand, LRLT has limitations in adult recipients, and one of the main difficulties is how to get grafts large enough for adult recipients without compromising the safety of the donor. Theoretically, a small-for-size graft can regenerate and eventually reaches the ideal liver size of the recipient [28–30]; however, the graft needs to provide immediate functions to cope with the metabolic needs of the recipient. The rate of regeneration may be affected by various factors existing preoperatively in the recipients as well.

Selecting the appropriate graft size is a very important factor for the successful transplantation. This value is dependent on the characteristics of donor and recipient and should be adjusted based on the pre-transplant conditions of the each recipient individually. Successful adult LRLT using a graft as small as 25% of the recipient's native liver weight has been reported [31]. However, the success of such a small-for-size graft depends on optimal peri-operative circumstances and the recipient will be potentially at risk of graft failure. Recent studies have demonstrated the grafts smaller than 40% of the recipient's native liver should be regarded as a marginal graft with a lower success rate [32]. We also reported that 1-year graft survival with 1.0 to 3.0% of graft-to-recipient weight ratio (GRWR) was 91.8% and, on the other hand, that with less than 0.8% was 59.7% [33]. These results are quite compatible to others in CLT [34,35]. Hyper-perfusion has been suspected to induce injury for small for size grafts and there are some experimental data supporting this theory [36–38].

Some groups have determined the minimum graft size required for recipients according to their pre-transplant conditions. For example, 30% of standard liver volume would be the limit for acute liver failure and 40% would be for pre-existing portal hypertension [39]. The graft weight might be also corrected by the degree of steatosis because fat is not functional and does not contribute to the restoration of liver mass [40].

3.2. Large-for-size graft

Large-for-size grafts in pediatric transplantation, more than 5% of GRWR, would be associated with other serious complications. Lower relative blood flow would attribute to poor blood supply to the graft and more frequent vascular complications [33]. Difficulty in abdominal wall closure is experienced sometimes in cases of excessively large grafts. Higher intra-abdominal pressure would induce the extrinsic compression of the vasculatures and will push up the diaphragm resulting in respiratory distress. Rejection is more frequent as well presumably due to the greater immunologic stimulus [33]. To address these issues, monosegment liver transplantation has been tried with satisfactory results [41,42]. In our institute, we started a new program of monosegment LRLT in 1999 and so far the initial results have been satisfactory.

4. RIGHT LOBE LRLT FOR ADULTS

4.1. Evolution of right lobe graft for adults

Early reports in adult LRLT with left lobe graft exhibited a poor outcome [43]. Shinshu's group in Japan followed by other groups reported the first successful adult LRLT in 1993 [44,45]. However, the overall results were still unsatisfactory and the limitation of the left lobe graft for adult recipients has been identified because left lobe from a relatively small donor does not meet the metabolic demand of a larger recipient [39]. To address this problem, many groups have had a great concern in LRLT using right lobe graft.

Our group reported the first success in right lobe LRLT in 1994 [46]. This case was not indicated for size matching but for anatomical variation in hepatic artery of the donor. We did not accept this technique immediately for LRLT in considering the safety of the donor. In 1997 Hong Kong's group reported their first case of adult LRLT using extended right lobe graft followed by 13 cases with 86% of graft survival [39,47,48]. At the same time, trials of right lobe LRLT for adult recipients were initiated in the United States and achieved 89% survival rate. These results were surprisingly better than those of left lobe graft for adults. In 1998, we started a new program using right lobe LRLT for adults, after experience with more than 350 cases of left lobe LRLT and 130 cases of right lobe LRLT were performed by November 2000. Based on our results in donor safety and recipient survival, we currently apply right lobe donation as a routine method for adult LRLT.

4.2. Donor safety

Donor safety is the most important issue in LRLT and special attention should be paid for it, especially in case of right lobe donation because of its complicated procedures. In our initial series with right lobe donation, the median blood loss during the operation was 330 ml and the median operation time was 6.7 hr [49]. Both of them were significantly greater than those of left lateral segmentectomy but did not have any statistical differences from those of left lobectomy. Post-operative liver function tests showed that peak levels of aspartate transaminoferase and total bilirubin in the donor after right lobectomy were significantly higher than those after left lateral segmentectomy and left lobectomy; however, they recovered rapidly to the normal level. Considering those results, the safety limits for the right lobe donation should be strict and careful donor selection may be necessary in right lobe LRLT.

In LRLT using the right lobe, the volume of the remnant liver is another major concern. The experiments in animal models demonstrated that 10% of viable liver mass was adequate for spontaneous recovery after hepatectomy [50] because regeneration of remnant liver begins immediately after liver resection until it reaches the ideal size [29,51–53]. Another study using magnetic resonance imaging (MRI) demonstrated that liver mass was almost completely restored after right lobe donation after only 2 weeks [54]. The lowest limit of the remnant liver, reported in the literature, ranges from 27% to 40% [55–57]. Volumetry using CT scan or MRI is necessary to estimate the residual liver volume preoperatively because there would be wide variations in the size of left lobe in each donor.

Another risk to the donor is biliary complications including stricture and leakage. In our initial series, biliary leakage occurred in 8% of donors after right lobe resection, which was higher than that occurring after left or left lateral donations. They were, however, all treated well with conservative or interventional therapies and the incidence of biliary leakage has recently decreased to 5% with some modifications in donor operation. Stricture in the remnant biliary tract occurred in just one out of 130 right lobe donation and he was successfully treated with PTCD and balloon dilatation.

4.3. Technical issues in right lobe LRLT

4.3.1. Vascular complications

Hepatic artery thrombosis (HAT) has been a critical problem in pediatric LRLT; however, the development of microsurgical technique could lead to the decrease of the incidence [58–61]. On the other hand, HAT is not common in right lobe LRLT because of the large caliber of the artery in the graft [40,51,52]. In our experience, only one case needed re-anastomosis of the hepatic artery for HAT in 130 cases of right lobe LRLT (data not published).

Venous drainage from the graft is one of the most important issues in right lobe LRLT. The procedures are divided into two categories; right lobe graft with middle and right hepatic vein, and with only right hepatic vein [39,40,46,62]. In case of right lobe graft with middle and right hepatic vein, preserving the middle hepatic vein is certainly favorable for the graft. Remnant medial segment in the donor will have little congestion because of the intrinsic network in the hepatic venous system [63,64]. The only potential risk could be the injury or stenosis of the left hepatic vein in the remnant liver by the closure of the orifice of the middle hepatic vein. Hong Kong's group has accepted this procedure and has reported 11 cases without any major complications [39,47,48]. They reconstruct the preserved middle hepatic vein to the recipient's middle hepatic vein in an end-to-end fashion. In another procedure, using the graft with only right hepatic vein, the drainage vein from a part of anterior segment is not reconstructed [40,49]. Our group has hired this method based on the data of MRI study, which demonstrated spontaneous disappearance of the initial vascular congestion detected in the part of anterior segment several weeks after the operation presumably due to formation of intra-hepatic venous shunt [40]. Large accessory hepatic vein, if exists, should be anastomosed to the inferior vena cava to augment the outflow of the graft. Korea's group routinely reconstructs the veins from the anterior segment using autologous vessels to preserve the outflow from the graft immediately after the reperfusion.

4.3.2. Biliary complications

The rate of biliary complication in right lobe LRLT was higher than whole liver transplantation and it was reported as high as 35% [23,40,65,66]. The bile leakage may occur from the cut surface of the graft to form a biloma. The smaller bile duct in the graft may make the anastomosis more difficult and may cause a stricture or leakage at the anastomotic site. In some cases, multiple hepatic duct will be encountered. In our initial data, the biliary complications were 15% in right lobe LRLT, which was almost the same incidence as that of whole liver transplantation [67]. Recently, we started duct-to-duct biliary reconstruction in right lobe LRLT. With this method, we can avoid Roux-en Y construction and bilioenteric continuity is preserved physiologically. Although the follow up period is less than 1 year, the initial results have been satisfactory.

5. FUTURE DIRECTIONS

LRLT has been expanding the territory to adult recipients by using right lobe grafts. With the initial favorable results, the application would be a great solution for organ donor shortage and would have a dramatic impact in reducing death of the patients on the waiting list. On the other hand, donor safety is always the top priority in LRLT and we should be sincerely careful in evaluation, operation and postoperative management of the donors. Further experience will improve surgical techniques, ensure donor and recipient safety, and eventually lead to fruitful outcome in LRLT.

REFERENCES

[1] United Network for Organ Sharing. Data. UNOS Annual Report 1999.

[2] Raia S, Nery JR, Mies S. Liver transplantation from live donors. Lancet 1989; 21: 497.

[3] Strong RW, Lynch SV, Ong TH, Matsunami H, Koido Y, Balderson GA. Successful liver transplantation from a living donor to her son. N Engl J Med 1990; 322: 1505–1507.

[4] Renz JF, Mudge CL, Heyman MB, Tomlanovich S, Kingsford RP, Moore BJ et al. Donor selection limits use of living-related liver transplantation. Hepatology 1995; 22: 1122–1126.

[5] Yamaoka Y, Morimoto T, Inamoto T, Tanaka A, Honda K, Ikai I et al. Safety of the donor in living-related liver transplantation – an analysis of 100 parental donors. Transplantation 1995; 59: 224–226.

[6] Inomoto T, Nishizawa F, Sasaki H, Terajima H, Shirakata Y, Miyamoto S et al. Experiences of 120 microsurgical reconstruction of hepatic artery in living related liver transplantation. Surgery 1996; 119: 20–26.

[7] Rogiers X, Broering DC, Mueller L, Burdelski M. Living-donor liver transplantation in children. Langenbecks Arch Surg 1999; 384: 528–535.

[8] Emond JC, Rosenthal P, Roberts JP, Stock P, Kelley S, Gregory G et al. Living related donor liver transplantation: the UCSF experience. Transplant Proc 1996; 28: 2375–2377.

[9] Morimoto T, Ichimiya M, Tanaka A, Ikai I, Yamamoto Y, Nakamura Y et al. Guidelines for donor selection and an overview of the donor operation in living related liver transplantation. Transplant Int 1996; 9: 208–213.

[10] Strong RW. Whither living donor liver transplantation? Liver Transplant Surg 1999; 5: 536–538.

[11] Sterneck MR, Fischer L, Nischwitz U, Burdelski M, Kjer S, Latta A et al. Selection of the living donor. Transplantation 1995; 60: 667–671.

[12] Morimoto T, Tanaka A, Ikai I, Yamamoto Y, Nakamura Y, Takada Y et al. Donor safety in living related liver transplantation. Transplant Proc 1995; 27: 1166–1169.

[13] Broelsch CE, Emond JC, Whitington PF, Thistlethwaite JR, Baker AL, Lichtor JL. Application of reduced size liver transplants as split grafts, auxiliary orthotopic grafts, living related segmental transplants. Ann Surg 1990; 212: 368–375.

[14] Heffron TG. Living related liver transplantation. Sem in Liver Dis 1995; 15: 165–172.

[15] Goldman LS. Liver transplantation using living donors: preliminary donor psychiatric outcomes. Psychosomatics 1993; 34: 235–240.

[16] Heffron TG, Langnas AN, Fox IJ, Mack D, Dhawan A, Kaufman S et al. Living related donor liver transplantation at the University of Nebraska Medical Center (1996). Transplant Proc 1996; 28: 2382.

[17] Sterneck M, Nischwitz U, Fischer L, Malago M, Rogiers X, Raedler A et al. Evaluation and morbidity of the living liver donor in pediatric liver transplantation. Transplant Proc 1995; 27: 1164–1165.

[18] Inomata Y. Liver transplantation – present status. J Jpn Surg Soc 1996; 97: 978–983.

[19] Tanaka A, Tanaka K, Itai T, Yanabu A, Sato B, Mori S et al. Living related liver transplantation across ABO blood groups. Transplantation 1994; 58: 548–553.

[20] Cacciarelli TV, So SK, Lim J, Concepcion W, Cox K, Esquivel CO. A reassessment of ABO incompatibility in pediatric liver transplantation. Transplantation 1995; 60: 757–760.

[21] Rogiers X, Schroeder T, Tuttlewski K, Broelsch CE. For the ILDR. First report of the international living donor liver registry. Presented at the 16th international congress of the transplantation society, Barcelona, Spain, August 25–30, 1996.

[22] Hashikura Y, Kawasaki S, Okumura N, Ishikawa S, Matsunami H, Ikegami T et al. Prevention of hepatic artery thrombosis in pediatric liver transplantation. Transplantation 1995; 60: 1109–1112.

[23] Cronin DC, Alonso EM, Piper JB, Newell KA, Bruce DS, Woodle E et al. Biliary complications in living donor liver transplantation. Transplant Proc 1997; 29: 419–420.

[24] Sanchez-Urdazpal L, Gores GJ, Ward EM, Maus TP, Buckel EG, Steers JL et al. Ischemic-type biliary complication after orthotopic liver transplantation. Hepatology 1992; 16: 49–53.

[25] Ueda M, Uemoto S, Inomata Y, Okajima H, Hashida T, Tanaka K et al. A proposal of FK506 optimal dosing in living related liver transplantation. Transplantation 1995; 60: 258–264.

[26] Inomata Y, Tanaka K, Egawa H, Uemoto S, Ozaki N, Okajima H et al. The evolution of immunosuppression with FK506 in pediatric living-related liver transplantation. Transplantation 1996; 61: 247–252.

[27] Hashikura Y, Kawasaki S, Matsunami H. Postoperative managemant and long-term outcome in living-related liver transplantation. Jpn J Transplant 1995; 30: 134.

[28] Van Thiel DH, Gavaler JS, Kam I, Francavilla A, Polimeno L, Schade RR et al. Rapid growth of an intact human liver transplanted into a recipient larger than the donor. Gastroenterology 1987; 93: 1414–1419.

[29] Kawasaki S, Makuuchi M, Ishizone S, Matsunami H, Terada M, Kawarazaki H. Liver regeneration in recipients and donors after transplantation. Lancet 1992; 339: 580–581.

[30] Starzl TE, Koep LJ, Weil R, Lilly JR, Putnam CV, Aldrete JA. Right trisegmentectomy for hepatic neoplasms. Surg Gynecol Obstet 1980; 150: 208–214.

[31] Lo CM, Fan ST, Chan JFK, Wei W, Lo RJW, Lai CL. Minimum graft volume for successful adult-to-adult living donor liver transplantation for fulminant hepatic failure. Transplantation 1996; 62: 696–698.

[32] Lo CM, Fan ST, Liu CL, Chan JK, Lam BK et al. Minimum graft size for living donor liver transplantation. Transplantation 1999; 68: 1112–1116.
[33] Kiuchi T, Kasahara M, Uryuhara K, Inomata Y, Uemoto S, Asonuma K et al. Impact of graft size mismatching on graft prognosis in liver transplantation from living donors. Transplantation 1999; 67: 321–327.
[34] Heffron TG. Living related liver transplantation. Semin Liver Dis 1995; 15: 165–172.
[35] De Ville De Goyet J, Otte JB. Cut-down and split liver transplantation. In: Busttil RW, Klintmalm GB, editors. Transplantation of the Liver. W.B. Saunders, 1996; pp. 481–496.
[36] Emond J, Renz J, Ferrell L, Rosenthal P, Lim R, Roberts J et al. Functional analysis of grafts from living donors. Implications for treatment of older recipients. Ann Surg 1996; 224: 544–554.
[37] Ku Y, Fukumoto T, Nishida T, Tominaga M, Maeda I, Kitagawa T et al. Evidence that portal vein decompression improves survival of canine quarter orthotopic liver transplantation. Transplantation 1995; 59: 1388–1392.
[38] Ueno S, Kobayashi Y, Kurita K, Tanabe G, Aikou T. Effect of prior portosystemic shunt on early hepatic hemodynamics and sinusoids following 84% hepatectomy in dogs. Res Exp Med 1995; 195: 1–8.
[39] Lo CM, Fan ST, Liu CL, Wei WI, Lo RJ, Lai CL. Adult-to-adult living donor liver transplantation using extended right lobe graft. Ann Surg 1997; 226: 261–270.
[40] Marcos A, Fisher RA, Ham JM, Shiffman ML, Sanyal AJ, Luketic VAC et al. Right lobe living donor liver transplantation. Transplantation 1999; 68: 798–803.
[41] Srinivasan P, Vilca-Melendez H, Muiesan P, Prachalias A, Heaton ND, Rela M. Liver transplantation with monosegments. Surgery 1999; 126: 10–12.
[42] Bonatti H, Muiesan P, Connelly S, Baker A, Mieli-Vergani G, Gibbs P et al. Hepatic transplantation in children under 3 months of age: a single centre's experience. J Pediatr Surg 1997; 32: 486–488.
[43] Haberal M, Bilgin N, Buyukpamukcu N, Tokyay R, Telatar H, Simsek H et al. Living donor hepatectomy in partial liver transplantation: surgical technique and results. Transplant Proc 1993; 2: 1899–1901.
[44] Hashikura Y, Makuuchi M, Kawasaki S, Matunami H, Ikegami T, Nakazawa Y et al. Successful living-related partial liver transplantation to an adult patient. Lancet 1994; 343: 1233–1234.
[45] Miwa S, Hashikura Y, Mita A, Kubota T, Chisuwa H, Nakazawa Y et al. Living-related liver transplantation for patients with fulminant and subfulminant hepatic failure. Hepatology 1999; 30: 1521–1526.
[46] Yamaoka Y, Washida M, Honda K, Tanaka K, Mori K, Shimahara Y et al. Liver transplantation using a right lobe graft from a living related donor. Transplantation 1994; 57: 1127–1130.
[47] Lo CM, Fan ST, Liu CL, Lo RJ, Lau GK, Wei WI et al. Extending the limit on the size of adult recipient in living donor liver transplantation using extended right lobe graft. Transplantation 1997; 63: 1524–1528.
[48] Fan ST, Lo CM, Liu CL. Technical refinement in adult-to-adult living donor liver transplantation using right lobe graft. Ann Surg 2000; 231: 126–131.
[49] Inomata Y, Uemoto S, Asonuma K, Egawa H, Kiuchi T, Fujita S et al. Right lobe graft in living donor liver transplantation. Transplantation 2000; 69: 258–264.
[50] Ganb J, Inversen J. Rat liver regeneration after 90% partial hepatectomy. Hepatology 1984; 4: 902–904.
[51] Park K, Lee S, Lee Y, Hwang S, Nam C, Choi K et al. Adult-to-adult living donor liver transplantation at Asian Medical Center, Seoul, South Korea. Transplant Proc 1999; 31: 456–458.

[52] Kawasaki S, Makuuchi M, Matsunami H, Hashikura Y, Ikegami T, Nakazawa Y et al. Living related liver transplantation in adults. Ann Surg 1998; 227: 269–274.

[53] Nakagami M, Morimoto T, Itoh K, Arima Y, Yamamoto Y, Ikai I et al. Patterns of restoration of remnant liver volume after graft harvesting in donors for living related liver transplantation. Transplant Proc 1998; 30: 195–199.

[54] Marcos A. Right lobe living donor liver transplantation: a review. Liver Transplant 2000; 6: 3–20.

[55] Fall ST, Lo CM, Liu CL, Yong BH, Chan JKF, Ng IOL. Safety of donors in live donor liver transplantation using right lobe grafts. Arch Surg 2000; 135: 336–340.

[56] Stone HH, Long WD, Smith RB III, Haynes CD. Physiological consideration in major hepatic resection. Am J Surg 1969; 117: 78–84.

[57] Kubota K, Makuuchi M, Kusaka K, Kobayashi T, Miki K, Hasegawa K et al. Measurement of liver volume and hepatic functional reserve as a guide to decision-making in resectional surgery for hepatic tumors. Hepatology 1997; 26: 1176–1181.

[58] Broelsch C, Whitington P, Edmond J, Heffroll T, Thistlethwaite J, Stevens L et al. Liver transplantation in children from living related donors. Ann Surg 1991; 214: 428–437.

[59] Kiuchi T, Inomata Y, Uemoto S, Asonuma K, Egawa H, Hayashi M et al. Living donor liver transplantation in Kyoto, 1997. Clin Transplant 1997; 191–198.

[60] Mori K, Nagata I, Yamagata S, Sasaki H, Nishizawa F, Takeda Y et al. The introduction of microvascular surgery to hepatic artery reconstruction in living-donor liver transplantation – Its surgical advantages compared with conventional procedures. Transplantation 1992; 54: 263–268.

[61] Emond J, Polastri R. Anatomical hepatectomy for resection or transplantation. Am J Surg 1996; 172: 29–34.

[62] Wachs M, Bak T, Karrer F, Everson G, Shrestha R, Trouillot T et al. Adult living donor liver transplantation using a right hepatic lobe. Transplantation 1998; 66: 1313–1316.

[63] Cheng Y, Huang T, Chen C, Chen T, Huang C, Ko S et al. Variations of the left and middle hepatic veins: Application in living related hepatic transplantation. J Clin Ultrasound 1996; 24: 11–16.

[64] Willd P, Douard R, Cugnenc P, Chevallier J. Anatomy of the common trunk of the middle and left hepatic veins: Application to liver transplantation. Surg Radiol Anat 1999; 21: 17–21.

[65] Reding R, de Goyet J, Delbeke I, Sokal E, Jamart J, Janssen M et al. Pediatric liver transplantation with cadaveric or living related donors: Comparative results in 90 elective recipients of primary grafts. J Pediatr 1999; 134: 280–286.

[66] Busuttil R, Gross J. Split liver transplantation. Ann Surg 1999; 229: 313–321.

[67] Seiler C. The bile duct anastomosis in liver transplantation. Dig Surg 1999; 16: 102–106.

Molecular Biology and Immunology in Hepatology
Edited by T. Tsuji, T. Higashi, M. Zeniya and K.-H. Meyer zum Büschenfelde

CHAPTER 25

Viral Cirrhosis and Hepatocellular Carcinoma in Relation to Living-Donor Liver Transplants

Takafumi Ichida

Niigata University, Third Department of Internal Medicine, Niigata, Japan

INTRODUCTION

The first cases of living-donor liver transplants involving children appeared in Japan in 1989. The first successful cases of living-donor liver transplants in adults making use of the regenerative power of the liver were seen in 1993 [1]. Later, living-donor liver transplants involving adults were conducted in a number of facilities, and the current case total is close to reaching 350 cases. Living-donor liver transplant serves to provide two adults with liver functions based on the regenerative capability of one liver; it is a life-saving treatment.

One reason for the rapid increase in cases of living-donor transplants conducted with adults is simply that there are large numbers of adults with liver disease in Japan. Many of these adults are suffering from chronic liver diseases with morbidity due to viral hepatitis. The use of transplant care where cases have lapsed into progressive and irreversible hepatic failure, such as decompensated cirrhosis and hepatocellular carcinoma, has yet to be established. Thus, this report involves a review of the clinical significance and problems associated with living-donor liver transplants relative to viral cirrhosis and hepatocellular carcinoma.

1. HEPATITIS B VIRUS (HBV)-POSITIVE CIRRHOSIS

Liver transplants from cadaveric donors have been conducted in patients with HBV-positive liver disease with the objective of examining fulminant hepatic failure as a result of acute infection as well as cirrhosis and hepatocellular carcinoma due to chronic infection. One finding from this work is that reinfection of HBV in the grafted liver is frequently noted, particularly in cases of cirrhosis. Pathologies such as rapid and severe hepatitis as well as fibrosing cholestatic hepatitis [2] are initiated, with fatal results [3,4]. Even when severe hepatitis is the result, the pathology is extremely poor when considering aspects like the advance of cirrhosis in the short-term. Of course, when progressive and serious hepatitis occurs after transplant with de novo HBV infection, as expected, the prognosis is poor [5]. In contrast, the reinfection rate after liver transplants associated with HBV-related fulminant hepatic failure is low; instead, active transplant accommodation is seen. Adaptation of transplants from cadaveric donors, which is based on the concept of equitable organ distribution, was first ruled out due to clinical findings such as post-operative HBV reinfection and high rates of early death for HBV-positive recipients excluding those suffering from fulminant hepatic failure. Nonetheless, immunological defense mechanisms against HBV reinfection after transplant were provided by means of administration of hepatitis B immunoglobulin (HBIG), or γ-globulin containing hepatitis B surface antigen, around 1987 [6,7]. Thus, transplant results for HBV-recipients improved, and then a reverse transcriptase inhibitor appeared in the form of lamivudine in 1995 [8]. In tandem with this development, the long-term prognosis for HBV-positive cirrhosis recipients today [9] is extremely favorable [10].

From 1987 to 1995, the transplant results in the US gave an overall 8-year survival rate of 58%, although the 8-year survival rate for HBV-positive recipients of liver transplants was only 47%. Because results as a whole were poorer, results of transplants involving malignancies were by far superior. Looking at recent European results [11], one can see that results for liver transplants in all cases yielded a 5-year survival rate of 67% after 1988; the 10-year survival rate was 61%. Of these findings, results for all cases of HBV-positive cirrhosis compare favorably; the 5-year survival rate was 68% and the 10-year survival rate was 61%, indicating the remarkable results the physicians in Europe have been able to achieve.

It is apparent that treatment with interferon, an antiviral agent used to combat reinfection with HBV, for the most part does not contribute to the betterment of that survival rate. Accordingly, the current consensus suggests that only HBIG and lamivudine can serve as treatment strategies to contribute to long-term survival after liver transplant for HBV cirrhosis. Overall strategies can be separated into preventative and treatment strategies, outlined below. Prophylaxis strategy has been described as consisting of: (1) continuous administration of lamivudine starting prior to the transplant and continuing after the transplant; (2) continuous administration of HBIG before the transplant; and (3) lamivudine administration before and after transplant with concurrent use of HBIG. In contrast, (4) lamivudine administration is the current treatment strategy for HBV-positive cases before transplant for prevention of recurrence after transplant.

1.1. Prophylaxis by means of HBIG

The first treatment tool used was HBIG, reported in 1987 [12], and by 1993 Samuel et al. [13], preventing almost 33% of post-operative reinfection by using HBIG. However, in 1994, the European consensus was resistance to use of this treatment due to problems preventing reinfection for HBV-DNA-positive cases [14]. Problems with HBIG were also cited in that: (1) there is a risk of an allergic reaction as a result of intravenous injection; (2) the pharmokinetics are complicated as well as expensive; and (3) there is a possibility of unknown viral infection because it is produced from human blood. Furthermore, the fact that the HBIG currently in use is not heat-treated is common knowledge.

TABLE 1

HBIG administration results

Source	Successful prophylaxis cases	Follow-up	Anti-Hepatitis B surface antigen titer
McGory et al. [15]	25/25	2–55 months	>500 (0–7), >25 (8–90), >100
Tchervenkov et al. [16]	12/13	9–56 months	>1000

TABLE 2

HBV prophylaxis by means of continuous lamivudine administration before liver transplant

Source	No. cases	HBV positivity	Amount of lamivudine administered	Before transplant administration period	After transplant follow-up period
Grellier et al. [17]	12	9 (75%)	100 mg	4 months	18–90 weeks
Lo et al. [18]	12	9 (75%)	100 mg	4 months	2–14 months
Perrillo et al. [19]	34	24 (71%)	100 mg	80 days	52 weeks
Niigata University	1	1 (100%)	100 mg	2 months	52 weeks

However, reinfection can be prevented if an appropriate antibody titer can be maintained. There are many cases where survival has been prolonged without a drop in QoL through the avoidance of HBV reinfection with continuous administration, albeit at a high price. Looking at recent reports (Table 1) indicates that the objective of prolonging survival can be achieved if appropriate hepatitis B surface antigen titer is maintained [15,16].

1.2. Prophylaxis by means of lamivudine administration

The effects of lamivudine on HBV cases were reported in 1995 [8], and long-term survival was achieved through the use of lamivudine independently and in combination with HBIG, by means of prevention of reinfection, which began immediately with lung transplant recipients [9]. At the same time, it underwent clinical application as an antiviral treatment that proved effective even during reinfection. Lamivudine was administered independently before transplant for prevention of reinfection. In about 70–75% of the cases where post-operative independent administration was performed, a decrease in the amount of anti-hepatitis B surface antigen and HBV-DNA was seen. The amount administered was 100 mg given from about 80 to 120 days before transplant, and administration also continued after the transplant (Table 2). Prevention of reinfection with independent administration was successful in 3/4 of the cases [17–19]. However, one problem is that variants in the YMDD arrangement appeared, but this factor was determined not to be a lethal pathology. Nonetheless, future investigation in relation to this variation is necessary.

1.3. Prophylaxis by means of lamivudine and combined use of HBIG

Markowitz et al. [20] administered 150 mg lamivudine before transplant, and the same amount in combination with HBIG after transplant. With the longest period of observation being 525 days, they reported that none of the 14 cases had anti-hepatitis B surface antigen antibodies and that there were no HBV-DNA-positive cases [20]. Gugenheim et al. [21] performed combined administration of 100 mg lamivudine and 10,000 International Units HBIG for four cases after transplant; and although HBV infection was present after 2 months, they reported not finding it at all later. Naomov et al. [22] substituted for the expensive HBIG by switching from HBIG to lamivudine only over the 6 months after transplant, and the clinical usefulness of this approach was noted.

In all recent reports, long-term follow-up was unsuccessful and led to difficulty in discussing the long-term prognosis. It is clear that HBV reinfection in a form like severe hepatitis after transplant is suppressed. Accordingly, a good long-term prognosis can be considered a result of the promise of the prophylaxis strategy. At this point, the most effective prophylaxis treatment strategies with respect to anti-hepatitis Be antigen antibodies and HBV-DNA-positive cases are priming with lamivudine before transplant, post-operative continuous administration, and where post-operative HBIG is positive for hepatitis B surface antigen.

1.4. Treatment with respect to cases of HBV infection after transplant using lamivudine

After considering the long-term prognosis, an important point to ascertain is an effective antiviral treatment strategy for cases of HBV infection occurring after liver transplant. Today, lamivudine is actively administered as an antiviral agent even after liver transplant. As a result, a similar prognosis for long-term survival as that for regular chronic hepatitis is being sought.

When Perillo et al. [23] administered lamivudine to HBV-positive recipients after transplant, they were successful in elimination of anti-hepatitis B surface antigen antibodies to 8%, elimination of anti-hepatitis Be antigen antibodies to 31%, and elimination of HBV-DNA to 60%. They also found that laboratory measures of liver function improved. While this research had only a short-term follow-up, it is a critical study [23] in terms of the expectations for long-term prognosis. At any rate, the importance of the finding that reinfection was not produced after liver transplant remains unchanged in both the clinical sense as well as for the QoL of recipients.

1.5. Future problems

Familial accumulation of viruses and liver disease is often seen with HBV. Accordingly, instances of living-donor transplants should primarily consist of candidate donors that are relatives, though the rate among families of HBV-positive individuals having liver disease is high and the existence of an appropriate donor is not favorable, compared with other disorders. In addition, there is also the problem of donors being positive for anti-hepatitis B core antigen antibodies. Initiation of HBV-positive hepatitis has

TABLE 3

Onset of hepatitis for anti-hepatitis B core-positive donor after living-donor liver transplant and regulation by means of HBIG

Source	Donor profile Anti-hepatitis B core	Recipient state		
		Hepatitis B		Prophylaxis by means of HBIG
Kyoto University [24]	Positive (n = 16)	15/16	(94%)	No
	Positive (n = 5)	0/5	(0%)	Yes
	Negative (n = 202)	0/202	(0%)	No
Shinshu University [25]	Positive (n = 6)	3/6	(50%)	No
	Positive (n = 1)	0/1	(0%)	Yes
	Negative (n = 50)	0/50	(0%)	No
Niigata University	Positive (n = 2)	0/2	(0%)	Yes

been determined to occur with many of these donors that are positive for anti-hepatitis B core antigen antibodies after a living-donor liver transplant [24,25], and HBIG and lamivudine administration is required (Table 3).

2. HEPATITIS C VIRUS (HCV)-POSITIVE CIRRHOSIS

2.1. HCV reinfection

HCV reinfection occurs at high rates after liver transplant for HCV-positive recipients. This infection is also noted extremely early after transplant, and in many cases HCV-RNA can be detected in blood 2–4 weeks post-transplant. However, not all HCV-positive recipients will turn HCV-RNA-positive after liver transplant, and approximately 5% avoid reinfection. Although a difference is cited in the reports, hepatitis is noted histologically in 14–72% of those reinfected [26,27]. The author investigated 20 cases of liver transplants from cadaveric donors overseas for Japanese. A search for HCV-positive recipients upon their return to Japan proved that all of the cases had HCV-positive chronic hepatitis after liver transplant [28,29].

HCV reinfection and hepatitis is initiated at high rates for HCV-positive recipients, and this fact may have some effect on liver transplant results. Assembling all of the research to this point, there is no significant difference between the 5-year survival rate for HCV-positive recipients after transplant and other non-HCV-positive recipients [30–34] (Table 4).

There are, nonetheless, cases where fibrosing cholestatic hepatitis is observed with HBV or cases where severe hepatitis is produced, and there are even cases involving a short-term transition to cirrhosis. The causes are unclear and a number of reports suggest a relationship for many of the factors (Table 5). Cases with high values for HCV-RNA before transplant [35] and post-operative hepatitis in cases of HCV genotype I [36–38] are thought to be related in terms of the degree of severity, while related factors like quasi-species of HCV [39,40] and recipient HLA-B1 or -DR antigen [41,42] and donor tumor necrosis factor (TNF)-α polymorphism [43] have been cited. As for changes after

TABLE 4

HCV-infected recipients, non-infected recipients, and variation in survival rates

Source	Recipient	1-Year survival rate	5-Year survival rate	P-value
Ferray et al. [30]	HCV ($n = 79$)	95%	80%	
	Non-HCV ($n = 106$)	98%	89%	NS
Gane et al. [31]	HCV ($n = 149$)	79%	70%	
	Non-HCV ($n = 623$)	75%	69%	NS
Boker et al. [32]	HCV ($n = 61$)		62%	
	Non-HCV ($n = 474$)		57%	NS
Casavilla et al. [33]	HCV ($n = 183$)	80%	75%	
	Non-HCV ($n = 556$)	78%	70%	NS
Ghobrial et al. [34]	HCV ($n = 183$)	86%	76%	
	Non-HCV ($n = 556$)	81%	71%	NS

TABLE 5

Appearance of infection after liver transplant, initiation of hepatitis, and severity-related factors

HCV viremia: high titer before liver transplant
HCV quasi-species
HLA-related factors
HLA B1, DRB1*04, DRB1 mismatch
HLA DRB3
Macrovascular steatosis
Donor TNF-α polymorphism
IgM anti-HCV core antibody
Genotype I
HLA class II-restricted CD4$^+$ T lymphocytes

the onset of hepatitis following transplant, the macro-vesicular steatosis of liver tissue [44] and anti-HCV core IgM [45–47] appear to be important indicators, and one theory argues that while immunosuppression is taking place, HLA class II-restricted CD4$^+$ T lymphocytes [48] form the basis of the hepatitis. Nonetheless, all of the necessary evidence has not been obtained, and there are even reports that genotype and HLA are not related [49,50]. Factors involved in the prediction of future HCV reinfection and increasing severity of hepatitis have not been elucidated and the current situation is simply one that does not allow definite conclusions.

2.2. *Prophylaxis for HCV re-infection*

HCV reinfection occurs at high rates after liver transplants for HCV-positive recipients, though it does not seem to affect survival rates. However, a transition to severe hepatitis and cirrhosis in a short period of time has been suggested recently, so HCV prophylaxis and treatment after liver transplant have been considered. Interferon-α that

TABLE 6

Treatment strategies with respect to recurrence of HCV after liver transplant and results

Source	Administered agent/duration	Cases	BR rate	PCR-positive	Tissue improvement	Rejection
Wright et al. [51]	IFN 3 μg × 3/week [a]	11	9%	0	0	0
Wright et al. [52]	IFN 3 μg × 3/week [b]	18	28%	0	0	4%
Ferray et al. [53]	IFN 3 μg × 3/week [a]	14	23%	0	14%	35%
Cattral et al. [54]	Ribavirin [a]	9	44%	0	22%	0
Gane et al. [55]	Ribavirin [a]	7	57%	0	57%	0
Bizollon et al. [56]	INF 3 μg × 3/week + ribavirin [a]	21	100%	48%	100%	0

[a] 6 months.
[b] 4 months.

TABLE 7

Prophylaxis with respect to HCV reinfection

Source	Prophylaxis	Graft hepatitis		Clearance of HV
Mazzaferro et al. [57]	INF 3 μg × 3/week + ribavirin	21	19%	42%
	INF 3 μg × 3/week	10	100%	20%
	No treatment	17	70.5%	0

Prophylaxis treatment was IFN 3 weeks after liver transplant, ribavirin 10 mg/kg/day started with meals.

serves as a treatment tool against reinfection of HCV-positive recipients was first used, but the results were poor [51,52] and there was suspicion as to whether rejection was being elicited [53]. However, recent years have seen the appearance of ribavirin and its administration in combination with interferon; when compared to independent administration [54,55], the combined administration has led to dramatic progress in treatment results [56]. Thus, it is thought to hold promise as part of the antiviral treatment strategy after transplant (Table 6). Of course, the ideal is to find no reinfection after liver transplant, and the main thrust is considering the administration of antiviral agents before transplant. However, a drop in platelets and a number of other complications make planned administration for liver transplant from a cadaveric donor difficult. Administration of interferon and ribavirin immediately after liver transplant is successful in the prevention of reinfection. Mazzafero et al. [57] reported limiting HCV reinfection to 42% immediately after liver transplant using combination therapy; however, the survival rate after 2 years was no different from that of the untreated group (Table 7).

2.3. Future problems

The time is coming when prevention of HCV reinfection will occur before liver transplant or immediately afterwards. To that end, appropriate anti-viral treatment with interferon before surgery will take place by means of planning and scheduling of surgery for live-donor liver transplants. Thus, the HCV positivity should be measured from levels in the blood and not in the liver. Prevention of HCV reinfection and early stage withdrawal of adrenocortical hormone after liver transplant will then be possible.

3. HEPATOCELLULAR CARCINOMA

3.1. Liver transplants and other treatments in terms of survival rates

In instances of hepatocellular carcinoma, deciding the superiority of treatment strategies after looking only at survival rates presents a problem. That is, long-term prolongation of life is possible with hepatocellular carcinoma if appropriate procedures are followed with respect to recurrence, which occurs at high rates. However, the results of the first treatment strategy used in those instances may be used to simply determine the survival rate. Moreover, conditions that are not fixed for applied standards will weaken the context of the survival rate itself.

When investigating conditions for survival rates in the US and Europe that have been affected by this bias, a disparity exists in that the 5-year survival rate for hepatocellular carcinoma cases as a whole is from 38 to 75% and the 10-year survival rate is from 24 to 45% depending on the facility.

Limiting the applicable cases to those such as the ones involving a small tumor diameter or short waiting time clearly improves the survival rate [11,58,59]. If the conditions for hepatocellular carcinoma satisfy all of the Milan Criteria, then the 5-year survival rate rises to 88%, and the survival rate with non-recurrence becomes 80%. When comparing hepatocellular carcinoma that does and does not satisfy the Criteria, a difference of 96 vs. 64% appears.

Even when comparing other treatment strategies, it is important to consider the liver transplant results. Yamamoto et al. [60] investigated the respective survival rates in conjunction with the patient's background among facilities where prospective patients for hepatic resection and liver transplant differ. In the investigation of the survival rates, it is difficult to detect a statistically significant difference among the two (Table 8), but one clear difference is that the survival rate with no recurrence for liver transplants from cadaveric donors is exceedingly high when compared to that for cases of hepatic resection (Table 9). Numerous other authors [61,62] have also reported similar findings. After 5 years of observation, the survival rate was not found to be significantly different, though high rates for the survival rate with non-recurrence have been clearly reported with cases of liver transplants from cadaveric donors. Comparative investigation is not possible, but one can simply look at the large number of cases reported for the survival rate involving a hepatocellular carcinoma treatment strategy. The Japan Liver Cancer Research Society's latest report [63] gives a 5-year survival rate of 65%, and a 10-year survival rate of 23%, with regard to hepatic resection. In contrast, the liver transplant results from the European Liver Transplant Registry (ELTR) are 50% for the 5-year survival rate and 40% for the 10-year survival rate; as was expected a difference in survival rates was not found. Ethanol local injection treatment and microwave incineration treatment are confined to the respective extent of the tumor;

TABLE 8

Survival rate for hepatic resection and liver transplant

Source	Surgery	5-Year survival rate	7-Year survival rate	10-Year survival rate
Yamamoto et al. [60]	Hepatic resection ($n = 294$) Liver transplant from cadaveric donor ($n = 270$)	47.1% 54.5%		24.4% 36.2% [a]
Figueras et al. [61]	Hepatic resection ($n = 35$) Liver transplant from cadaveric donor ($n = 85$)	51% 60% [b]		
Llovet et al. [62]	Hepatic resection ($n = 77$) Liver transplant ($n = 87$)	51% 52%		
Japan Liver Cancer Research Society [63]	Hepatic resection ($n = 21{,}025$)	64.9%	34.8%	23.3%
ELTR [11]	Liver transplant from cadaveric donor ($n = 2395$)	50%		40%

[a] $P = 0.40$.
[b] $P = 0.34$.

TABLE 9

Survival rate with non-resurgence for hepatic resection and liver transplant

Source	Surgery	5-Year survival rate	7-Year survival rate
Yamamoto et al. [60]	Hepatic resection ($n = 294$) Liver transplant from cadaveric donor ($n = 270$)	53.9% 14.3%	44.4% 7.2% ($P < 0.0001$)
Figueras et al. [61]	Hepatic resection ($n = 35$) Liver transplant from cadaveric donor ($n = 85$)	31% 60% ($P < 0.027$)	

thus, comparative investigation of cases conforming to the Milan Criteria and PEIT, PMCT, and RFA must be conducted.

3.2. Liver transplants and other treatments in terms of cases of mortality

Even though surgical techniques and peri-operative/post-operative management for liver transplants are improving, the mortality rate in the surgical period following liver transplant is still extremely high. Yamamoto et al. [60] pointed out that the mortality rate within 30 days and within 150 days for liver transplant is significantly high when compared to corresponding rates for hepatic resection (Table 10). An investigation of cases involving adult living-donor liver transplants in Japan also found that the

TABLE 10

Investigation of mortality during the surgical period after living-donor liver transplant in Japan

	Mortality rate in 30 days	Mortality rate in 150 days	Overall mortality rate
Hepatocellular carcinoma ($n = 18$)	0	3 (16.7%)	5 (27.8%)
Cirrhosis ($n = 22$)	2 (9.0%)	6 (27.3%)	6 (27.3%)
Cases as a whole ($n = 308$)	28 (9.1%)	59 (19.2%)	68 (22.1%)

TABLE 11

Comparative investigation of mortality during surgical period for cirrhosis complicating hepatocellular carcinoma

	Mortality rate in 30 days	Mortality rate in 150 days
Liver transplant from cadaveric donor ($n = 270$)	22 (7.8%)	49 (17.3%)
Hepatic resection ($n = 294$)	4 (1.4%)	17 (5.8%)

From Yamamoto et al. [60].

majority of overall cases of mortality occur within 150 days (Table 11). Recurrence of hepatocellular carcinoma serves as one cause of the mortality rate in the surgical period following liver transplant, with links to risks like post-operative infection, arterial occlusion, stenosis of the bile duct, impaired blood flow, and acute immunological rejection. Compared to hepatic resection, the mortality rate in the surgical period following liver transplant is high. Nonetheless, performing appropriate patient selection like that described by the Milano group [58] has been reported to keep the mortality rate in the surgical period following liver transplant low. Thus, this variation is likely to disappear with progress in management during the surgical period and appropriate patient selection. However, the differences between hepatic resection and liver transplant as it appears today are decisive.

3.3. Liver transplants and other treatments in terms of applicable standards

The expression ‘appropriate patient for liver transplant’ is another way of describing the establishment of applicable standards for liver transplant. The Milan Criteria [58] (Table 12) and UNOS standards [64] (Table 13) are almost the same. The basic approach focuses on the diameter and number of tumors and the presence or absence of vascular infiltration.

Other reports follow the same idea [65]; of course, the fibrolamellar type of hepatocellular carcinoma has the best prognosis and results [66], but this is a special instance. An interesting finding is that the liver transplant survival rate for hepatocellular carcinoma with cirrhosis as part of underlying liver disease and that for uncomplicated hepatocellular carcinoma differ. Detailed investigation of liver transplant results with respect to hepatocellular carcinoma from ELTR indicates that the 5- and 10-year survival rates for 952 cases of incidental hepatocellular carcinoma and small incidental

TABLE 12

Milan Criteria

Single hepatocellular carcinoma, individual maximum diameter within 5 cm
Multiple tumor within three nodes, individual maximum diameter within 3 cm
Excluding vascular infiltration and lymph node infiltration

From [58].

TABLE 13

UNOS Criteria

1.	Tumor factor criteria Tumor 1 node maximum diameter within 1.9 cm (T1) Tumor 1 node maximum diameter 2–5 cm (T2) Tumor 2–3 nodes maximum diameter within 3 cm (T2)
2.	General conditions Macroscopic vascular infiltration, excluding extrahepatic metastasis
3.	Other conditions Non-applicable hepatic resection cases

From [64].

hepatocellular carcinoma and 1842 cases of hepatocellular carcinoma complicated with cirrhosis yield almost the same results (5-year 56 vs. 54% and 10-year 45 vs. 45%). However, the 5- and 10-year survival rates for 554 cases of hepatocellular carcinoma uncomplicated with cirrhosis are extremely low at 38 and 28% [11]. This finding is not simply based on factors such as the diameter or number of the hepatocellular carcinoma tumor; it is instead due to the difference in biological characteristics, such as the nature of vascular infiltration in hepatocellular carcinoma uncomplicated with cirrhosis. There are critical phenomena for the future as part of medical care involving liver transplants in patients with hepatocellular carcinoma. One point is whether hepatic resection or local treatment is recommended for hepatocellular carcinoma with appropriate standards. Hepatocellular carcinoma that develops after cirrhosis accounts for a majority of hepatocellular carcinoma cases in Japan, and the minimum goal is to exceed the survival rates from 5 to 10 years from the Japan Liver Cancer Research Society (Table 14). This is because liver transplants must treat hepatocellular carcinomas as well as cirrhosis.

3.4. Recurrence of hepatocellular carcinoma after transplant

Recurrence of hepatocellular carcinoma after transplant is the metastasizing of hepatocellular carcinoma tumor cells in the recipient to the liver transplanted from the donor. As a result, the hepatocellular carcinoma presents anew in the liver that was transplanted. Essentially, it is best to think of this as metastasis. Factors in the US and Europe for comprehensive determination are a small diameter or number of tumors,

TABLE 14

Japan Liver Cancer Research Society's cases of single tumor onset and Stage 1 respective treatment results

	5-Year survival rate	7-Year survival rate	10-Year survival rate
Survival rate for cases of single tumor onset			
Hepatic resection ($n = 14{,}727$)	53.4%	39.2%	27.8%
PEIT ($n = 2525$)	46.3%	30.6%	–
TAE ($n = 5162$)	25.9%	15.2%	–
PMCT ($n = 259$)	79.4%	–	–
Survival rate with maximum tumor diameter of 2 cm or greater			
Hepatic resection (>2 cm) ($n = 3888$)	63.3%	45.1%	30.6%
PEIT (1–2 cm) ($n = 1849$)	48.1%	36.4%	–
PMCT (1–2 cm) ($n = 147$)	84.0%	–	–

Revised from [63].

a lack of vascular infiltration, or when there are good results when the carcinoma is encapsulated. For results to be called good, recurrence of hepatocellular carcinoma, accounting for the majority of deaths, must not be observed. Not observing recurrence means that the hepatocellular carcinoma has halted inside nodes and that intrahepatic and extrahepatic metastasis has not occurred. Of course, extrahepatic metastasis is adequately detected before surgery, and cases where this characteristic is not found are selected. However, non-observance cannot be decided merely with diagnostic images, as micrometastasis can be assumed to be quite frequent. In a report of the Japan Liver Cancer Research Society, there is a low rate of finding infiltration of the portal vein or hepatic vein as well as intrahepatic or extrahepatic metastasis during surgery. However, this frequency is generally quite high as determined during autopsy (Table 15). That is, the hepatocellular carcinoma seen at the autopsy stage is thought to be the same as that at the terminal stage of progressive hepatocellular carcinoma. About half of the cases that lapse into this stage are thought to be due to extrahepatic metastasis. Even though it cannot be seen with diagnostic imaging, it will lead to a failure in liver transplant accommodation. Accordingly, it is best to think of this stage for hepatocellular carcinoma liver transplant as being at the same degree of progress as that for the accommodation stage for resection.

TABLE 15

Frequency of vascular infiltration and intrahepatic metastasis during surgery and during autopsy

	During surgery	During autopsy
Extrahepatic metastasis	69/4431 (1.6%)	258/568 (45.4%)
Intrahepatic metastasis	1108/4344 (25.5%)	
Lymph node metastasis	85/4226 (2.0%)	153/484 (31.6%)
Portal infiltration	567/4051 (14.0%)	290/460 (63.0%)
Hepatic vein infiltration	195/3934 (5.0%)	147/416 (35.3%)

Revised from [63].

In addition, about half of the cases will display extrahepatic metastasis even with rapidly progressive hepatocellular carcinoma, which is outside the applicable range for liver transplants from cadaveric donors in the US and Europe. In contrast, it is possible to handle living-donor liver transplants while maintaining that probability. No doubt liver transplant should be considered the ultimate treatment strategy with respect to progressive hepatocellular carcinoma that cannot be treated with either hepatic resection or surgical means. As for medical care involving liver transplant, living-donor liver transplant [12] will be considered before liver transplant from a cadaveric donor. The reason for this is that strict distribution of donor organs is carried out with liver transplants from a cadaveric donor to make effective use of a small number of donors in a fair, equitable, and rational manner. Practical medical care is to consider the benefit of the persons concerned for living-donor liver transplant where a number of relatives and principally immediate family can provide organ donation. Of course there are numerous opinions to the contrary, but there is no courage in sitting idly by and waiting for death to come with respect to hepatocellular carcinoma that cannot be forestalled. Is it not the purpose of modern medical care to take the challenge to do whatever can be done?

To summarize, the fact that hepatocellular carcinoma can recur is noted in the blood or if tumors cells that are present in the liver spread to other organs beyond the liver as part of hepatocellular carcinoma; vascular infiltration leading to circulation throughout the body can be assumed. In other words (1) the existence of micrometastasis before surgery cannot be detected, (2) a situation with tumor cell immunosuppressant agents after liver transplant in which metastasis, occupation, and proliferation of the grafted liver occur, and (3) tumor cell dissemination during surgery, are thought to be the causes of recurrence. In any event, early stage hepatocellular carcinoma, where vascular infiltration that causes tumor cells to circulate outside the liver is not present, is not considered to be recurrent. However, recurrence is seen in the lung in about half of the instances, the remainder being mostly liver and bones. The former is suggested to be present after surgery, while the latter is thought to be caused by drifting of circulating tumor cells to the transplanted liver. Liver transplant is performed in a situation where clinical diagnosis of extrahepatic metastasis is not or cannot be rendered due to vascular infiltration as part of hepatocellular carcinoma, lymph node metastasis, and peritoneal tumor dissemination. Due to the use of immunosuppressive agents after surgery, the dominant organ that is the source of metastasis or recurrence of hepatocellular carcinoma in the donated liver can be seen.

Accordingly, the preferred situation for liver transplant is one in which the hepatocellular carcinoma does not actually bring about extrahepatic metastasis. Either there is no method of treatment for previously existing hepatocellular carcinoma or the liver transplant is conducted as treatment continues, so a struggle must be undertaken. To that end, appropriate chemotherapy after liver transplant and active medical care are critical according to the authors. In general, chemotherapy is the first step; the correct combination of medical treatment like TAE treatment or PEIT regularly in use before and after surgery can permit long-term survival. However, there is currently no appropriate regimen for chemotherapy and systemization of effective medical care and chemotherapy is not conducted.

3.5. Future problems

Progressive hepatocellular carcinoma that deviates from the Milan Criteria and applicable standards from UNOS, is often noted. That is, treatment for recurrence is repeated after the first stage of treatment for hepatocellular carcinoma; in the end, there are many levels of cases leading to Stage IVa conditions. Many are hepatitis virus-positive hepatocellular carcinomas, with multicentric onset from chronic liver diseases. Appropriate consideration for liver transplants in relation to these conditions does not appear to be happening in Japan. To that end, medical care involving liver transplants is progressing using the same methods as with liver transplants from cadaveric donors in the US and Europe so as to obtain just those results. At a minimum, (1) a reduction in the amount of immunosuppressive agents used, (2) prevention of reinfection with the hepatitis virus using antiviral agents, and (3) creation of chemotherapy programs are vital necessities.

In each individual case, various schemes must be formulated, so this work will not end merely with the publication of numbers of cases of living-donor liver transplants. Future research will, in fact, examine options in relation to this area.

REFERENCES

[1] Ichida T, Matsunami H, Kawasaki S et al. Living related donor liver transplantation from adult to adult for primary biliary cirrhosis. Ann Intern Med 1995; 122: 275–276.

[2] Davis SE, Portmann BC, O'Grady JG et al. Hepatic histological findings after transplantation for chronic hepatitis B virus infection, including a unique pattern of fibrosing cholestatic hepatitis. Hepatology 1991; 13: 150–157.

[3] Todo S, Demetris AJ, Van Theil DH et al. Orthotopic liver transplantation for patients with hepatitis B virus-related liver disease. Hepatology 1991; 13: 619–626.

[4] Belle SH, Beringer KC, Detre KM. Recent findings concerning liver transplantation in the United States. In: Cecka JM, Terasaki PI, editor. Clinical Transplants. LA, USA: UCLA Tissue Typing Laboratory, 1997; pp. 15–29.

[5] Chazouilleres O, Mamish D, Kim M et al. 'Occult' hepatitis B virus as source of infection in liver transplant recipients. Lancet 1994; 343: 142–146.

[6] Lauchart W, Muller R, Pichlmayr R. Immunoprophylaxis of hepatitis B virus reinfection in recipients of human liver allografts. Transplant Proc 1987; 19: 2387–2388.

[7] Samuel D, Bismuth A, Mathieu D et al. Passive immunoprophylaxis after liver transplantation in HBsAg positive patients. Lancet 1991; 337: 813–816.

[8] Dienstag JL, Perrillo RP, Schiff EF et al. A preliminary trial of Lamivudine for chronic hepatitis B infection. New Engl J Med 1995; 333: 1657–1661.

[9] De Man RA, Niester HGM, Fevery J et al. Evaluation of limiting dilution PCR of HBV-DNA decrease in a double-blind randomized six month trial of Lamivudine for chronic hepatitis B: implications for the application in liver transplant recipients. AASLD single topic symposium: liver transplantation for chronic viral hepatitis, 1995: 10 (abstract).

[10] Ichida T, Satoh Y, Kashida H. Long term follow-up study of HBV positive recipient after liver transplantation. Kan Tan Sui 2000; 41: 131–138. (In Japanese.)

[11] European Liver Transplant Association. In: European Liver Transplant Registry, Data analysis booklet 05/1968–12/1999.

[12] Lauchart W, Muller R, Pichlmayr R. Long-term immunoprophylaxis of hepatitis B virus reinfection in recipients of human liver allograft. Transplant Proc 1987; 19: 4051–4052.

[13] Samuel D, Muller R, Alexander G et al. Liver transplantation in European patients with the hepatitis B surface antigen. New Engl J Med 1993; 329: 1842–1847.

[14] Muller R, Samuel D, Fassati LR et al. 'EUROHEP' consensus report on the management of liver transplantation for hepatitis B virus infection. J Hepatol 1994; 21: 1140–1143.

[15] McGory RW, Ishitani MB, Oliveira WM et al. Improved outcome of orthotopic liver transplantation for chronic hepatitis B cirrhosis with aggressive passive immunization. Transplantation 1996; 61: 1358–1364.

[16] Tchervenkov JI, Tector AJ, Barkun JS et al. Recurrence-free long-term survival after liver transplantation for hepatitis B using interferon alpha pre-transplant and hepatitis B immune globulin posttransplant. Ann Surg 1997; 226: 356–369.

[17] Grellier L, Mutimer D, Ahmed M et al. Lamivudine prophylaxis against reinfection in liver transplantation for hepatitis B cirrhosis. Lancet 1996; 348: 1212–1215.

[18] Lo CM, Fan ST, Lai CL et al. Lamivudine prophylaxis in liver transplantation for hepatitis B in Asia. Transplant Proc 1999; 31: 535–536.

[19] Perrillo RP, Schiff ER, Dienstag JL et al. Lamivudine for prevention of recurrent hepatitis B after liver transplantation: final results of a U.S./Canadian multicenter trial. Hepatology 1999; 30: 222A.

[20] Markowitz JS, Martin P, Conrad AJ et al. Prophylaxis against hepatitis B recurrence following liver transplantation using combination Lamivudine and hepatitis B immune globulin. Hepatology 1999; 28: 585–589.

[21] Gugenheim J, Baldini E, Ouzan D et al. Good results of Lamivudine in hepatitis B surface antigen-positive patients with active viral replication before liver transplantation. Transplant Proc 1999; 31: 554–555.

[22] Naomov NV, Lopes R, Crepalid G et al. Randomized trial of Lamivudine versus hepatitis B immunoglobulin for prophylaxis of HBV recurrence after liver transplantation. J Hepatol 1999; 50(S): 51.

[23] Perrillo R, Rakela J, Dienstag J et al. Multicenter study of Lamivudine therapy for hepatitis B after liver transplantation. Hepatology 1999; 29: 1581–1586.

[24] Uemoto S, Sugiyama K, Marusawa H et al. Transmission of hepatitis B virus from hepatitis B core antibody-positive donors in living related liver transplantation. Transplantation 1998; 65: 494–499.

[25] Kiyosawa K. Liver transplantation. Jpn J Intern Med 2000; 89: 473–479. (In Japanese.)

[26] Bizollon T, Mutimer D, Ducerf C et al. Hepatitis C virus recurrence after liver transplantation. Gut 1999; 44: 575–578.

[27] Teixeira R, Pastacaldi S, Papatheodoridis GV et al. Recurrent hepatitis C after liver transplantation. J Med Virol 2000; 61: 443–454.

[28] Ichida T. Clinical aspects of HCV after organ transplantation. Annual Report of Intractable Hepatic Diseases by Ministry of health and Welfare 1995. 1996; pp. 112–115.

[29] Ichida T. Clinical problems of cadaveric liver transplantation for Japanese recipients. Acta Hepatol Jpn 1997; 38: 129–133. (In Japanese.)

[30] Ferray C, Gigou M, Samuel D et al. The course of hepatitis C virus infection after liver transplantation. Hepatology 1994; 20: 1137–1143.

[31] Gane EJ, Portmann BC, Naoumov NV et al. Long-term outcome of hepatitis C infection after liver transplantation. New Engl J Med 1996; 334: 815–820.

[32] Boker KHW, Dalley G, Bahr MJ et al. Long-term outcome of hepatitis C virus infection after liver transplantation. Hepatology 1997; 25: 203–210.

[33] Casavilla FA, Rakela J, Kapur S et al. Clinical outcome of patients infected with hepatitis C virus infection on survival after primary liver transplantation under tacrolimus. Liver Transplant Surg 1998; 4: 448–454.
[34] Ghobrial RM, Farmer DG, Baquerizo A et al. Orthotopic liver transplantation for hepatitis C. Outcome, effect of immunosuppressant, and causes of re-transplantation during an 8-year single-center experience. Ann Surg 1999; 6: 824–833.
[35] Charlton M, Seaberg E, Wiesner R et al. Predictors of patient and graft survival following liver transplantation for hepatitis C. Hepatology 1998; 28: 823–830.
[36] Pageaux GP, Ducos J, Mondain AM et al. Hepatitis C virus genotypes and quantification of serum hepatitis C virus RNA in liver transplant recipients: relationship with severity of histological recurrence and implications in the pathogenesis of HCV infection. Liver Transplant Surg 1997; 3: 501–505.
[37] Costes V, Durand L, Pageaux GP et al. Hepatitis C virus genotypes and quantification of serum hepatitis C RNA in liver transplant recipients. Relationship with histologic outcome of recurrent hepatitis C. Am J Clin Pathol 1999; 111: 252–258.
[38] Casino C, Lilli D, Rivanera D et al. Recurrence of hepatitis C virus infection after orthotopic liver transplantation: role of genotypes. New Microbiol 1999; 22: 11–18.
[39] Pessoa MG, Browej N, Berenguer M et al. Evolution of hepatitis C quasi-species in patients with severe cholestatic hepatitis after liver transplantation. Hepatology 1999; 30: 1513–1520.
[40] Pelletier SJ, Raymond DP, Crabtree TD et al. Pre-transplantation hepatitis C virus quasi-species may be predictive of outcome after liver transplantation. Hepatology 2000; 32: 375–381.
[41] Belli LS, Zavaglia C, Alberti AB et al. Influence of immunogenetic background on the outcome of recurrent hepatitis C after liver transplantation. Hepatology 2000; 31: 1345–1350.
[42] Cotler SJ, Gaur LK, Gretch DR et al. Donor–recipient sharing of HLA class II alleles predicts earlier recurrence and accelerated progression of hepatitis C following liver transplantation. Tissue Antigens 1998; 52: 435–443.
[43] Rosen HR, Lentz JJ, Rose SL et al. Donor polymorphism of tumor necrosis factor gene: relationship with variable severity of hepatitis C recurrence after liver transplantation. Transplantation 1999; 68: 1898–1902.
[44] Pelletier SJ, Jezzoni JC, Crabtree et al. Prediction of liver allograft fibrosis after transplantation for hepatitis C virus: persistent elevation of serum transaminase levels versus necroinflammatory activity. Liver Transplant 2000; 6: 44–53.
[45] Crespo J, Carte B, Lozano JL et al. Hepatitis C virus recurrence after liver transplantation: relationship to anti-HCV core IgM, genotype, and level of viremia. Am J Gastroenterol 1997; 92: 1458–1462.
[46] Negro F, Giostra E, Rubbia-Brandt L et al. IgM anti-hepatitis C virus core antibodies as marker of recurrent hepatitis C after liver transplantation. J Med Virol 1998; 56: 224–229.
[47] Casino C, Lilli D, Rivanera D et al. Diagnosis value of anti-hepatitis C virus core immunoglobulin M in recurrence of HCV infection after orthotopic liver transplantation. J Clin Microbiol 1999; 37: 2726–2728.
[48] Rosen HR, Hinrichs DJ, Gretch DR et al. Association of multispecific CD4(+) response to hepatitis C and severity of recurrence after liver transplantation. Gastroenterology 1999; 117: 926–932.
[49] Shuhart MC, Bronner MP, Gretch DR et al. Histological and clinical outcome after liver transplantation for hepatitis C. Hepatology 1997; 26: 1646–1652.

[50] Vargas HE, Laskus T, Wang LF et al. The influence of hepatitis C virus genotypes on the outcome of liver transplantation. Liver Transplant Surg 1998; 4: 22–27.
[51] Wright HI, Gavaler JS, Van Thiel DH et al. Preliminary experience with alpha-2b-interferon therapy of viral hepatitis in liver allograft recipients. Transplantation 1992; 53: 121–124.
[52] Wright TL, Combs C, Kim M et al. Interferon alpha therapy for hepatitis C virus infection after liver transplantation. Hepatology 1994; 20: 773–779.
[53] Feray C, Samuel D, Gigou M et al. An open trial of IFN alpha recombinant for hepatitis C after liver transplantation: antiviral effects and risk of rejection. Hepatology 1995; 22: 1084–1089.
[54] Cattral MS, Krajden M, Wanless IR et al. A pilot study of ribavirin therapy for recurrent hepatitis C virus infection after liver transplantation. Transplant 1996; 61: 1483–1488.
[55] Gane EJ, Tibbs CJ, Ramage JK et al. Ribavirin therapy for hepatitis C infection following liver transplantation. Transplant Int 1995; 8: 61–64.
[56] Bizollon T, Palazzo U, Ducerf C et al. Pilot study of the combination of alpha interferon and ribavirin as therapy of recurrent hepatitis C after liver transplantation. Hepatology 1997; 26: 500–504.
[57] Mazzafero V, Regalia E, Pulvirenti A et al. Prophylaxis against HCV recurrence after liver transplantation. Effect of interferon and Ribavirin combination. Transplant Proc 1997; 29: 519–521.
[58] Mazzaferro V, Regalia E, Doci R et al. Liver transplantation for the treatment of small hepatocellular carcinoma in patients with cirrhosis. New Engl J Med 1996; 334: 693–699.
[59] Llovet JM, Bruix J, Fuster J et al. Liver transplantation for treatment of small hepatocellular carcinoma: the TMN classification dose not have prognostic power. Hepatology 1998; 27: 1572–1577.
[60] Yamamoto J, Iwatsuki S, Kosuge T et al. Should hepatomas be treated with hepatic resection or transplantation? Cancer 1999; 86: 1151–1158.
[61] Figueras J, Jaurrieta E, Valls C et al. Resection or transplantation for hepatocellular carcinoma in cirrhotic patients: outcomes based on indicated treatment strategy. J Am Coll Surg 2000; 190: 580–587.
[62] Llovet JM, Fuster J, Bruix J et al. Intention-to-treat analysis of surgical treatment for early hepatocellular carcinoma: resection versus transplantation. Hepatology 1999; 30: 1434–1440.
[63] Japanese Study group of Liver Cancer. 14th Annual Report-long term follow-up study, 1999.
[64] Ichida T, Iwatsuki S, Kakumu S. UNOS selection criteria and order of priority for the candidate of liver transplantation. Jpn J Gastroenterol 2001; 98: 1–7. (In Japanese.)
[65] Figueras J, Jaurrieta E, Valls C et al. Survival after liver transplantation in cirrhotic patients with and without hepatocellular carcinoma: a comparative study. Hepatology 1997; 25: 1485–1489.
[66] Houben KW, McCall JL. Liver transplantation for hepatocellular carcinoma in patients without underlying liver disease: a systematic review. Liver Transplant Surg 1999; 5: 91–95.

Index